CEN Study Guide 2022-2023

New Outline + 700 Test Questions and Detailed Answer Explanations for the Certified Emergency Nurse Exam (Includes 4 Full-Length Practice Tests)

Table of Contents

Introduction

Note: This guide uses the new revised outline and is intended for those who are taking the exam after January 18, 2022.

A certified emergency nurse (CEN) is a registered nurse who is formally trained to work in emergency rooms (ERs). CENs are often described as the cornerstone of ERs. This is because there are generally more CENs than physicians, and CENs spend the most time with patients. CENs make quick decisions, multitask and carry out their nursing responsibilities in a high-pressure environment like the ER.

The Purpose of a Certified Emergency Nurse

1. Acute resuscitation – Patients who present to the ER often have their initial contact with an emergency nurse. CENs can provide acute resuscitation to patients with acute diseases or acute exacerbations of chronic or debilitating diseases. Acute resuscitation follows the principles of airway, breathing and circulation. Other aspects of acute resuscitation include the provision of drugs and elimination of toxic substances.
2. Nursing care – CENS can make nursing diagnoses, create nursing care plans and provide nursing interventions. This is because CENs are RNs with formal training in the principles of physiology, pathology and pharmacology.
3. Patient education – CENS educate patients on the nature of their conditions and the purpose of the nursing care provided. All these are required for patient awareness, primary health education and informed consent. CENs also educate patients' primary caregivers and relatives.

4. Advocacy – CENs advocate for the welfare of their patients. This is because they care not only for a patient's medical condition but also religious, social, emotional and psychological needs.
5. Collaboration – CENs collaborate with other members of the health team, including physicians, phlebotomists, nursing assistants, licensed practical nurses and physiotherapists.
6. Supervision – CENs are responsible for supervising the work of junior members of the nursing team, including nursing assistants, nursing students and licensed practical nurses.

Education Requirements

A CEN is a registered nurse who has passed the NCLEX-RN exam and the BCEN exam. The following is a general summary of the trajectory of CEN professional preparation.

1. Qualify for the NCLEX-RN exam

To take the NCLEX-RN exams, you are expected to have a diploma in nursing or a bachelor of science in nursing.

2. Become a registered nurse

To become a registered nurse, you must first pass the National Council Licensure Examination for Registered Nurses (NCLEX-RN), a licensing exam administered by the National Council of State Boards of Nursing to assess the skills of entry-level registered nurses. It is a computerized adaptive test consisting of 75 to 265 questions answered over six hours.

3. Work experience

It is ideal to have at least two years of experience in the ER before taking the licensing exam for emergency nursing.

4. Licensing and certification

Licensure as a CEN is offered only by the Board of Certification of Emergency Nursing (BCEN). Registered nurses who wish to become CENs must take this exam. Details of the exam will be discussed in full in this book.

Career Options

Career options in hospital settings

CENs work in ERs and attend to all cases that cut across the five major specialties: medicine, pediatrics, psychiatry, obstetrics and gynecology, and surgery. They can also work in subspecialties after obtaining additional board certification. To become licensed subspecialists, CENs are expected to obtain the necessary clinical experience, obtain recommendations and pass a specialty exam. Subspecialties are varied, including flight nursing, pediatric emergencies, ground transportation and obstetric emergencies.

Career options outside hospital settings

CENs can work in any institution offering care to acute cases. Some of these institutions include correctional facilities, air ambulances, crisis intervention centers, burn centers, geriatric centers, community settings and rural areas.

Remuneration

The median annual salary of a CEN is $66,000. Salary ranges from $53,000 to $79,000 depending on the location, type of facility and career experience.

1. Location – Currently, the highest average salary a CEN can earn is in Los Angeles, California ($81,696). This is followed by Phoenix, Arizona ($70,687), Houston, Texas ($69,399), Denver, Colorado ($63,066), and finally, Dallas, Texas ($62,153). CENs in urban areas earn more than their counterparts in rural areas. However, before considering employment in an urban area, you should consider the impact that rent, transportation, food and other necessities will have on your income.
2. Experience – The salary of a CEN increases as the individual grows in experience. Entry-level CENs have an average salary of $53,665; CENs in the early stage of their careers earn an average of $58,240 per year; those in the mid-stage of their career earn $65,580 per year; experienced CENs earn about $73,400 per year and those in the late phase of their career earn about $79,000 per year.

Pros and Cons of Being a Certified Emergency Nurse

Pros

1. Fast job growth– The demand for RNs will continue to rise. Demand is projected to rise by 18 percent in 2023. More demand brings better working conditions, better remuneration and increased opportunities for explosive career growth.
2. Job satisfaction – Like other health-related services, emergency nurses provide direct service to people. As such, it can be deeply rewarding to use

your skills, time and expertise to save lives. Apart from the rewarding experience, CENs make friends and form meaningful and satisfying relationships.

3. Remuneration – The remuneration of CENs is above average, even for entry-level CENs. This advantage alone makes emergency nursing a lucrative option for most people. Furthermore, due to the increasing demand for registered nurses, salaries are projected to increase in the coming years.

Cons

1. Long hours – Emergency nurses work long hours that may include 12-hour shifts, night shifts and call duties. They also work every day of the week, all year round, weekends, during summer holidays and on national holidays.
2. Emotional and physical burnout – Like other health workers, CENs are vulnerable to emotional and physical burnout. This is because providing care to sick people is demanding. The career of an emergency nurse involves a lot of physical activity, carrying, lifting and pushing in a high-pressure environment. Also, CENs provide emotional support and compassion to all their patients, including the difficult ones. They have to deal with the loss of their patients, even after putting in maximum effort to save their lives. They have to make split-second decisions in critical cases and emergencies.
3. Exposure to biohazards – CENs are vulnerable to biohazards like needle-prick injuries, infected aerosols, infected contact surfaces and radiation. Biohazards are serious and can be life-threatening. Sometimes they may be difficult to prevent, even in the most professional of settings.

Traits of a Successful Certified Emergency Nurse

1. Ability to work in a high-pressure environment – An emergency nurse is expected to manage different kinds of patients, from the acutely ill to patients with chronic conditions. The numerous needs of these patients can be tedious, and a successful emergency nurse is skilled in applying the principles of prioritization, therapeutic communication and delegation.
2. Decision-making – The CEN must make quick and accurate decisions when and where they are needed.
3. Leadership and administration – The CEN is responsible for assessing patients and creating nursing plans for them. This means that the CEN is responsible for the outcome of all nursing care.
4. Empathy – The CEN should have empathy for both patients and their caregivers. Empathy makes it easy to use therapeutic communication techniques to convey and receive information.
5. Team player – The successful CEN is a team player and collaborator who knows how to function with other members of the health team and collaborate with the supervising physician or surgeon.

What Is the CEN Exam?

The Certified Emergency Nursing Exam is the only licensing exam used in certifying emergency nurses in the United States. This exam is created and administered by the Board of Certification of Emergency Nursing (BCEN). Apart from the CEN exams, the BCEN also offers certifications in Certified Pediatric Emergency Nurse (CPEN), Certified Flight Emergency Nurse (CFEN), Certified Transport Emergency Nurse (CTEN) and Trauma Certified Emergency Nurse (TCEN).

For more than 40 years, the BCEN has been committed to providing certified emergency nurses who can guarantee the safety of the public. To do this, the BCEN uses a set of standardized clinical and task-oriented skills that can verify the proficiency of an average entry-level emergency nurse in the United States, the District of Columbia and all US territories. Apart from administering certification exams, the BCEN also provides resources to certified emergency nurses for ongoing and continuous learning, improves employer-employee relationships via their employer resources and programs and provides scholarships and other resources for nursing students. The BCEN takes pride in its ability to provide services that are diverse, nondiscriminatory and inclusive.

The CEN exams provided by the BCEN are validated by the Accreditation Board of Specialty Nursing Certifications (ABSNC). This board is the sole accreditor for certifying specialty nurses. The accreditation provided by the ABSNC means that the BCEN has fulfilled all the requisite requirements in developing, implementing and maintaining certification exams.

Eligibility Requirements

1. Education – All candidates are expected to have either a diploma or baccalaureate degree in nursing and also licensure as registered nurses. As stated earlier, this licensure is administered after passing the NCLEX-RN exam.
2. Work experience – All candidates are expected to have a minimum of two years of working experience in an ER.

Pass Rates

Pass rates of the CEN exams from January 1, 2020 through December 31, 2020:

Program	Delivered Exams	Passed Exams	Failed Exams	Recertification	Total Certificates
CEN	6,836	3,750	3,086	6,452	40,367

Passing Standard

The test plan for the CEN exam is created by a team of certified and practicing emergency nurses. These nurses come from all geographical regions of the United States and work with groups of analysts to ensure that the questions are psychometrically sound and written in an understandable format. Thereafter, the passing standard is approved by the BCEN's board of directors. Passing standards are based on job and practice analyses obtained from surveys and research. The board approves questions only after the questions are assessed for level of cognitive distribution, use of integrated concepts and distribution based on the CEN-specific content area. This evaluation and analysis is done every five years.

How to Register for the CEN Exam

Application

Application is done solely online on www.bcen.org. You can register by following these steps:

1. Create a profile – This is required for new users. Old users can log in using their usernames and passwords. Remember to use a valid email address.
2. Confirm eligibility – You must meet the requirements for eligibility. International candidates with an equivalent RN license outside the United States will need evaluation by the BCEN International Credential Evaluation. To do this, contact CGFNS, the verification board for BCEN, and upload your transcripts and license for verification. This verification requires an application form and a $250 application fee. Evaluation is also required for recertification.
3. Fill out the application form – On the BCEN dashboard, click on **Certifications** and select **CEN** exam. Fill out the form and make payment via check, credit card or ECheck/ACH.

Notification

After successful registration, which includes payment and uploading of the necessary documents, you will receive a notification email that acknowledges payment. The email will contain the 90-day period in which you can take the exam. The email will also provide information on how to schedule your exam with PSI and links to the student handbook.

Scheduling an exam

To schedule your exam, click on the **Schedule Exam** icon on the BCEN dashboard. You will be automatically directed to the PSI website. On the PSI website, first-time exam takers must create an account. To schedule the exam, you must use the ID number provided in the notification email. After you schedule the exam, Pearson VUE will send an email that confirms the scheduled test date and time, phone number and address for the test center, and directions to the test venue.

Rescheduling and canceling the exam

To reschedule an exam, you must do so at least 48 business hours before the scheduled date. This must be done via the Pearson VUE website. Failure to do so leads to the automatic cancelation of the exam. To take another exam, you must reapply and pay new application fees. You must reschedule within the 90-day window provided in your original notification email.

To cancel the exam, log in to your BCEN account and click on the **Schedule/Manage Exam** icon. Reschedules must be done promptly because PSI assigns seating arrangements on a first-come, first-served basis. If you do not reschedule promptly, the exam will be automatically canceled. There are no refunds if you do not reschedule or cancel your test appointment in advance. Refunds are also not given if a request to opt out from the exam is made after the 90-day window has expired. Refunds are given only if you cancel within the 90-day window and have never made a scheduling appointment with PSI.

Application Fees

You can pay via credit card, check or money order. Payment is made via a voucher program, discounted fees for members of the Emergency Nursing Association (ENA) or individual payment.

1. Voucher plans – Voucher plans are nonrefundable and are valid for 12 months. They are used for bulk applications and can be used for initial tests, retake tests and recertification exams. Eleven to 20 test vouchers are sold at $190 each; if 21 or more vouchers are purchased, they are $185 each.
2. Discounted fees – These discounts are given to members of the ENA. In this case, the initial exam costs $230; retake exams cost $200 and recertification exams cost $210.
3. Individual payment – For individuals, the initial cost of the exam is $370; retake exams are $340; and recertification exams cost $350. Military personnel have a discounted fee of $195 for initial, retake and recertification exams.

Renewal of Certificate

CENs are required to recertify every four years. To do so, log in to your BCEN account and click on the **Recertification** tab. Choose your desired mode of recertifying, fill out the application form and pay the fee. There are two options for recertification.

Option 1: Recertification by CEM attestation

In this mode, CENs are expected to:

1. Have a current CEN certification
2. Have a current and unencumbered RN license, or an RN equivalent for the United States and its territories
3. Have achieved at least 100 contact hours of continuing education within the validity of their license (60 minutes is equivalent to 1 contact hour).

Option 2: Recertification by exam

In this mode, you are required to apply for and take a recertification exam as long as you have a current CEN certification and have a current and unencumbered RN licensure equivalent for the United States and its territories. Recertification fees are discussed above.

Acceptable forms of continuing education include accredited provider courses like PALS, ACLS, ABLS, ATLS, GENE, NRP, ATCN and NRP, among others. Teaching activities, such as clinical presentations, lectures and seminars, are not eligible if they were done as a requirement for the faculty's expected job performance.

1. Academic credit – You are expected to have at least a C in content suitable for CEN. In this case, a one-semester course is equivalent to 15 contact hours; one trimester course is equivalent to 12 contact hours, and one quarter course is equivalent to 10 contact hours.
2. Preceptorship – For a preceptorship to be deemed eligible, you must have college credits. A maximum of 15 contact hours is accepted for preceptorship. One semester preceptorship is equivalent to 15 contact hours; one trimester preceptorship is equivalent to 12 contact hours, and one quarter preceptorship is equivalent to 10 contact hours.

3. Authoring – The content must be peer-reviewed and related to emergency nursing. An article is equivalent to five contact hours; a chapter/module is equivalent to 10 contact hours, and a textbook is equivalent to 50 contact hours.
4. Poster presentation – One poster is equivalent to five contact hours. It is usually not accredited.

Retake Policies

There are no restrictions on the number of times you can retake the test. However, you must wait 90 days before retaking it.

What to Expect on the Exam Day

<u>What to do</u>

1. Check-in – You must be present at the designated testing center at least 30 minutes before your scheduled time. This is to enable you to verify your identity during recheck, identify your seat and be comfortably settled before the exam begins. If you arrive more than 15 minutes after the exam starts, you will not be allowed to take it. Items that are prohibited from the testing center include reference materials like books, papers and dictionaries; personal items like purses; garments like headwear, hoodies, veils and coats; and briefcases. Pearson and the BCEN will not take responsibility for any missing or stolen items, so these items should be left at home or in your vehicle.
2. Identification – Temporary means of identification are usually not accepted at the testing center. ID must be government-issued and must match the first and last names you used when registering for the exam. Acceptable government IDs are international passports, visas, driver's

licenses and state/province ID cards. All these IDs must have your photo on them. If you do not have an approved ID, you will not be allowed to take the exam. You will be listed as having missed the appointment, and no refunds will be made. Before the exam begins, you are expected to confirm your name and the nature of the exam being taken and must agree to the rules and regulations of PSI and BCEN.

Mode of exam delivery

The CEN exams are administered via a testing facility or live remote proctoring (LRP).

CBT exams are offered in testing centers via PSI. All the scheduling processes of PSI are discussed above. If an exam is disrupted due to weather or an emergency that impacts the test center, all candidates will be contacted within two days to reschedule their exams.

With LRP, you do not have to go to a testing center to take the exam. You can take it remotely in a secure area. This exam is supervised in real time and is the same as the CBT exam offered in testing centers.

Requirements for LRP

You must check in no later than 30 minutes before the exam commences. After checking in, you will be asked to download a secure browser, run a system check of the microphone and webcam, scan your work area and test environment, present an approved government ID card and take a photograph. After this process is completed, the proctor will launch the exam. You are allowed two blank papers for your exam. These papers must be shown to the proctor before the start of the exam and must be destroyed after the exam in the presence of the proctor.

Exam length

The CEN exam lasts three hours. It has 175 multiple-choice questions. Of those questions, 150 are scored and 25 are not. You will be unable to differentiate a scored question from an unscored question. Five practice questions are given before the start of the test to help you get familiar with the interface.

Exam breaks

There are no formal breaks, but you can take as many breaks as needed. However, additional time will not be given to finish the exams. Breaks must not exceed 15 minutes. If they do, you risk cancelation of the exam. You must obtain expressed consent from the testing center staff or proctor. You are not allowed to pick up personal belongings during a break unless you need access to scheduled medication. Also, you are expected to show your approved ID before and after any breaks. If you are taking your exam via LRP, you will be required to rescan your work area and environment after returning from breaks.

Test Accommodation

If you require testing accommodations, you must fill out the Test Accommodations Form in the exam application. The BCEN will assess your request based on the information provided on the form and offer standard and nonstandard test accommodations as needed.

Security Procedures

Testing facilities

Testing centers are supervised by both audio and visual surveillance systems. Additional security is provided by the testing center staff to ensure that candidates do not violate the rules and regulations governing the exam. Staff are at liberty to assign seats to candidates, separate suspicious candidates from other test takers and use table dividers to dissuade candidates from cheating. Failure to comply with a staff member's instructions can lead to the cancelation of your exam.

LRP exams are also monitored by visual and audio surveillance systems. Footage of the exams is kept for at least 30 days.

Rules and Regulations

Testing facilities

1. You are not allowed to communicate verbally or in other formats with other test takers once you enter the examination hall.
2. You are not permitted to copy, duplicate, communicate or transmit the test content for any reason. Copying and duplicating test content is a violation of the PSI's security policy. Violation can put you at risk of being disqualified from the exam and reported to the BCEN and security officials.
3. Electronic devices of any kind are banned from the exam hall.

4. Personal items and effects are banned from the exam hall. Store these items in a safe place before entering the hall. PSI is not liable for any missing or stolen property.
5. Abusive behavior toward the staff is prohibited. You are expected to be courteous and professional. Respect the staff, and follow the exam's rules and regulations. Candidates who are abusive to the staff are at risk of forfeiting the exam and being reported to the BCEN and security personnel.
6. Third parties are prohibited from entering the examination room.
7. You are prohibited from leaving the building or using telephones during the examination.

Live remote proctoring

Software systems are used to monitor candidates during the exam. Proctors who suspect violations can pause the exam. In cases of major violations, they have the right to cancel the exam. In such instances, the candidate's scores will be withheld and reported to the BCEN. The following are the rules and regulations of the LRP exam:

1. You are required to have a web camera, speakers, microphone and stable internet connection for the exam.
2. You are not allowed to communicate with the proctor or other third parties during the exam.
3. You are not allowed to reproduce, copy or transmit the test content in any format. Copying and duplicating test content is a violation of the PSI's security policy. Violation can put you at risk of being disqualified from the exam and reported to the BCEN and security officials.

4. Apart from the testing computer, electronic devices of any kind are banned from the exam.
5. You are expected to scan your work area and environment before the exam commences and after returning from a break.
6. You must present an approved government ID before the exam. Military IDs are not allowed.
7. Abusive behavior toward the proctor is prohibited. You are expected to be courteous and professional, respect the staff and follow the exam's rules and regulations. Candidates who are abusive to the staff are at risk of forfeiting the exam and being reported to the BCEN and security personnel.
8. You are at liberty to communicate with the proctor no later than 30 minutes before the commencement of the exam.
9. You are not allowed to leave the camera's view or use any form of an electronic device besides the computer during the examination.
10. Your hands and work area must be seen at all times. You are not allowed to talk during the exam.

How the Exam Is Developed

BCEN uses three principles in producing psychometrically sound test content. They are:

1. Test constriction – Role delineation studies are used to evaluate relevant and up-to-date practice every four to five years. In these studies, emergency nurses from diverse geographical regions of the United States are surveyed. The exam committee members use the results of the surveys to create test questions that are feasible and valid.
2. Item development – In this step, experts in emergency nursing are hired as members of the examination committee. These experts are from diverse

geographical, practice and demographic regions of the United States. Experts are also hired based on clinical experience, qualifications and skills. They are then trained in the principles of writing CEN test questions.

3. Analysis – In this stage, quality-control testing is done on test items. The data from this analysis are evaluated based on reliability, discrimination level, difficulty and performance.

How the Exam Is Scored

The Angoff technique is used to determine pass/fail status. Statistical equating is also used to match the difficulty of the exam to the pass rates and adjust the passing score based on the exam's overall difficulty. The BCEN has the liberty to make corrections on any erroneous pass/fail status. Students who pass the exams are given their certificate and a wallet card within 15 days of getting their scores. Certificates are valid for four years. Test reports are either pass or fail. This status is derived from the raw scores of correct answers. Score reports are given by the testing staff in the testing center. Score reports are also sent to the candidate's email. Students who used the LRP form of the test will get their scores at the end of the exam. In this case, a pass or fail is shown on the screen. Score reports are also sent to their emails.

Students who do not pass the exams are sent a candidate performance report containing their raw scores in each component of its outline. Candidates can reapply and retake the exam after 90 days.

Cancelation of Scores

The BCEN can cancel or withhold scores if a candidate is guilty of a violation of rules and regulations. The following can lead to cancelation of test scores:

1. Falsifying information during application
2. Falsifying documents required by the BCEN
3. Having an encumbered RN license during the application or during the time of the test
4. Misrepresenting certification
5. Cheating or conspiring to cheat during the exam.

Please note that the BCEN performs a detailed investigation into allegations of misconduct, misrepresentation and noncompliance. You can appeal disciplinary actions and decisions. The appeals process is described on the BCEN's website.

Confidentiality of the Candidates

Score reports and certificates are not given to third parties. More information on confidentiality is provided on the BCEN's website.

Tips on How to Pass the CEN Exam

Passing the CEN exam requires a combination of preparation, organization and mental attitude. Adequate preparation has a lot to do with the type of resource materials you prepare with, the amount of time you spend preparing and the capacity of your recall.

How to choose the right resource material

Here are a few things to consider before choosing the right study material for your exams:

1. Relevance – Your study material should be relevant to the exam. To increase your chances of selecting relevant study material, you can buy resources that are recommended by tutors, colleagues and peers who have taken and passed the exams.
2. Revised – How current is your study material? The BCEN reviews the CEN exams every five years. Therefore, your study material should be current, updated and revised to reflect the current BCEN standard.
3. Cost –Beware of outrageously expensive materials. There are good study materials available that are reasonably priced. Highlights – Your study material should give highlights on the distribution of test questions and priority areas to focus on. Focused concentration is a characteristic of effective studying. The right study material should help you narrow your reading to specific and key areas.
4. Comprehensive rationales – Your study material should give comprehensive rationales for test questions and their answers. This fine-tunes your critical thinking and helps you identify subtle words and distinctions you did not notice before.
5. Organized – Your study material should be organized methodically. Study materials that break down bulky segments into outlines and sections improve your recall. Haphazard study materials can slow down your preparation process.

Chapter 1: Cardiovascular Emergencies

There are 19 questions in this section. Topic areas are:

Acute coronary syndrome

1. STEMI – This is called ST-elevation myocardial infarction. It is a serious form of a heart attack in which a major coronary vessel is completely blocked, and a portion of the heart does not receive a blood supply.
2. NSTEMI – A non-ST-elevated myocardial infarction is not as serious as a STEMI because there is a temporal or partial blockage of the coronary artery.
3. Angina pectoris – This includes Prinzmetal variant, unstable and stable angina.
4. Complications – These include arrhythmias, heart failure, aneurysm, myocardial rupture, mural thrombosis, pericarditis, cardiogenic shock, disorders of the papillary muscle and postmyocardial infarction syndrome.

Aneurysm and dissection

1. Aortic dissection – This is the passage of blood through a false pocket between the tunica intima and tunica media. Causes include atherosclerosis, malignant hypertension, acquired connective tissue disorders, hereditary connective tissue disorder, iatrogenic causes from aortic catheterization and aortic valve surgery and trauma. Clinical features are tearing pain in the precordial area that can spread to the scapular; severe hypotension; syncope; arterial pulse deficits between the two limbs and features of impaired perfusion (stroke, paraplegia, renal insufficiency and myocardial and intestinal infarction). It is often fatal. Treatment requires rapid resuscitation with beta-blockers to control blood pressure and immediate surgery.

2. Aortic aneurysm – This includes thoracic or abdominal aneurysms. Causes include atherosclerosis; uncontrolled hypertension; family history of aneurysms; white race; male sex; older patients and most significant of all, cigarette smoking. It is often asymptomatic. Clinical features are usually from compression of surrounding structures or rupture. Major complications are embolization, rupture and DIC. Treatment modalities are management of blood pressure and cessation of smoking. Surgical interventions are the insertion of an endovascular stent.

Cardiopulmonary arrest

This is the arrest of mechanical activity of the heart and consequent reduction of cardiac output. It requires rapid intervention to reduce the risk of death. Causes in adults are mainly from primary diseases of the heart, especially coronary artery disease. Other causes are pulmonary embolism, metabolic derangement, hemorrhage of the splanchnic circulation and trauma. Causes in infants are obstruction of the airway, drowning, sudden infant death syndrome and smoke inhalation. Treatment includes immediate CPR and treatment of the underlying cause.

CPR in adults

1. Airway and breathing – This includes assessment, clearing and opening of the airway; use of mouth-to-mouth resuscitation in nonhospital settings; ventilating with a bag and mask and inserting oropharyngeal or nasopharyngeal airways where appropriate. Endotracheal intubation may be indicated. Note that compression and use of a defibrillator are prioritized over the airway.
2. Circulation – Chest compressions are done until defibrillation is performed. Chest compressions must be interrupted for at least 10

seconds. In adults, the compressions are done to a depth of five to six centimeters (1.9 to 2.5 inches). During the compressions, the ER nurse must notice as the chest recoils during the release phase before starting again. Open chest cardiac compressions may be done for patients with penetrating trauma to the chest. In some facilities, mechanical chest compression devices are used to eliminate errors due to fatigue.

3. Defibrillation – Ventricular fibrillation and pulseless ventricular tachycardia are shockable and therefore amenable to defibrillation. Defibrillation with direct current cardioversion is more effective than the use of antiarrhythmic drugs. In this procedure, defibrillation pads are positioned in between the clavicle and the second intercostal space, just over the fifth intercostal space. About 120 to 200 joules of energy are used, to a maximum of 360 joules.
4. Drugs – These include adenosine, atropine, calcium chloride, calcium gluconate, dopamine, dobutamine, glucose, epinephrine, naloxone, magnesium sulfate, norepinephrine, procainamide and others.

Dysrhythmias

1. Atrial fibrillation – Afib (AF) is a common type of arrhythmia. There are absent waves before the QRS complex. The heart rate is also irregular.
2. First-degree heart block – This is a sinus rhythm in which the PR interval lasts more than 0.2 seconds due to prolonged transmission from the atria to the ventricles.
3. Second-degree AV heart block – This includes Mobitz Type I (Wenckebach) or Mobitz Type II. In Mobitz Type I block, the PR interval lengthens progressively until the QRS complex drops. In Mobitz Type II, there is an intermittent drop in the QRS complex that is not typical of the

Type I pattern. Also, in the Mobitz Type II block there is no rapid progression to a complete heart block.

4. Third-degree heart block – This is called a complete heart block. There is a discontinuity between the P and QRS waves. The P-P intervals are usually regular, but they are not related to the QRS complexes.
5. Ventricular tachycardia – Another name for this is Vtach (VT). There are widened QRS complexes, absent P waves and an abnormal rate that is more than 100 per minute. This rhythm can quickly turn into ventricular fibrillation and death.
6. Ventricular fibrillation – Another name for this arrhythmia is Vfib, or VF. There is a chaotic wave pattern that has no pulse. VF may respond to electrical defibrillation.
7. Paroxysmal ventricular tachycardia – This presents as a narrow QRS complex. In some cases, wide QRS complex, retrograde P waves may also be seen. There is also rapid and regular tachycardia.
8. Sick sinus syndrome – There are numerous possible presentations on ECG, including sinus arrest, sinus bradycardia, sinoatrial block and bradycardia-tachycardia syndrome.
9. Torsades de Pointes – This presents with a long QT interval and irregular and rapid QRS complexes that look like they are twisting around the ECG baseline
10. Premature beats – This is also called premature ventricular contraction. It presents as broad QRS complexes that are more than 1,200 ms with associated discordant T-wave and ST-segment changes. These beats occur faster than normal for the incoming sinus wave.
11. Atrial fibrillation/atrial flutter – This is a supraventricular arrhythmia. There is a saw-toothed flutter that is characteristically seen on the ECG, which are multiple P waves that appear for each of the QRS complexes.

Endocarditis

1. Infective endocarditis – This is an infection of the endocardium by staphylococci or streptococci. Fungal infections are rare. Risk factors are underlying abnormality of the endocardium leading to the formation of vegetations, and bacteremia from IV drug abuse. Clinical features are low-grade fever, chills, night sweats, weakness, weight loss, murmur and cutaneous manifestations. Diagnosis is via Duke's criteria.

Duke's Criteria

1. Major criteria – Two positive blood cultures of implicated organisms. Blood cultures must be collected more than 12 hours apart. Positive serologic response to Coxiella burnetii or at least one positive blood culture for Coxiella burnetii. Echocardiographic findings of endocarditis, including cardiac abscess; new onset of valvular regurgitation; new onset of dehiscence of a prosthetic cardiac valve; presence of an oscillating mass on the valves or other structures surrounding the valves.
2. Minor criteria – History of IV drug abuse, a temperature that is greater than or equal to 38.3°C and features of vascular occurrences like Janeway lesions, conjunctival petechiae, intracranial hemorrhage or arterial or septic pulmonary embolism. Evidence of immunologic occurrence may manifest as glomerulonephritis, Roth's spots, Osler nodes and rheumatoid factor. Diagnosis is made in the presence of two major criteria, or one major and three minor criteria or zero major and five minor criteria.
3. Noninfective endocarditis – This is characterized by the formation of sterile thrombin, fibrin and platelet plugs on the cardiac valves. Causes include cardiac catheterization and autoimmune disorders like SLE and antiphospholipid syndrome. It is also seen in patients with chronic

diseases like carcinomas of the pancreas or lungs, tuberculosis, and osteomyelitis. Diagnosis is via blood cultures and echocardiography.

Heart failure

1. Right ventricular heart failure – There is an increase in systemic venous pressure due to the backflow of blood from the IVC and SVC. This increase causes movement of fluid from the intravascular space into the tissue space. Affected patients present with pedal and/or sacral edema, distended neck veins and ascites. Patients also have tender hepatomegaly, which may manifest with hyperbilirubinemia, elevated hepatic enzymes and prolonged prothrombin time. Patients with chronic RVF have malabsorption syndromes.
2. Systolic heart failure – It is characterized by decreased cardiac output and increased pulmonary venous pressure. Increased pulmonary venous pressure leads to increased hydrostatic pressure in the capillary bed and consequent pulmonary edema. Patients often present to the ER anxious and restless with cyanosis, breathlessness and chest pain. Patients must first be placed in the cardiac position and promptly managed with IV Lasix, supplemental oxygen, anticoagulants and anxiolytics.
3. Heart failure with reduced ejection fraction – It is characterized by left ventricular dysfunction with an increase in diastolic volume and reduction in ejection fraction less than or equal to 40 percent. Causes include dilated cardiomyopathy, myocardial infarction and myocarditis. These conditions predominantly affect systolic function.
4. Heart failure with preserved ejection fraction – This is known as diastolic heart failure that causes an increase in end-diastolic pressure on exertion or at rest. End-diastolic volume is often preserved. The ejection fraction is more than 50 percent. It is often caused by conditions that stiffen the

ventricles and make them unable to relax. Some causes include valvular disease, hypertrophic cardiomyopathy, constrictive pericarditis and amyloidosis.

Hypertension

Drugs for hypertension

1. Adrenergic agonists – Clonidine, methyldopa and guanfacine stimulate alpha 2 adrenergic receptors in the brain stem and reduce the activity of the sympathetic nervous system. Due to their central action in the nervous system, they cause depression, drowsiness and lethargy. Methyldopa is safe to use in pregnancy.
2. Angiotensin-converting enzyme inhibitors – They prevent the conversion of angiotensin I to angiotensin II (which releases bradykinin, causes vasoconstriction and stimulates the release of aldosterone). These drugs reduce resistance in peripheral vessels without causing reflex tachycardia. They are not recommended for initial therapy in Blacks. The most significant side effect is a dry cough. Angioedema is a potential and serious side effect. These drugs also increase potassium and creatinine levels. Examples are captopril, enalapril, lisinopril and fosinopril.
3. Angiotensin II receptor blocker – These drugs inhibit the stimulation of angiotensin II receptors and therefore inhibit activation of the Renin-angiotensin system. ARBs should not be used with an ACEI. They are useful in hypertensive patients with diabetic nephropathy. They are contraindicated in pregnancy. Examples are telmisartan, losartan, valsartan and candesartan.
4. Calcium channel blockers – They prevent the action of calcium on smooth muscles and therefore reduce resistance in peripheral blood vessels. The dihydropyridines are very effective vasodilators that may cause reflex

tachycardia. Examples are amlodipine, nifedipine, felodipine and nicardipine. The nondihydropyridines reduce heart rate, myocardial contractility and atrioventricular conduction. They are not used in patients with atrioventricular block caused by left ventricular failure. Examples are verapamil and diltiazem.

5. Diuretics – These drugs reduce preload by reducing plasma volume. Examples are potassium-sparing loop diuretics like furosemide and torsemide. Thiazide-type diuretics include hydrochlorothiazide, chlorothiazide, hydroflumethiazide and indapamide. These diuretics are potassium-wasting diuretics and cause hypokalemia. Potassium-sparing diuretics include amiloride and spironolactone. Side effects of these drugs are hyperkalemia, gynecomastia (spironolactone), nausea and GIT disturbances.
6. Direct vasodilators – These drugs work directly on peripheral blood vessels without affecting autonomic nervous system activity on the blood vessels. Examples of these drugs are hydralazine and minoxidil. Side effects of these drugs are tachycardia, headaches and edema. These drugs increase the risk of angina in patients with coronary artery disease.
7. Nitrates – These include sodium nitroprusside and nitroglycerin. They are potent vasodilators that reduce afterload. Side effects of nitrates are rebound hypertension, reflex tachycardia and postural hypotension. These drugs must not be taken with phosphodiesterase 5 inhibitors (sildenafil).

Pericardial tamponade

This is a cardiac emergency caused by an accumulation of blood in the pericardial sac. This sac constricts the heart and prevents it from relaxing during diastole. If left untreated, patients can die from obstructive shock. It is caused by either blunt or penetrating trauma to the chest. However, penetrating trauma is a more common cause. Clinical features include Beck's triad of hypotension, distended neck veins and muffled heart sounds. Other features are pulsus paradoxus and shock. The

Beck's triad may not easily be confirmed in a noisy and busy ER. This is because patients often present with multiple trauma, and hypotension can blunt distension of the neck veins. Also, a muffled heart sound may not readily be appreciated. Treatment is immediate pericardiocentesis under ECG monitoring, followed by thoracotomy if the patient does not respond to the initial procedure. This procedure must be done in the operating room as soon as possible.

Pericarditis

1. Acute pericarditis – Causes include autoimmune infections (mostly viral); inflammation; trauma; myocardial infarction (Dressler's syndrome); radiation therapy; uremia; cancer and drugs (isoniazid, hydralazine, phenytoin, anticoagulants and procainamide).
2. Subacute pericarditis – This has the same causes as acute pericarditis but lasts longer (from days to weeks).
3. Chronic pericardial effusion – Causes are hypothyroidism (myxedema) and metastases from breast and lung carcinomas, sarcoma, lymphoma, melanoma and leukemia.
4. Transient constrictive pericarditis – May be idiopathic. Also caused by infection or inflammation postpericardiotomy.
5. Fibrosis of the pericardium – It is sequelae of purulent pericarditis, tuberculosis, MI, carcinoma or a disorder of the connective tissue. It can also be a complication of hemopericardium caused by insertion of pacemakers, cardiac catheterization, insertion of a central venous line or rupture of a thoracic aortic aneurysm.

6. Clinical features – Features of inflammation (hyperpyrexia, malaise, weakness and night sweats); features of pericardial effusion (muffled heart sounds, cardiac dullness and change in the cardiac silhouette on chest X-ray); pleurisy, chest pain; tachypnea; pericardial friction rub; nonproductive cough and cardiac tamponade in massive pericardial effusion. Constrictive pericarditis presents as features of elevated ventricular and diastolic pressures, and features of congestion of the peripheral venous system (pedal edema, hepatomegaly and distension of neck veins). A pericardial knock may also be heard.
7. Treatment – Symptomatic treatment with NSAIDs, corticosteroids and colchicines; pericardiocentesis for relief of effusions; resection for pericardial fibrosis and use of triamcinolone to prevent the proliferation of fibrotic tissue. Definitive treatment is the management of the underlying cause.

Peripheral vascular disease

1. Peripheral arterial disease – This is caused by atherosclerosis and occlusion of the vessels in the lower limbs. It may be asymptomatic in mild cases, but patients may also present with intermittent claudication. Clinical features are intermittent claudication, which patients describe as an aching, burning or heavy sensation in their thighs, calves, hips or buttocks. This pain is worsened by activity and relieved by rest. On examination, the affected limb shows dependent rubor, and pale and atrophic hairless skin in chronic cases. The leg may be cyanotic and diaphoretic. In severe cases, patients present with peripheral arterial ulcers on the heel or toes. The ulcers are tender and have dry, black and necrotic tissue. Treatment includes removal of risk factors, treatment of

underlying cause (smoking cessation, use of antilipids, weight loss and diet modification) and drug therapy with antiplatelet drugs, analgesics and ACEIs. Surgical intervention includes percutaneous transluminal angioplasty, revascularization and sympathectomy for amputation in severe cases.

2. Raynaud's syndrome – It is characterized by vasospasms of arteries in the hands due to cold or emotional stress. Clinical features are paresthesia in the affected hand, characterized by burning, tingling or cold sensations and pain, and change in color, characterized by pallor, cyanosis or rubor. Secondary Raynaud's syndrome can cause ulcerative changes. Treatment is avoidance of triggers, use of relaxation techniques, cessation of smoking and use of calcium channel blockers. In secondary causes, surgical debridement of the wound may be indicated.

Peripheral venous disorders

1. Deep venous thrombosis – This is a primary cause of pulmonary embolism. It is characterized by the formation of blood clots in the deep veins of the lower limbs. Risk factors include obesity; age greater than 60 years; cigarette smoking; cancers; use of estrogen agonists like tamoxifen; heart failure; hypercoagulability disorders; immobilization, trauma to the limbs; presence of a venous catheter; nephritic syndrome; use of oral contraceptives or estrogen replacement therapy; prior history of thromboembolism; pregnancy and myeloproliferative neoplasms like polycythemia, sickle cell anemia and trauma. Clinical features are asymptomatic in small veins. In bigger veins, they may present as edema, tenderness and erythema of the affected side. Patients may present with fever or features of pulmonary embolism and thromboembolism.

Treatment modalities include anticoagulation therapies, use of thrombolytic drugs or IVC filter. Surgery is required in severe cases. Prevention modalities include early mobilization of surgical patients, prophylactic use of anticoagulants in at-risk patients and use of pneumatic compression.

2. Arteriovenous fistula – This is an abnormal communication between an artery and a vein. It can be congenital or acquired from trauma. It presents as symptoms and signs of arterial or venous insufficiency. Treatment modalities are the use of percutaneous occlusion techniques and surgery.
3. Varicose veins – This is the dilation of superficial veins in the lower limbs. They are often asymptomatic. However, patients may complain of pain, hyperesthesia and paresthesia in the affected limb. Treatment modalities include compression stockings and surgery.

Thromboembolic diseases

1. Disseminated intravascular coagulation – This is excessive generation of thrombin in the blood, leading to embolism. When the clotting factors are exhausted, bleeding ensues. Causes are obstetric complications (abruptio placentae, eclampsia, severe preeclampsia or embolism of amniotic fluid, a retained product of conception and severe maternal sepsis); septicemia caused by gram-negative microorganisms; adenocarcinomas of the pancreas and prostate; shock; snake envenomation; intravascular hemolysis; tissue damage from burns or frostbite and complications of prostate surgery.
2. Myeloproliferative disorders – This is essential thrombocythemia caused by a primary increase of platelets; polycythemia vera caused by a primary

increase of red blood cells, white blood cells and/or platelets; primary myelofibrosis and chronic myeloid leukemia.

3. Thrombotic disorders – Genetic causes include protein C deficiency, protein S deficiency, protein Z deficiency, antithrombin deficiency and mutation of Factor V. Acquired causes are antiphospholipid antibodies; heparin-induced thrombocytopenia; hyperhomocysteinemia; severe sepsis; oral contraceptives; stasis of venous blood; tissue trauma; cancers of the lung, stomach, colon and pancreas; and atherosclerosis.

Treatment options for thromboembolic disorders

1. Antiplatelets – Prevent aggregation of platelets. Examples include aspirin, a COX-2 inhibitor that prevents the synthesis of prostaglandins and leukotrienes. Others include clopidogrel, an ADP receptor inhibitor; phosphodiesterase inhibitors like cilostazol; glycoprotein IIB/IIIA inhibitors like abciximab and tirofiban; and thromboxane inhibitors.
2. Thrombolytics – These drugs encourage lysis of blood clots. Examples are streptokinase, which increases secretion of plasmin required in breaking down thrombin; and recombinant tissue plasminogen activators like alteplase, reteplase and urokinase, which activate the conversion of plasminogen to plasmin.
3. Anticoagulants – This includes warfarin, low-molecular-weight heparin, unfractionated heparins, Factor Xa inhibitors like apixaban and edoxaban and Factor IIa inhibitors like dabigatran.

Cardiovascular Trauma

1. Aortic disruption – This is rupture of the aorta following blunt or penetrating chest injury. Clinical features are pulse deficits of the upper extremities, chest pain, systolic murmur, hoarseness, hypotension and

shock. Treatment modalities are acute resuscitation with fluids and supplemental oxygen, and stabilization of blood pressure with a beta-blocker. Definitive treatment is emergency repair or insertion of an endovascular stent.

2. Myocardial contusion – Caused by blunt cardiac injury. Patients may present with arrhythmias in severe cases.
3. Rupture of the ventricles – Often fatal, although patients with smaller tears may present with cardiac tamponade. It is typically caused by a blunt cardiac injury.
4. Disruption of valves – Patients often present with murmurs and features of heart failure. It is typically caused by blunt trauma to the chest.
5. Septal rupture – Patients may also present with heart failure. It is typically caused by blunt trauma to the chest.
6. Commotio cordis – Caused by blunt trauma to the precordium in patients without underlying cardiovascular comorbidity. Patients present with sudden cardiac arrest. It causes ventricular fibrillation and is often fatal.

Cardiogenic Shock and Obstructive Shock

1. Obstructive shock – Caused by extrinsic factors that impair filling or emptying of the heart. Mechanism includes:

   A. Mechanical obstruction to ventricular filling – Cardiac tamponade, clot, or tumor in the atria; tension pneumothorax and compression of the IVC or SVC.

   B. Mechanical obstruction to ventricular emptying – Pulmonary embolism.

2. Cardiogenic shock – Reduced cardiac output due to an intrinsic cardiac disorder. Mechanism includes:

A. Inefficient contractility of the myocardium – Myocardial ischemia, myocarditis, myocardial infarction and certain drugs that induce arrhythmias.
B. Abnormal cardiac rhythm – All the examples of dysrhythmias.
C. Structural disorders of the cardiomyocytes – Mitral or aortic regurgitation, rupture of the interventricular septum and malfunction of the prosthetic valve.

Chapter 2: Respiratory Emergencies

There are 18 test questions in this section. Content areas are:

Aspiration

1. Causes – Swallowing impairment from neurologic and neuropathic diseases; impaired consciousness or cognition; severe vomiting; enteral feeding tubes; endotracheal tubes; oropharyngeal and nasopharyngeal airways and gastroesophageal reflux disease.
2. Clinical features – Dyspnea, fever, cough, and chest pain. Features of chemical pneumonitis from aspiration of caustic poisoning include hemoptysis, fever, pinky frothy sputum, wheezing and diffuse crackles.
3. Treatment – Supportive treatment with supplemental oxygen and assisted ventilation. Antibiotic therapy with beta-lactamase inhibitors or clindamycin for patients with chemical pneumonitis. Abscesses in the lungs are treated with IV antibiotics and percutaneous drainage.

Asthma

1. Risk factors – Male sex; non-Hispanic blacks; exposure to allergens (dust, cold, dander and pollen) diet and chronic exposure to irritants.
2. Clinical features – Patients with mild to moderate cases experience chest tightness, breathlessness, wheezing and cough. Symptoms are often worse during sleep. On presentation, signs include wheezing, tachypnea, pulsus paradoxus, tachycardia and breathlessness evidenced by the use of accessory muscles of respiration. Patients with severe exacerbations present with altered consciousness, cyanosis and a silent chest. In chronic cases, patients have barrel-shaped chests and hyperinflated lungs.
3. Treatment

A. Acute resuscitation with supplemental oxygen and NIPPV for patients with cyanosis and metabolic acidosis.
B. Inhaled bronchodilators – Bronchodilation with beta-agonists like salbutamol and albuterol, and acetylcholine receptor antagonists like ipratropium bromide. Nebulized bronchodilators are used for children.
C. Intravenous corticosteroids – These are used to reduce inflammation and mucus plug formation in the respiratory tract.
D. Magnesium sulfate – This is used for bronchodilation.

Chronic obstructive pulmonary disease (COPD)

1. Chronic bronchitis – This is characterized by a chronic productive cough that lasts for at least three months in two consecutive years. Smoking is the predominant risk factor for chronic bronchitis. Patients with chronic bronchitis are referred to as blue bloaters, with characteristic cyanosis, edema, chronic productive cough, leg swelling and pulmonary hypertension.
2. Emphysema – Characterized by progressive destruction of the lung parenchyma with loss of elastic recoil, radial airway traction and alveoli septa. Patients with emphysema are typically referred to as pink puffers, with cachectic appearance, pursed-lip breathing, dome-shaped chest and use of accessory muscles of respiration.

Infections

1. Community-acquired pneumonia – This pneumonia is contracted outside the hospital. The most common causative pathogens are Streptococcus pneumonia; Haemophilus influenza; atypical bacteria like Legionella species; Chlamydia pneumonia; viruses and Mycoplasma pneumoniae.

2. Nosocomial pneumonia – This is hospital-acquired pneumonia. Risk factors include immunosuppression, intubation, old age, immobility and sepsis. Nosocomial pneumonia is contracted by inpatients 48 to 72 hours after being admitted. It is generally caused by a bacterial infection rather than a virus. Implicated bacteria include rod-shaped, gram-negative organisms like Pseudomonas aeruginosa, Klebsiella pneumoniae and Enterobacter spp; gram-positive bacteria like Staphylococcus aureus; and Haemophilus influenzae. Implicated viruses include influenza and respiratory syncytial virus and cytomegalovirus.
3. Empyema – This is the collection of pus/abscesses in the lungs. Risk factors include pulmonary tuberculosis and other infectious suppurative lung diseases.
4. Ventilator-associated event – This is a new or progressive and persistent radiographic abnormality that develops in a patient on mechanical ventilation or within 48 hours of mechanical ventilation. This patient must also demonstrate one or more systemic signs, like fever, leukopenia or leukocytosis. It can also include altered mental status in patients more than 70 years of age and have the following pulmonary criteria: dyspnea, rales, new-onset cough, increased respiratory secretions, impaired oxygenation and bronchial breath sounds.

Inhalation injuries

Irritant gas inhalation injury

1. Cause – These gases dissolve in water in the respiratory tract and cause inflammation. They include sulfur dioxide, hydrogen sulfide, ozone, ammonia, chlorine, nitrogen dioxide, phosgene and chloramine, which is created by mixing toilet cleaners with bleach. Acute exposure in large

doses is most often from industrial accidents. Water-soluble gases like hydrogen chloride and sulfur dioxide quickly dissolve in the upper airway and stimulate acute inflammatory response, while less soluble gases like ozone and phosgene do not stimulate an acute response until they are properly dissolved in the respiratory tract. They cause a delayed inflammatory response.

2. Clinical features – Immediate response includes coughing, retching, hemoptysis, wheezing and chest pain. Irritant gases also irritate the eyes and nose. About two weeks after exposure, some patients experience bronchiolitis obliterans caused by plugging of the airways with granulation tissue. This can lead to acute respiratory distress syndrome. Complications are acute respiratory distress syndrome, superseding bacterial infection, sepsis and pulmonary fibrosis.
3. Treatment
    A. Removal from exposure and decontamination.
    B. Supportive management of symptoms – supplemental oxygen, inhaled bronchodilators and systemic corticosteroids.
    C. In severe cases, patients are managed with mechanical ventilation and inhaled epinephrine.

Smoke inhalation

1. Causes – Often an acute complication of burns from exposure to fire.
2. Clinical features – Cough, stridor and wheezing from local irritation; confusion, coma and lethargy from hypoxia; features of carbon monoxide poisoning; headache; weakness; nausea and confusion.
3. Treatment –Supportive with supplemental oxygen and mechanical ventilation. Hyperventilation or use of hyperbaric oxygen is required for carbon monoxide poisoning.

Obstruction

Obstruction of the airway due to narrowing and remodeling (e.g., asthma, COPD, alpha-1-antitrypsin deficiency). Other causes of obstruction include tumors of the respiratory tract, pneumothorax, hemothorax, abscess and others.

Pleural effusion

This is an accumulation of fluid within the pleural space. Causes are varied and classified as either transudates or exudates. Diagnosis is clinical and confirmed by chest X-ray. However, thoracocentesis and analysis of the pleural fluid are needed to diagnose the cause. Treatment modalities include thoracocentesis, pleurectomy and chest tube drainage.

Pneumothorax

1. This is the accumulation of air in the pleural space. Types include primary pneumothorax, which occurs in young men with a tall and thin habitus. There is typically no underlying lung disease.
2. Secondary spontaneous pneumothorax occurs in patients with underlying pulmonary pathology.
3. Traumatic pneumothorax occurs as a result of blunt or penetrating trauma to the chest wall.
4. Iatrogenic pneumothorax occurs as a result of surgical interventions like thoracocentesis, transthoracic needle aspiration, mechanical ventilation and others.

Noncardiac Pulmonary edema

1. Causes – Cardiogenic cause from left ventricular heart failure from decompensated heart failure, acute coronary syndrome, arrhythmias or valvular disease. Noncardiogenic causes include fluid overload, drowning, aspiration pneumonitis, respiratory distress syndrome, allergic reactions and acute kidney injury.
2. Clinical features – Chest tightness, difficult breathing, chest pain, worsening cyanosis, diaphoresis and anxiousness. Patients with cardiogenic causes present with cardiovascular symptoms like murmurs, distended neck veins, hypertension and hepatomegaly.
3. Treatment
    A. Place the patient in the high Fowler's position for relief of chest symptoms. This position causes gravitational movement of fluid to the lower lobes of the lung.
    B. Administer supplemental oxygen. Unresolved cases will require mechanical ventilation.
    C. IV Lasix for cardiogenic causes of pulmonary edema
    D. IV morphine to reduce work of breathing
    E. IV inotropes for patients in heart failure
    F. In noncardiogenic causes, the underlying causes are treated.

Pulmonary embolus

1. Cause – Deep vein thrombosis is the most common cause of pulmonary embolism. An embolus is most often released from the deep veins of the legs. However, embolus can come from the central veins of the chest via central lines and thoracic outlet syndromes and the veins in the arm. Risk factors for deep vein thrombosis are further discussed in the section on peripheral venous disorders under cardiovascular emergencies.

2. Clinical features – They include chest pain, difficulty breathing, cough, hemoptysis, symptoms of shock in massive embolism, hypotension, tachypnea, tachycardia and features of right ventricular heart failure. Patients may also present with localized features of deep vein thrombosis.
3. Treatment
    A. Acute resuscitation with supplemental oxygen and mechanical ventilation where indicated.
    B. Rapid dissolution of clots with systemic thrombolytic drugs or catheter-directed therapy.
    C. Anticoagulation therapy.
    D. Prevention of further embolism by controlling and modifying risk factors.

Respiratory distress syndrome

1. Cause – Increased hydrostatic pressure in the alveolar capillaries (pulmonary edema), increased permeability of the alveolar capillaries, diffuse alveolar hemorrhage, right to left cardiac shunts as seen in congenital cyanotic heart diseases and Eisenmenger syndrome.
2. Clinical features – Difficulty breathing, anxiety, restlessness, cyanosis, altered sensorium, diaphoresis, tachycardia, tachypnea, crackles, distended neck veins, cardiac arrhythmias and death.
3. Treatment – Mechanical ventilation treatment of underlying cause.

Respiratory Trauma

Flail chest

1. Cause – Fracture of more than three adjacent ribs from blunt or penetrating trauma. The broken ribs move paradoxically during breathing (i.e., inward during inspiration and outward during expiration).
2. Treatment
    A. Acute resuscitation and stabilization for patients with multiple injuries
    B. Supportive management of symptoms – IV analgesia for pain relief, supplemental oxygen and mechanical ventilation where indicated and IV fluids.
    C. Surgery may be required for specific patients.

Hemothorax

1. Cause – Accumulation of blood within the pleural space due to penetrating injuries that lacerate the lung, internal mammary artery or intercostal vessels.
2. Clinical features – In large hemothoraces, patients present with difficulty breathing. On examination, there are decreased percussion notes and breath sounds on the affected side. These may not be easily elicited in patients with multiple injuries. Patients may also present with hypovolemic shock.
3. Treatment
    A. Acute resuscitation with oxygen, mechanical ventilation, IV fluids, vasopressors and blood products where indicated.
    B. Chest tube thoracostomy.
    C. Thoracotomy in select cases.

Pneumothorax

1. Cause – Penetrating or blunt trauma to the chest. Patients may also present with hemithorax. Clinical features of traumatic pneumothorax are

difficulty breathing tachypnea, pleuritic chest pain and tachycardia. On examination, there are hyperresonant sounds on percussion and crackles when the affected side is palpated (subcutaneous emphysema). There may also be a Hamman sign caused by air in the mediastinum. In tension pneumothorax, patients may present with hypotension, distension of the neck veins and tracheal deviation. The affected area is also tense and distended.

2. Treatment
    A. Acute resuscitation with IV fluids, supplemental oxygen and mechanical ventilation where indicated.
    B. Immediate thoracentesis and chest tube thoracostomy.

Pulmonary contusion

1. Causes – Blunt or penetrating chest trauma.
2. Clinical features – Chest pain, difficulty breathing and tenderness of the chest wall. Complications are acute respiratory distress syndrome and pneumonia.
3. Treatment
    A. Acute resuscitation with mechanical ventilation where indicated.
    B. Supportive management with analgesics and supplemental oxygen.

Pulmonary hypertension

Pulmonary hypertension occurs when pressure increases significantly in vessels that carry blood from the heart to the lungs. There is lots of muscle that grows on the walls of blood vessels that lead to the lungs.

Chapter 3: Neurological Emergencies

There are 18 test questions in this section. Contents areas are:

Neurological disorders

Multiple sclerosis

1. Clinical features – Paresthesia is the most common early feature of multiple sclerosis. Paresthesia can affect the upper and/or lower extremities, and also the trunk or a part of the face. Paresthesia is associated with muscle weakness. Visual disturbances are also early signs. They include optic neuritis, scotomas and internuclear ophthalmoplegia. Other clinical features are vertigo; disturbance of gait; bladder dysfunction characterized by hesitancy, frequency, urgency, retention or incontinence; and disturbances of cognition and mood. Patients also have motor signs like brisk tendon reflexes, positive Babinski sign and ankle clonus. Cerebellar symptoms include vertigo, nystagmus, ataxia and slurred speech.
2. Treatment – Corticosteroids and immunomodulators to slow down the immune response, baclofen to treat muscle spasticity, analgesia with Gabapentin or tricyclic antidepressants and symptomatic management.

Myasthenia gravis

1. Cause – This is a neuromuscular disorder caused by autoimmune destruction of acetylcholine receptors.
2. Clinical features – The most common symptoms are ptosis, double vision and muscle weakness that worsens as the day progresses. Some patients may experience bulbar symptoms like dysphagia, choking and regurgitation. In severe cases, patients experience myasthenic crisis

characterized by quadriparesis and respiratory distress that requires urgent mechanical ventilation.

3. Treatment – Involves the use of anticholinesterase drugs, corticosteroids, plasma exchange, IV immune globulin and thymectomy.

Guillain-Barré syndrome

This is an acute polyneuropathy disease characterized by muscle paresis and loss of sensation in distal extremities.

1. Cause – It is an autoimmune disease often triggered by infections with any of these; herpes virus, campylobacter jejuni, mycoplasma species and enteric viruses.
2. Clinical features – The most common symptom is flaccid paralysis of the extremities. It is accompanied by paresthesia and starts from the legs before moving to affect the arms. The paralysis lasts for weeks before spontaneously resolving. The urethral and rectal sphincters are not affected. In severe cases, affected patients have respiratory failure due to the paresis of muscles of respiration. Some patients may also experience severe hypotension due to loss of autonomic control.
3. Treatment – This is a medical emergency that requires prompt support of respiration and treatment in the ICU with plasma electrophoresis or IV immune globulin.

Headache

This includes primary and secondary headache disorders.

1. Migraine – This is a primary headache disorder that is episodic, severe and lasts four to 72 hours. Migraine headaches are throbbing, lateral and worsened by activity. Migraines are typically accompanied by other

symptoms like nausea, vomiting, photophobia and auras. Treatment is with dihydroergotamine, antiemetics, triptans and analgesics.

2. Cluster headache – This is a primary headache disorder that is characterized by very severe headaches that are unilateral in the periorbital or temporal region, with accompanied ipsilateral autonomic features such as lacrimation, nasal congestion, ptosis and rhinorrhea.
3. Tension-type headache – This is a primary headache disorder that is characterized by mild and generalized headaches, nausea, vomiting and photophobia. The pain is mild and not as incapacitating as other kinds of headaches.
4. Secondary headaches:
    A. Acute angle-closure glaucoma – This causes unilateral headaches in the orbital or frontal region. The headaches are associated with vomiting, conjunctival redness, decreased vision and halos. Diagnosis is made by tonometry.
    B. Encephalitis – Patients experience headaches that are associated with fever, neurologic deficits, altered mental states and seizures. Diagnosis is done by CSF analysis and brain CT scan.
    C. Giant cell arteritis – Headaches in this disorder are throbbing, unilateral, and associated with fever, night sweats, jaw pain, proximal myalgias and tenderness of the temporal artery.
    D. Idiopathic intracranial hypertension – This is also called pseudotumor cerebri. Headache is migraine-like, with associated tinnitus, papilledema, loss of peripheral vision and diplopia.
    E. Medication overuse headache – This headache is triggered by overuse of analgesics for a headache disorder. Headache is chronic, with varying bouts of intensity. Location is also variable and is usually present as soon as the patient awakes.

F. Postlumbar puncture headache – This headache is intense and caused by reduced CSF pressure and volume after lumbar puncture. Headache is worsened when the patient elevates the head either by standing or sitting and is associated with vomiting and neck pain. These postures stretch the meninges and worsen the pain. The pain is alleviated only by placing the patient in a supine position.

Increased intracranial pressure (ICP)

Intracranial pressure is the pressure exerted on brain tissue. Normal pressure in an adult is 7 to 15 mmHg. Disturbances in CSF production and drainage mean arterial pressure and cerebral blood flow autoregulation can increase intracranial pressure.

1. Cause – Mass effect from brain tumors, hydrocephalus, hematoma, cerebral hemorrhage, cerebral abscess and cerebral contusions. Cerebral edema can be a complication of fulminant liver failure, hypertensive encephalopathy, hypertensive encephalopathy, uremic encephalopathy and hypercapnia. Cerebral edema can also be caused by increased venous pressure from thrombosis in the venous sinus, heart failure and obstruction of the jugular veins. Another cause is craniosynostosis.
2. Clinical features – Headaches, altered consciousness, projectile vomiting, ocular palsies and papilledema. Patients also present with the Cushing's triad, which is characterized by widened pulse pressure (systolic hypertension), irregular breathing and bradycardia. Herniation of brain tissue is an acute complication of raised ICP.
3. Treatment
   A. Elevate the head of the bed to 30° to improve the venous return from the brain and reduce cerebral edema.

B. Hyperventilate with supplemental oxygen to induce hypocapnia and vasoconstriction, and reduce cerebral edema. The aim is to reduce PCO2 to about 30 mmHg. This can reduce ICP by about 30 percent.
C. Use hypertonic fluids like IV mannitol to induce movement of water from the tissues into the intravascular space. Mannitol is usually given with IV furosemide to prevent hypertension and pulmonary edema.
D. Use diuretics like acetazolamide – Control of blood pressure in severe hypertension with short-acting antihypertensives like IV labetalol, nicardipine or hydralazine.
E. Use corticosteroids for vasogenic cerebral edema.
F. Decompressive craniotomy in some cases.

Meningitis

1. Cause – Most-implicated bacteria in neonates and infants are group B Streptococcus, gram-negative bacteria (especially E. coli) and listeria monocytogenes. In older infants, children and young adults, the most implicated organisms are Neisseria meningitidis, Streptococcus pneumoniae and Haemophilus influenzae (in the nonimmunized population). The most implicated organisms in older adults are Streptococcus pneumoniae and Neisseria meningitides. The most common viruses are enteroviruses. Other causes are varicella-zoster and herpes simplex virus type 2 (HSV-2). Noninfectious causes include autoimmune disorders like SLE, Bechet's syndrome and rheumatoid arthritis. Anti-inflammatory drugs like cyclosporine, azathioprine and NSAIDs; some antibiotics like isoniazid, ciprofloxacin and penicillin; carbamazepine and ranitidine. Subacute and chronic meningitis are caused by mycobacterium tuberculosis, HIV, toxoplasma gondii, rickettsiae and spirochetes.

2. Clinical features – Altered sensory, fever, neck stiffness, focal nerve deficits and features of raised intracranial pressure. In meningococcal meningitis, clinical features are more severe and include petechial rashes, DIC and Waterhouse-Friderichsen syndrome. Acute complications are seizures, focal nerve deficits, raised ICP, brain herniation, respiratory depression and sepsis. Late-onset complications are hydrocephalus, seizure disorders and nerve deficits.
3. Treatment – Definitive treatment of the underlying cause based on results of CSF analysis. Supportive treatment of symptoms: antipyretics, anticonvulsants, osmotic diuretics for raised ICP, corticosteroids, fluid input and output monitoring and provision of nutrition.

Seizure disorders

1. Causes: In patients less than two years, fever, birth injuries, hereditary neurological disorders and congenital or acquired metabolic disorders.
2. Ages 2–14: Idiopathic.
3. Adults: Alcohol withdrawal, trauma, strokes, idiopathic causes.
4. Older people: Strokes and tumors.

Classification

1. Generalized-onset seizures – Includes motor and nonmotor (absence seizures). In this disorder, the seizure begins from neurons in both cerebral hemispheres. Patients lose both consciousness and awareness. Patients with generalized motor seizures have bilateral motor activity and are classified into a tonic clinic, clonic, tonic, myoclonic-atonic, infantile spasms, myoclonic, atonic and myoclonic-tonic-clonic seizures. Generalized nonmotor seizures include typical absence seizures, atypical

absence seizures, eyelid myoclonia and myoclonic seizures. Absence seizures occur in children.

2. Focal onset seizures – These seizures stake in one cerebral hemisphere or subcortical structures. They include focal aware seizures, also called simple partial seizures, and focal impaired awareness seizures, also called complex partial seizures. Focal onset motor seizures include atonic, clonic, automatisms, epileptic spasms, myoclonic, hyperkinetic and tonic seizures.
3. Focal onset nonmotor seizures – Also classified based on the earliest presenting symptom: autonomic dysfunction involving GI changes, temperature changes, sexual arousal, palpitations and piloerection, behavioral arrest, cognitive dysfunction, emotional dysfunction and sensory dysfunction.
4. Unknown-onset seizures – These seizures are classified based on ambiguity in their origins. They can be motor or nonmotor. Unknown motor seizures include epileptic spasms and tonic-clonic seizures. Unknown onset nonmotor seizures include behavior arrest.

Treatment

Treatment of the underlying cause, avoidance of situations where seizure disorders are life-threatening, anticonvulsant therapy and surgery.

Stroke

1. Ischemic stroke – This makes up 80 percent of stroke cases. Causes are lacunar infarcts in the cerebral circulation, cardioembolism, atherosclerosis of large vessels and cryptogenic.
2. Hemorrhagic stroke – This makes up 20 percent of all stroke cases. They include intracerebral hemorrhage and subarachnoid hemorrhage.

3. Risk factors – In ischemic stroke, modifiable risk factors are atherosclerosis, diabetes mellitus, dyslipidemia, cigarette smoking, obesity, alcoholism, psychosocial stress, hypercoagulability and vasculitis. Nonmodifiable risk factors are a history of stroke, family history of stroke, race, age and sex. In hemorrhagic stroke, the etiology of subarachnoid hemorrhage includes trauma to the head and ruptured aneurysms. Risk factors for intracerebral hemorrhage are rupture of atherosclerotic arteries, congenital aneurysms, vascular malformations, blood dyscrasia, vasculitis, excessive anticoagulation and hemorrhagic infarction.
4. Clinical features – Altered sensorium, hypertension, features of end-organ damage and raised ICP.
5. Principles of management: Management is supportive and occurs in a stroke center. It includes:
    A. Acute resuscitation
    B. Antihypertensive therapy in severe hypertension and end-organ dysfunction
    C. Antiplatelet therapy for ischemic stroke
    D. Surgical interventions for hemorrhagic strokes
    E. Treatment of hyperthermia, hyperglycemia/hypoglycemia
    F. Physiotherapy.

Transient ischemic attack (TIA)

This is a transient and sudden loss of neurologic deficits that lasts less than an hour. Risk factors are the same for ischemic stroke. Treatment includes eliminating modifiable risk factors for strokes.

Head and Spinal Cord Trauma

Head Trauma (Traumatic brain injury)

1. Cause – Motor vehicle accidents, falls, sports-related accidents and assaults.
2. Clinical features – Patients present with features of a brain hemorrhage. Depth of injury is measured via the Glasgow Coma Scale.
3. Treatment – Acute resuscitation and assessment of injuries, supportive management of symptoms and complications and surgery.

Spinal Cord Trauma (Spinal injuries)

1. Spinal cord injury – The most common cause is motor vehicle accidents, followed by falls.
2. Vertebral injuries – This includes fractures that can involve the lamina, pedicles, vertebral body and transverse processes. Other injuries include dislocations and subluxations.
3. Cauda equina injury – Injury to the conus medullaris, which is at L1. Lesions to this part of the spinal cord mimic conus medullaris syndrome.

Neurogenic Shock

This is also called vasogenic shock. It is a loss of autonomic function due to trauma to the spinal cord. It is often caused by trauma above T6. Clinical features are hypotension, bradycardia, hypothermia, loss of temperature regulation and respiratory failure.

Chapter 4: Gastrointestinal, Genitourinary, Gynecology and Obstetrical Emergencies

There are 18 questions in this section of the test. Content areas include:

A. Gastrointestinal

Acute abdomen

1. Causes – Obstruction by a hypertrophied lymphoid tissue, fecalith, worms or foreign bodies.
2. Clinical features – Fever, anorexia and vomiting, abdominal pain, rebound tenderness, psoas sign, obturator sign and Rovsing's sign.
3. Treatment – Appendectomy, which must be done quickly to reduce the risk of perforation and peritonitis.

Peritonitis

Inflammation of the peritoneal cavity.

Appendicitis

Inflammation of the vermiform appendix.

Bowel perforation

This occurs when a hole forms in the small intestine's walls, or the colon's walls. This is dangerous because the material inside the intestine can move through to the abdomen and cause an infection.

Cyclic vomiting syndrome

Cyclic vomiting syndrome happens when someone has continuous vomiting sessions without any apparent reason. These sessions can go on for hours or even days during which there may be periods of relaxation. Sessions usually start and end around the same time of the day with similar intensities. This syndrome is more common in children.

Bleeding

Upper GI bleeding

1. Causes – The most common cause is duodenal ulcer, followed by esophageal varices. Other causes are erosive gastritis, gastric ulcers, Mallory-Weiss tear, arteriovenous malformations, erosive esophagitis, hemobilia, tumors of the gastrointestinal stromal and angioma.
2. Clinical features – Hematemesis, melena stools or hematochezia in severe cases. Patients can also present with signs of hypovolemic shock, tachycardia, pallor, hypotension and syncope.
3. Treatment – Acute resuscitation with intravenous fluids and oxygen where indicated for patients with shock; definitive treatment depends on the cause.

Lower GI bleeding

1. Causes – Anal fissures, angiodysplasia, colorectal cancer, internal hemorrhoids, colonic polyps, Crohn's disease and ulcerative colitis.
2. Clinical features – Hematochezia, constipation, diarrhea, abdominal cramps, intestinal bloating and symptoms of hypovolemic shock.
3. Treatment – Acute resuscitation for those in cardiovascular collapse; treatment of the underlying cause.

Cholecystitis

1. Cause – Most common cause is cholelithiasis. Impacted gallstones cause bile stasis, inflammation of the mucosa of the gallbladder and superseding bacterial infection. If left untreated, there is a high risk of necrosis and

gallbladder perforation. Causes of acalculous cholecystitis include total parenteral nutrition, prolonged fasting, critical illness, vasculitis and immune deficiency. This form of cholecystitis is thought to be caused by bile stasis, infection and ischemia.

2. Clinical features – Biliary colic characterized by right hypochondrial pain; tenderness in the right hypochondrium, which can be elicited by the Murphy's sign; low-grade fever and nonspecific symptoms like nausea, anorexia, malaise and vomiting. Complications include perforation, peritonitis and gallstone pancreatitis.
3. Treatment – Supportive treatment of symptoms, IV fluids, antibiotics and analgesia. Definite treatment is cholecystectomy.

Cirrhosis

Advanced stage of hepatic fibrosis is characterized by regenerative nodules of hepatic tissue that is surrounded by fibrotic tissue.

1. Causes – Alcohol liver disease; nonalcoholic fatty liver disease; chronic hepatitis B and hepatitis C infection; primary sclerosing cholangitis; primary biliary cholangitis; autoimmune hepatitis and drugs like tolbutamide, amiodarone, isoniazid, methyldopa and methotrexate.
2. Clinical features – Stigmata of chronic liver disease, which include jaundice, ascites, pedal edema, skin atrophy, testicular atrophy, gynecomastia, Dupuytren contracture, parotitis, lanugo hair, finger clubbing, paronychia, caput medusae, xanthelasma, asterixis, pallor and petechiae rashes. Complications are a result of decompensated liver failure. They include esophageal varices, rectal varices, caput medusae, hepatic encephalopathy, thromboembolism, portal hypertension, hepatorenal syndrome, hepatopulmonary syndrome, spontaneous bacterial peritonitis and others.

3. Treatment
    A. The definite treatment is a liver transplant.
    B. Supportive management of symptoms, which includes reduced protein intake, bowel sterilization, use of motility drugs like Dulcolax to prevent constipation, restriction of the use of sedatives in patients with decompensated liver failure and transjugular intrahepatic portosystemic shunts in patients with portal hypertension.

Diverticulitis

1. Risk factors – Red meat, cytomegalovirus infection and previous history of diverticulitis.
2. Clinical features – Pain in the left lower quadrant of the abdomen. The pain can also be in the right lower quadrant or suprapubic area. In some patients, there are palpable masses in the sigmoid colon. Other features are fever, nausea and urinary frequency or urgency. Complications are peritonitis; bowel obstruction; fistula, which may present as fecaluria, pneumonitis, infection of the abdominal wall or passage of feculent vaginal discharge.
3. Treatment – Antibiotic therapy with empiric antibiotics for anaerobic and aerobic bacterial infection, percutaneous drainage of the abscess and surgery for patients with peritonitis or intestinal obstruction.

Esophageal varices

1. Causes – Portal hypertension from decompensated liver failure. In this condition, portal pressure is higher than that in the inferior vena cava. This causes shunting of blood via venous collateral in the esophagus,

fundus of the stomach and rectum. These varices have a risk of rupturing and causing severe upper GI bleeding.

2. Clinical features – Features of upper GI bleeding; hematemesis, which is painless, severe and sudden. Complications include hypovolemic shock and hepatic encephalopathy.
3. Treatment
   A. Immediate resuscitation: airway, IV fluids, blood products and vasopressors where indicated
   B. Endoscopic banding
   C. Sclerotherapy
   D. Use of IV octreotide
   E. Mechanical compression with Sengstaken-Blakemore tube
   F. Transjugular intrahepatic portosystemic shunts for persistent bleeding.

Foreign bodies

1. Esophageal – Most common cause is impacted food that is not properly chewed, steaks, fishbones and hot dogs. Infants and toddlers have a high risk of choking on small, round foods like candies, sweets, peas, peanuts and pieces of cut fruits and vegetables. Complications include perforation of the esophagus and obstruction.
2. Gastric – Gastric bezoars are undigested materials that accumulate in the stomach to form stone-like materials. Examples are phytobezoars, which are made from undigested fruit and vegetable seeds, peels or fiber; diospyrobezoars made from accumulation of persimmon fruit; trichobezoars made of hair; lactobezoars made of milk protein and pharmacobezoars made of drugs. Bezoars can also be made of inorganic substances like Styrofoam cups and tissue paper. Risk factors include

patients with psychiatric disorders, gastric bypass surgery, infants, elderly patients, diabetes mellitus and hypochlorhydria.

3. Intestinal – This includes foreign objects in the esophagus and stomach that migrate to the intestine, body packing or body stuffing with heroin or cocaine and other substances.
4. Rectal – This includes swallowed foreign bodies, fecaliths, gallstones, vaginal pessaries, surgical materials, sex toys, urinary calculi and drug packets.

Hepatitis

1. Causes – Infectious causes include hepatitis A, B, C, D and E viruses; cytomegalovirus; yellow fever; infectious mononucleosis; amebiasis; malari and schistosomiasis. Other causes include alcohol, hypercholesterolemia, autoimmune disorders, genetic diseases of the liver and infiltrative diseases like amyloidosis and sarcoidosis.
2. Clinical features – Depends on the cause. Examples are jaundice, pruritus, pale stools, dark-colored urine, fever, malaise and anorexia. Patients may also present with stigmata of chronic liver disease.
3. Treatment – Treatment of underlying cause. Hepatitis A and E infections are often short-lived and require no antibiotic treatment, just supportive management of symptoms. Hepatitis B infection is chronic and has no treatment. It is, however, preventable with a vaccine. Hepatitis C infection is treatable with direct-acting antivirals like telaprevir, simeprevir, sofosbuvir, dasabuvir, ombitasvir, daclatasvir and others. Removal of risk factors (e.g., alcohol, offending drugs) and use of antilipids for fatty liver disease. Supportive management including nutrition, IV fluids for rehydration, cholestyramine for pruritus and management of complications in patients with chronic liver disease.

Intussusception

1. Causes – Mostly idiopathic. Risk is higher in males, during the peak season of viral enteritis, young children and old formations of rotavirus vaccine. Other risk factors include cystic fibrosis, Merkel's diverticulum, gastrointestinal polyps and lymphoma.
2. Clinical features – Colicky abdominal pain is the earliest symptom. Other symptoms are lethargy, dehydration and passage of currant jelly-like stool. In complicated cases, the patient presents with intestinal obstruction, perforation or peritonitis.
3. Treatment – Air enema for reduction of the bowel. Surgical interventions for failed air enemas.

Obstructions

1. Causes – The most common causes include hernias, tumors and adhesions. Other causes are foreign body impaction, volvulus, fecal impaction and intussusception.
2. Clinical features – Abdominal cramps and vomiting. Patients with complete obstruction experience obstipation, while patients with partial obstruction experience diarrhea. Bowel sounds are hyperactive. Absent bowel sounds indicate peritonitis. In complicated cases, patients present with shock. Obstructions of the large intestine are milder than obstructions of the small intestine. Patients present with constipation, vomiting and abdominal cramps. A mass may be palpable.
3. Treatment

   It is a surgical emergency. Treatment modalities include:

   A. Placing the patient on NPO
   B. Nasogastric suction
   C. Fluid and electrolyte replacement via IV fluids

D. Measurement of fluid input and output (via urethral catheter)
E. IV antibiotics
F. Definitive treatment is surgical exploration, resection and anastomosis where appropriate.

Pancreatitis

1. Causes – The most common causes are alcoholism and gallstones. Other causes are viral infections with mumps, cytomegalovirus and coxsackievirus B, metabolic causes like hypercalcemia, hypertriglyceridemia, trauma, pancreatic cancer and others.
2. Clinical features – Upper abdominal pain, nausea, vomiting, hypotension and fever. Significant findings are Cullen and Turner signs. In complicated cases, patients have paralytic ileus, peritonitis, infection and sepsis with multiple organ dysfunction.
3. Treatment – Supportive management of dehydration, hypoglycemia, infections and pain. Patients need adequate nutrition via an enteral feeding tube. Adequate pain relief.

Gastrointestinal trauma

1. Causes – Blunt injuries (e.g., direct blow to the abdominal wall from falling on an object or impact from a moving vehicle). The spleen is the most affected organ, followed by the liver and small intestine. Patients may also present with other multisystemic injuries. Penetrating injuries include stab wounds and gunshot injuries. If injuries do not affect the peritoneum, injuries to the organs are unlikely.
2. Clinical features – Abdominal pain is the cardinal symptom. On inspection, there may be open wounds and bleeding in penetrating trauma or ecchymoses in blunt trauma. Patients with abdominal distension may

have a severe hemorrhage. On palpation, there is tenderness with signs of peritonitis. There may be gross bleeding on digital rectal examination. Patients may be in hypovolemic shock characterized by hypotension, tachycardia, altered sensorium and diaphoresis.

3. Treatment – Acute resuscitation with IV fluids, oxygen, vasopressors and blood products as indicated. Emergency exploratory laparotomy.

B. Genitourinary

Genitourinary infections

Pyelonephritis

1. Cause – Most often caused by enteric gram-negative bacteria. Risk factors include female sex, obstructive uropathy, urethral catheterization, chronic constipation and menopause.
2. Clinical features – Patients with uncomplicated cases present with fever, flank/lower abdominal pain, anorexia, nausea, vomiting, dysuria and hematuria. Patients with complicated cases present with symptoms of acute kidney injury: oliguria, hypertension and fluid retention.
3. Treatment – Treatment with empiric intravenous antibiotics until results of bacterial culture and sensitivity are obtained. Supportive management of pain and other symptoms. Management of acute kidney injury in patients who present with it. Treatment of the underlying cause and elimination of risk factors.

Epididymitis

1. Cause – Causes of bacterial epididymitis are Chlamydia trachomatis and Neisseria gonorrhea in most males less than 35 years (gram-negative coliform bacteria are the most implicated bacteria in males who are older than 35 years). These organisms are often seen in patients with obstructive uropathy or retained catheters. Nonbacterial causes of epididymitis are viruses like cytomegalovirus and fungi like Blastomyces and actinomycetes. Noninfectious causes are trauma and retrograde flow of urine.
2. Clinical features – Scrotal pain is the cardinal symptom. Other features are fever, nausea, anorexia and vomiting. Patients also experience irritative

urinary symptoms: frequency, urgency, incontinence, dysuria and hematuria. In complicated cases, patients present with septic shock.
3. Treatment – Supportive management, which includes bed rest, elevation of the scrotum, analgesia and antibiotic therapy.

Orchitis

1. Cause – Infections that are localized to just the testes are mainly caused by viruses (e.g., mumps). Other causes are leprosy, tuberculosis, varicella-zoster infection, coxsackievirus infection and congenital syphilis.
2. Clinical features – Testicular pain, edema and induration. Patients may also experience systemic symptoms like fever, nausea, vomiting and myalgias. On testicular examination, there is tenderness and induration of the testes and scrotal skin.
3. Treatment – Antibiotics for bacterial causes. Supportive measures with analgesia for viral causes.

Priapism

1. Causes – Drugs used to treat erectile dysfunction (sildenafil, phentolamine, alprostadil, and papaverine); hematologic disorders like leukemia, sickle cell anemia and lymphoma; and advanced prostate cancer. Also implicated are beta-blockers, antipsychotics, anticoagulants, oral hypoglycemic agents, lithium and recreational drugs like cocaine and amphetamine.
2. Clinical features – Persistent, painful and abnormal erection without sexual desire.
3. Treatment

   For ischemic priapism:

A. Aspiration of blood from the corpora cavernosa with a nonheparinized syringe
B. Intracavernous injection of phenylephrine
C. Irrigation with normal saline
D. Creation of a surgical shunt for unresponsive cases
E. For patients with sickle cell anemia, management of vaso occlusive crisis is required.

For nonischemic priapism:

A. Conservative measures – Analgesia and cold compression with ice packs
B. For unresponsive cases, surgery is required.

Renal calculi

1. Causes – Risk factors for calcium calculi are hypercalciuria from hypocitraturia, renal tubular acidosis, hyperoxaluria, primary hyperparathyroidism, vitamin D poisoning, hyperthyroidism and multiple myeloma. Other causes of calcium calculi are vitamin C hypervitaminosis and hyperuricosuria. Cystine calculi are caused by cystinuria, while magnesium ammonium phosphate calculi are caused by chronic urinary tract infections.
2. Clinical features – Renal colic with nausea and vomiting. Patients may present with symptoms of urinary tract infection and/or symptoms of obstructive uropathy.
3. Treatment – Analgesia for prompt relief, IV fluids, use of alpha-receptor blockers to enhance passage of the calculus, removal via endoscopy, management of urinary tract infections and obstructive uropathy as indicated.

Testicular torsion

1. Cause – Anomalies in the development of the tunica vaginalis and spermatic cord cause incomplete fixation of the testis to the tunica vaginalis. Torsion is common in males ages 12 to 18 years with such anomalies. It is most likely to occur in the left testis.
2. Clinical features – Severe testicular pain accompanied by nausea and vomiting. On inspection, the testes are tender, swollen and indurated. They may be elevated and horizontal. Cremasteric reflex on the affected testis is absent.
3. Treatment – Analgesia for prompt relief, manual detorsion and emergency surgery for failed detorsion.

Genitourinary trauma

Bladder trauma

1. Cause – Blunt or penetrating trauma to the pelvis, perineum or suprapubic region of the abdomen. Blunt trauma is the most common cause following a vehicle crash, an external blow to the abdomen or a fall. Patients are also likely to have pelvic fractures. The bladder can also be injured during pelvic surgeries, especially abdominal hysterectomy, excision of a pelvic mass and caesarean section. Risks increase when there is fibrosis from surgery, after radiation exposure and when the tumor to be excised is extensive.
2. Clinical features – Suprapubic pain, urine retention and hematuria. Patients may also present with abdominal distension, peritonitis and hypovolemic shock. Complications are urine ascites, persistent hematuria, infections and sepsis, incontinence and formation of a fistula.
3. Treatment – Drainage with a catheter, exploration and surgical repair.

Urinary retention

1. Cause – Bladder outlet obstruction, impaired contractility of the bladder, anticholinergics, fecal impaction and in patients with neurogenic bladder: multiple sclerosis, diabetes and Parkinson's.
2. Clinical features – Feeling of incomplete voiding, frequency, suprapubic swelling and suprapubic pain. In complicated cases, patients present with symptoms of urinary tract infections and/or obstructive uropathy.
3. Treatment – Prompt relief of symptoms via urethral/suprapubic catheterization. Treatment of underlying cause.

C. Gynecology

Dysfunctional uterine bleeding

Dysfunctional uterine bleeding is caused by ovulatory disorders.

1. Causes – Causes of anovulatory abnormal uterine bleeding include structural causes of hypothalamic dysfunction (e.g., hypothalamic tumors); irradiation; traumatic brain injury; genetic disorders affecting the hypothalamus; infiltrative disorders; functional causes of hypothalamic dysfunction (e.g., eating disorders); depression; drugs like cocaine; malnutrition; obesity; excessive exercise; diets; food fads and chronic diseases. Also implicated are disorders of the pituitary and ovaries, as well as endocrine abnormalities. Causes of ovulatory abnormal uterine bleeding include endometriosis, polycystic ovarian syndrome and inadequate stimulation of the endometrium with progesterone.
2. Clinical features – Polymenorrhea, which is a menstrual cycle that is less than 21 days; menorrhagia, which is bleeding that lasts for more than seven days; metrorrhagia, which is bleeding in between periods; and menometrorrhagia, which is increased bleeding and bleeding in between periods. Patients may also experience painful menstruation and premenstrual symptoms.
3. Evaluation – Patients who present to the ER with active bleeding should have a hematocrit and complete blood count and coagulation profile, a pregnancy test and an obstetric ultrasound scan. Other tests include endometrial sampling, hormone profile, STI screening, hysteroscopy, liver function test and Pap smear screening where indicated.
4. Treatment
    - A. Acute resuscitation in women with active bleeding and hypovolemic shock
    - B. Correction of iron deficiency anemia

C. Treatment of underlying cause.

Gynecological infections

Vaginitis

1. Causes – In children, the most common cause is infection by flora in the gastrointestinal tract due to improper wiping after urination and poor perineal hygiene. Other causes are foreign bodies in the vagina; certain soaps and bubble baths; tight, nonbreathable underwear; sexual abuse and obesity (candida vaginitis). Common causes in women of reproductive age are bacterial vaginosis, which is triggered by the destruction of lactobacillus in vaginal flora and proliferation of opportunistic bacteria. Risk factors are douching, multiple sexual partners, poor hygiene, menstrual blood and semen. All these reduce the acidity of the vagina. Trichomonas vaginitis, which occurs through sexual contact. Candidal vaginitis, which is caused by disruption of the vaginal flora; use of tight, nonbreathable underwear; obesity; excess heat and humidity; tampons and chronic use of antibiotics. In postmenopausal women, the most common cause is atrophic vaginitis caused by decreased estrogen secretion, decreased acidity of the vagina and disruption of vaginal flora. Other causes are poor perineal hygiene, urine and fecal incontinence.
2. Clinical features – Abnormal vaginal discharge, which is associated with fever, pruritus, dysuria, dyspareunia and erythema of the labia majora and minora.
3. Treatment – Symptomatic relief of itching; treatment of underlying cause.

Cervicitis

1. Causes – The most common causes are sexually transmitted chlamydia trachomatis and Neisseria gonorrhoeae. Other implicated organisms are

Trichomonas vaginalis, herpes simplex virus and mycoplasma. Noninfectious causes include foreign bodies, allergens, chemicals and the performance of gynecologic procedures.

2. Clinical features – The most common symptoms are vaginal discharge, dyspareunia and vaginal bleeding during intercourse or in between periods. Other symptoms are dysmenorrhea, dysuria and vaginal itching. Significant findings on examination are cervical erythema and edema, oozing of mucopurulent discharge and cervical friability.
3. Treatment
   A. Empirical antibiotics based on clinical features, then appropriate antibiotics after retrieving results of microscopy, culture and sensitivity.
   B. Contact tracing and treatment of all sexual partners.
   C. Re-evaluation after three months.

Pelvic inflammatory disease (PID)

1. Causes – Most common causes are chlamydia and Neisseria gonorrhoeae. Other microorganisms are Mycoplasma, gram-negative bacilli, Streptococcus agalactiae, Haemophilus influenzae and Ureaplasma spp. Risk factors include multiple sexual partners, previous history of PID, younger age, douching and low socioeconomic status. Complications include hydrosalpinx, Fitz-Hugh-Curtis syndrome, scarring of the fallopian tubes, increased risk of ectopic pregnancies and tubo ovarian abscess.
2. Clinical features – Features of vaginitis, cervicitis and salpingitis.
3. Treatment – Empirical antibiotic therapy, screening and treatment of STDs and contact tracing where appropriate.

Ovarian disorders

Ovarian cysts

1. Causes – Follicular cysts from Graafian follicles, and corpus luteum cysts.
2. Clinical features – Are typically asymptomatic. Patients with ruptured cysts present with lower abdominal pain, features of peritonitis and hypovolemic shock. In adnexal torsion, patients present with severe lower abdominal pain, nausea, and vomiting. On cervical examination, cervical motion tenderness is positive and the adnexal mass may be palpable.
3. Treatment – Acute resuscitation for patients with rupture or adnexal torsion. The definite treatment is exploratory laparotomy with cystectomy, salpingectomy and salpingotomy as indicated.

Ovarian torsion

This condition is cause for an emergency. It is also called adnexal torsion and happens when an ovary becomes curled around the tissues surrounding it. In other cases, the fallopian tube can be curled as well. The patient who has this condition will be in severe pain because there will be no blood supply to the above-mentioned organs during ovarian torsion.

Ovarian Rupture

This "rupture" is usually a normal part of a woman's periods. During ovulation, the egg is released from the cyst and this is referred to as the "rupture". However, sometimes there can be complications that may require surgery.

Sexual assault and battery

This includes rape; inappropriate, nonconsensual touching or holding and the use of threats.

1. Risk factors – Females are most at risk of sexual assaults.

2. Clinical features – Victims of rape may present to the ER. Clinical presentations include genital and extragenital injuries, psychological symptoms, features of sexually transmitted diseases, PIDs and cervicitis. On evaluation, the patient may have PTSD, be pregnant or have hepatitis or HIV infection.
3. Evaluation – The initial response is to provide safety for patients who present to the ER with their partners who may be perpetrators of the assault. For rape victims, the goals of evaluation are medical evaluation and prompt treatment of injuries and STDs. Patients should also be screened for pregnancy, and appropriate measures taken to prevent pregnancy and STDs. Forensic evidence should be collected with the patient's consent to legal intervention. Crisis intervention should be recommended to all patients. The sexual assault rape team should be consulted where available.

Gynecological trauma

This has been discussed under bladder trauma in Genitourinary Emergencies.

D. Obstetrical

Abruptio placenta

1. Causes – Risk factors are older maternal age, trauma to the abdomen, hypertension, chorioamnionitis, polyhydramnios, premature rupture of membranes, vasculitis, tobacco use, cocaine use and maternal thrombotic disorders.
2. Clinical features – Vaginal bleeding of dark or bright red blood. In patients with retroplacental hemorrhage, there will be no or slight vaginal bleeding. Patients may present with hypovolemic shock in severe bleeding. The uterus is rigid and tender and there may be signs of fetal distress. Complications include hemodynamic instability, hypovolemic shock, DIC in the patient and fetal compromise. Fetomaternal transfusion can cause Rh sensitization.
3. Treatment
    A. Acute resuscitation with oxygen, IV fluids, vasopressors and blood products where indicated.
    B. In severe hemodynamic compromise and fetal distress, prompt delivery is required by emergency caesarean section. For pregnancies less than 37 weeks, IV dexamethasone is given to hasten the maturity of the fetal lungs. Vaginal delivery can be attempted in pregnancies greater than 37 weeks if the patient is hemodynamically stable, fetal heart rate is reassuring and there are no contraindications to vaginal delivery.
    C. Modified rest is indicated for hemodynamically stable patients with reassuring fetal heart rate and pregnancies that are less than 37 weeks.

Ectopic pregnancy

1. Risk factors – History of previous ectopic pregnancies, history of PIDs, assisted reproduction, intrauterine contraceptive devices, previous tubal surgeries, history of induced abortion, cigarette smoking and multiple sexual partners.
2. Clinical features – Presentation in the ER is due to ruptured ectopic pregnancy. Features include severe lower abdominal pain and vaginal bleeding. To rule out a diagnosis of ruptured ovarian cysts, a pregnancy test is done. Patients are likely to present with features of hypovolemic shock and peritonitis.
3. Treatment
   A. Acute resuscitation with IV fluids, supplemental oxygen and blood products where indicated
   B. Definitive treatment is emergency laparotomy with salpingotomy or salpingectomy where appropriate.

Emergent delivery

A. Indications for emergency caesarean section:
   1. Antepartum hemorrhage with maternal hemodynamic stability and fetal compromise
   2. Obstructed labor
   3. Eclampsia/severe preeclampsia
   4. Chorioamnionitis with hemodynamic instability and fetal compromise.

B. Indications for induction of labor are the same for emergency caesarean sections. However, the risk of fetal compromise and maternal hemodynamic instability are lower.

C. Contraindications to induction are:
   1. Previous caesarean section

2. Previous myomectomy
3. Placenta previa
4. Abnormal fetal presentation
5. Cephalopelvic disproportion.

D. Techniques for induction are:
1. Vaginal misoprostol
2. Vaginal prostaglandin E2
3. Insertion of intracervical balloon catheters
4. Sweeping of the cervix and amniotomy
5. Intravenous infusion of oxytocin.

E. Complications of caesarean section
1. Postpartum hemorrhage
2. Damage to the bladder, intestine and surrounding structures.
3. Anesthetic complications
4. Sepsis.

F. Complications of induction of labor
1. Uterine hyperstimulation and uterine rupture
2. Fetal distress
3. Water retention and oxytocin from intravenous oxytocin.

Hemorrhage (i.e. Postpartum bleeding)

1. Causes – The most common cause of postpartum hemorrhage is uterine atony. Risk factors for uterine atony are grand multiparity, multiple gestations, polyhydramnios, fetal macrosomia, congenital anomalies, precipitate labor, anesthesia and chorioamnionitis. Other causes of hemorrhage are uterine rupture, retained products of conception, cervical tears, episiotomies, inversion of the uterus, bleeding disorders and coagulopathies, uterine fibroids and involution of the placenta.

2. Clinical features – Vaginal bleeding. Patients rapidly go into hypovolemic shock.
3. Treatment
    A. Prompt resuscitation with IV fluids and blood products.
    B. Stimulation of uterine contractions with intravenous oxytocin. IV ergot alkaloids are used in severe bleeding. Ergot alkaloids are contraindicated in patients with cardiovascular disease.
    C. Bimanual uterine massage and manual evacuation of the uterus.
    D. In cases of atony, tamponade with balloon Foley catheters.
    E. Cervical tears and episiotomies are promptly repaired.
    F. In cases of uterine rupture, immediate laparotomy with repair. If repair is impossible, a hysterectomy is done.

Hyperemesis gravidarum

1. Cause – Hormonal. Increased levels of estrogens and beta HCG. Morning sickness is a usual occurrence in the first and second trimesters.
2. Clinical features – In hyperemesis gravidarum, there is severe vomiting that causes dehydration, electrolyte derangement, ketosis and weight loss. Patients present with features of hypovolemic shock. Complications are fatty degenerative changes in the liver, Wernicke encephalopathy and Mallory-Weiss tears.
3. Treatment
    A. Nil per oral
    B. Resuscitation with IV fluids, usually Ringer's lactate and dextrose saline. During infusion of dextrose, IV thiamine is added to prevent Wernicke encephalopathy.
    C. Correction of electrolyte derangement

D. IV antiemetics: doxylamine, promethazine, ondansetron or metoclopramide
E. Commencement of small, non-spicy meals and oral multivitamins for patients who can tolerate oral foods
F. Symptomatic treatment of jaundice
G. Termination of pregnancy may be considered for patients with worsening symptoms.

Neonatal resuscitation

1. Indications – Birth asphyxia characterized by Apgar score less than 7 in the first one minute of life.
2. Preparation – Identification of perinatal risk factors like gestational age less than 36 weeks or greater than 41 weeks, operative vaginal delivery, fetal compromise during labor or delivery, emergency caesarean delivery, obstructed labor and meconium-stained fluid. Preparation also includes the provision of necessary equipment and the presence of at least one person skilled in resuscitation.
3. The fetus should be given warmth and quickly assessed for an APGAR score. They should be dried for warmth and stimulation. Suctioning with a bulb syringe is also used for infants with aspiration or obstruction of the airway. The cord should be clamped, and babies who do not require resuscitation are quickly given to their mother to establish skin-to-skin contact.
4. Ventilation and oxygenation – For babies who require resuscitation, stimulation is given via flicking the soles or rubbing the back. Suctioning is not used as a form of stimulation. If the APGAR score is low in the next one minute of stimulation, positive pressure ventilation is administered

via bag and mask. The neonate is placed in the appropriate position and the appropriate cuff is used.

5. Intubation and chest compression – Infants with heart rates less than 100 bpm should be quickly intubated and chest compressions commenced at the rate of three compressions to one breath. In 60 seconds, a total of 90 compressions and 30 breaths should be given. An assistant is used in this stage.
6. Drugs – If the heart rate remains below 60 bpm, epinephrine is given via the endotracheal tube.
7. Fluids – If the neonate does not respond to resuscitation, volume expanders like 0.9 percent saline are given and compression and ventilation are recommenced again. Pneumothorax should be ruled out.

Placenta previa

1. Causes – Older maternal age, multiple gestation, previous caesarean section or myomectomy, multiparity, smoking and uterine abnormalities.
2. Clinical features – Sudden and painless vaginal bleeding. The blood is often bright red. There may be no fetal compromise even in the face of maternal hemodynamic instability. Apart from antepartum hemorrhage, other complications of placenta previa are prelabor rupture of membranes, fetal malpresentation, intrauterine growth restriction, postpartum hemorrhage and increased risk of placenta accreta.
3. Treatment
    A. Acute resuscitation in patients with hemodynamic instability. For pregnancies greater than 37 weeks, an emergency caesarean section is done.

B. For a first episode of mild bleeding before 36 weeks, the mother is placed on total bed rest. If the mother is stable and pregnancy is greater than 36 weeks, emergency caesarean section is done.
C. IV dexamethasone is given to patients with pregnancies less than 34 weeks to expedite maturity of the fetal lungs.
D. RhoGam is given to rhesus-negative patients to protect the fetus against isoimmunization.

Postpartum infection

1. Risk factors – Chorioamnionitis, prolonged rupture of membranes, caesarean delivery, prolonged labor, invasive fetal monitoring, frequent cervical examination, anemia, postpartum hemorrhage, bacterial vaginosis, low socioeconomic status and young maternal age. The most implicated organisms are anaerobes, gram-positive cocci and gram-negative bacteria. The endometrium is the most infected, although the myometrium and parametrium may also be involved.
2. Clinical features – Foul-smelling lochia, fever, lower abdominal pain, uterine tenseness, fever, malaise and anorexia. The patient may present with features of septic shock.
3. Treatment – Acute resuscitation with IV fluids and blood products where indicated. Empirical antibiotic therapy with broad-spectrum antibiotics, clindamycin and gentamicin. Amoxicillin may be added.

Preeclampsia, eclampsia, HELLP syndrome

1. Risk factors – Nulliparity, multiple gestation, hypertension, older or very young maternal age, obesity, family history of preeclampsia, previous history of preeclampsia and thrombotic disorders.

2. Clinical features – Fluid retention, facial puffiness, excessive weight gain, proteinuria and hypertension. In severe preeclampsia, patients experience visual disturbances, epigastric pain, severe headaches, confusion, difficulty breathing and oliguria. In eclampsia, patients have seizures, altered neurologic deficits and coagulopathies.
3. Treatment
    A. Acute resuscitation for patients with hemodynamic instability
    B. Control of blood pressure with IV labetalol or IV hydralazine, which are safe to use in pregnancy
    C. Control of seizures or prevention of seizures with IV magnesium sulfate. According to the Pritchard regimen, a loading dose of 4 g is given IV over 20 minutes, followed by 10 g given intramuscularly, 5 g in each buttock. A maintenance dose is given IM 5 g every 4 hours until 24 hours after delivery or until the last seizure, whichever occurs last. According to the Zuspan regimen, a loading dose of 4 g is given IV over 20 minutes followed by a maintenance dose of 1 to 2 g every hour via an infusion pump. The patient must be monitored for magnesium sulfate toxicity.
    D. Definitive treatment is delivery of the fetus or termination of pregnancy. IV dexamethasone is given to expedite the maturity of the fetal lungs.

Preterm labor

1. Causes – Chorioamnionitis, prelabor rupture of membranes, multiple gestations, abnormalities of the fetus, congenital malformations, pyelonephritis, sexually transmitted infections, cervical insufficiency and previous history of preterm labor.
2. Treatment

A. Corticosteroids to hasten the maturity of fetal lungs in pregnancies less than 34 weeks
B. Conservative management with bed rest, tocolytics and hydration
C. Empirical antibiotics to treat group B Streptococci are used until results of culture and sensitivity are obtained. Tocolytics include magnesium sulfate, prostaglandin inhibitor and calcium channel blockers. Tocolytics are not used for first-line treatment.

Threatened/spontaneous abortion

1. Causes – Cervical insufficiency, congenital malformations not compatible with life, viral infections (e.g., cytomegalovirus, rubella virus, parvovirus and herpes virus), uterine anomalies and major trauma to the uterus. Risk factors include older maternal age, substance abuse disorders, cigarette smoking, poorly controlled diabetes mellitus or hypertension and thyroid disorders.
2. Clinical features – Vaginal bleeding and cramping abdominal pain. In spontaneous abortion, the cervical os is opened, and there may be complete expulsion of the fetus. In patients with threatened abortion, the cervical os is closed. If products of conception are retained, sepsis may set in.
3. Treatment
   A. Acute resuscitation for patients with hemodynamic instability
   B. Analgesia for pain relief
   C. For threatened miscarriage, the patient is placed on bed rest and observed.
   D. In spontaneous abortion, the uterus is examined via ultrasound for retained products of conception. If completely expelled, uterine evacuation is not done. If there are retained products of conception,

the uterus is evacuated via suction curettage for pregnancies less than 12 weeks, dilatation and evacuation for pregnancies 12 to 23 weeks or induction of labor for pregnancies greater than 23 weeks.

Obstetric trauma

A. Uterine rupture

1. Cause – Overdistension of the uterus, multiple gestations, polyhydramnios and fetal anomalies. Overstimulation with uterotonics, internal or external fetal version, prolonged obstructed labor and iatrogenic perforation of the uterus. Risk for rupture increases in women with previous caesarean section, myomectomies or open maternal-fetal surgery.
2. Clinical features – Hemorrhagic shock, persistent vaginal bleeding, fetal bradycardia, variable deceleration, floating fetal head and severe abdominal pain.
3. Treatment – Emergency laparotomy with a uterine repair. Subtotal or total hysterectomy is done in intractable hemorrhage.

Chapter 5: Mental Health Emergencies

There are 11 questions in this section of the exam. Content areas are:

Aggressive and violent behavior

1. Causes of agitation include psychotic episodes, substance use disorder, acute mania, delirium, delusional disorders, schizophrenia and intoxication with alcohol or recreational drugs.
2. Risk increases when a patient has had a prior history of agitation.
3. Treatment and evaluation should be simultaneous. The principle of management is to ensure the patient's safety and safety of others by putting the patient in a separate room, using therapeutic communication techniques and using physical or chemical restraints where necessary.

Anxiety disorders

1. Generalized anxiety disorder – Patients have an excessive display of worry or anxiety that lasts for days for a minimum of six months. Sources of anxiety are health, social interactions, work and other life activities. Symptoms include restlessness, agitation, fatigue, lack of concentration, insomnia, muscle tension and others.
2. Panic disorder – Affected individuals have recurrent and unexpected sudden episodes of panic attacks and unexpected episodes of intense fear that build up quickly. Attacks can be expected or caused by triggers. Symptoms include palpitations, sweating, shaking, difficulty breathing/fast breathing, hyperventilation, feeling of doom and feelings of things going out of control.
3. Phobia-related disorders – A phobia is an intense fear of specific situations or/and objects. In phobias, the fear is out of magnitude to the danger caused by the object/situation. Symptoms include excessive worry,

anxiety, panic or feeling of impending doom. There are different types of phobias, some of which are the fear of heights, spiders, blood, flying and others.

4. Social anxiety disorder – This is also known as social phobia. Affected individuals have a deep fear of social situations. They worry that their actions may be negatively interpreted by others. This leads to embarrassment, worry, and avoidance of social gatherings. Affected people are worried that their actions or behaviors caused by their anxiety will be unacceptable to others, thereby making them embarrassed.
5. Separation anxiety disorder – Affected individuals are afraid of being separated from people they are attached to. This is often seen in young children, but it can also be seen in adults. Affected individuals may experience nightmares of separation from their attachment figures. They may also experience physical symptoms when separated or when anticipating a separation.

Mood Disorders

Bipolar disorder

1. This disorder is characterized by alternating episodes of mania and depression. However, patients may have a predominance of one or the other.
2. Classification of bipolar disorders includes
   A. Bipolar I disorder, which is characterized by at least one full-fledged manic episode and usually depressive episodes
   B. Bipolar II disorder, which is characterized by major depressive episodes with at least one hypomanic episode and no full-fledged manic episodes

C. Unspecified bipolar disorder, which has clear bipolar features that do not meet the specific criteria for other bipolar disorders.

Depression

1. This disorder is characterized by severe and persistent sadness that interferes with function.
2. Classification of depression includes

   A. Major depressive disorder, which is a persistent depressive disorder that lasts for more than two years, even with medication

   B. Other specified or unspecified depressive disorder

   C. Classification by etiology, which includes premenstrual dysphoric disorders, depressive disorder due to another medical condition and substance/medication-induced depressive disorder.

Homicidal and Suicidal ideation

Homicidal ideation

1. This refers to the contemplation of homicide. Risk factors are personality disorders, psychosis, delirium and substance-induced disorders.
2. Homicidal ideation also occurs in patients with no psychiatric disorder.

Suicidal ideation

This includes completed suicide and attempted suicide.

1. Completed suicide – This is a suicidal act that results in death.
2. Attempted suicide – This is a nonfatal but injurious act that is self-directed and intended to result in death. It may or may not cause injury.

Nonsuicidal self-injury (NSSI) – This is a self-inflicted injurious act that is not intended to cause death. The causes of suicidal behavior include depression;

other mental disorders like schizophrenia and bipolar disorder; alcohol and substance abuse; previous suicide attempts; unemployment; economic repression; personality disorders; impulsivity; traumatic childhood experiences; family history of suicide; mental disorders and others.

Thought Disorders

Psychosis

1. Patients with brief psychotic disorder experience hallucinations, delusions and other symptoms for at least one day. These symptoms last less than a month.
2. Causes are stressful events, pre-existing personality disorders and conditions like SLE. Treatment is the same as treatment given for schizophrenia.

Schizophrenia

1. Schizophrenia is a disorder that occurs in the brain.
2. Symptoms include erratic speech, hallucinations and delusions and slow thinking.

Situational crisis

1. This refers to sudden and stressful situations that disrupt the normal activity of an individual. The characteristics of a situational crisis are the presence of a stressful event, the inability of the individual to cope with the event and intervention.
2. Examples of situational crises are natural disasters, family disruption, life events like divorce or losing a child, the death of a loved one, suicide and economic changes.

Overdose and ingestions

Acetaminophen overdose

1. Features – Nausea, vomiting, abdominal cramps, hepatomegaly, pancreatitis and hepatic failure.
2. Treatment
   A. Use of activated charcoal within four hours of ingestion
   B. Use of the antidote N-acetylcysteine within eight hours of ingestion
   C. Supportive management of gastroenteritis and liver failure
   D. Liver transplantation may be needed in rapidly progressive liver failure.

Aspirin poisoning

1. Features – Nausea, vomiting, hyperventilation and tinnitus. Patients also present with confusion, fever, seizure and restlessness. In severe cases, patients can deteriorate to acute renal failure, rhabdomyolysis and respiratory failure.
2. Treatment
   A. Activated charcoal if ingested within four hours of presentation
   B. Fluid and electrolyte replacement
   C. Alkaline diuresis with sodium bicarbonate
   D. Hemodialysis in severe poisoning.

Opioid overdose

1. Clinical features – Respiratory depression, apnea, miosis, hypotension, delirium, bradycardia, hypothermia and urinary retention.
2. Treatment
   A. Acute resuscitation
   B. Mechanical ventilation

C. Intravenous naloxone.

Iron poisoning

A common cause of accidental poisoning in children.

1. Clinical features – Acute onset presentation include nausea, hematemesis, diarrhea and abdominal cramps. Late-onset presentations include shock, metabolic acidosis, seizures and coagulopathy. Complications are liver failure and gastric outlet obstruction.
2. Treatment – Whole bowel irrigation with polyethylene glycol, an osmotic laxative and use of IV deferoxamine in severe poisoning.

Anxiolytic poisoning

1. Clinical features – Depressed superficial reflexes, ataxia, impaired coordination, nystagmus, confusion, respiratory depression and death. Treatment – Supportive with mechanical ventilation. Use of flumazenil, a benzodiazepine receptor antagonist.

Chapter 6: Medical Emergencies

There are 14 questions in this section of the exam. Content areas are:

Allergic reactions and anaphylaxis

1. Atopic and allergic reactions are all classified under type 1 hypersensitivity reaction, which is mediated by IgE immune response.
2. Examples of atopic disorders are atopic dermatitis, urticaria, angioedema, latex allergies, allergic rhinitis and others.
3. Anaphylaxis is an acute and life-threatening form of IgE-mediated hypersensitivity reaction.
   A. Causes are allergens in drugs (insulin, beta-lactam antibiotics, streptokinase); foods (nuts, eggs and seafood); latex; animal venom and blood transfusion.
   B. Clinical features range from urticaria, flushing, pruritus, rhinorrhea, diarrhea, dizziness, syncope and wheezing to more serious complications like shock, angioedema, cyanosis and respiratory failure.
   C. Treatment is with IV epinephrine, and acute resuscitation with IV fluids, oxygen and vasopressors when necessary. Oral antihistamines are given for pruritus, and nebulized beta-agonists are given for respiratory symptoms.

Hematologic Disorders

Hemophilia

1. This includes Von Willebrand disease, a bleeding disorder caused by a deficiency of the Von Willebrand factor. Screening tests reveal a slightly prolonged PTT and normal platelet count.
2. Diagnosis reveals low amounts of Von Willebrand factor.

3. Treatment is replacement therapy with factor VII and desmopressin.
4. Other examples of coagulation disorders are hemophilia A and B, which are genetic bleeding disorders that are caused by a deficiency of factor VIII or IX. Screening reveals a prolonged PTT, normal prothrombin time and platelet count. A confirmatory diagnosis test reveals a deficiency of clotting factors VIII/IX. Treatment involves clotting factor replacement.

Thrombocytopenia

This is a reduced amount of platelets in the blood. Causes are varied and include reduced or absent megakaryocytes (as seen in myelosuppressive and chemotherapy drugs); leukemias; paroxysmal nocturnal hemoglobinuria decreased platelet production (as seen in alcohol-induced thrombocytopenia, folate and cobalamin deficiency); myelodysplastic syndromes and HIV-associated thrombocytopenia.

It also occurs with sequestration of platelets in the spleen (as seen in cirrhosis, sarcoidosis and Gaucher disease); myelofibrosis; immunologic destruction of platelets (as seen in connective tissue disorders); antiphospholipid antibody syndrome; drug-induced thrombocytopenia; lymphoproliferative disorder; nonimmunology-mediated destruction of platelets (as seen in systemic diseases like hepatitis, DIC and pregnancy); hemolytic uremic syndrome and dilutional causes like massive RBC transfusion.

Leukemia

This includes acute and chronic lymphocytic leukemia and acute and chronic myeloid leukemia.

A. These malignancies primarily involve white blood cells.

B. Risk factors are exposure to ionizing radiation; atomic bombs; chemicals like pesticides and benzene; previous treatment with antineoplastic drugs; some genetic conditions like Fanconi anemia; Down syndrome; Bloom syndrome; ataxia-telangiectasia; viral infections with Epstein-Barr virus and a history of hematologic disorders like myelodysplastic and myeloproliferative syndromes.

Sickle cell crisis

This is a hemoglobinopathy characterized by chronic hemolytic anemia.

A. Sickle cell disease is an autosomal recessive disease that leads to the formation of sickle-shaped red blood cells that stick to one another and occlude blood vessels. These red blood cells are susceptible to hemolysis and therefore give the patient chronic hemolytic anemia.

B. Clinical features include chronic anemia, vaso occlusive crisis, organ ischemia and major systemic complications.

C. Diagnosis is done via electrophoresis and sickling tests.

Treatment is supportive with blood transfusion, adequate hydration, antibiotics, adequate analgesia and the use of prophylactic hydroxyurea. Definitive treatment is bone marrow transplantation.

Electrolyte and fluid imbalance

1. Hyperkalemia – Acute kidney injury, chronic kidney injury, use of potassium-sparing diuretics, rhabdomyolysis, burns, hemolysis and others.
2. Hypokalemia – Gastroenteritis, laxative abuse, malabsorption, fistula, colostomy, hyperglycemia, hyperaldosteronism, renal tubular acidosis, metabolic alkalosis, total parenteral nutrition, dialysis, plasmapheresis and others.

3. Hypernatremia – Dehydration, iatrogenic causes, excessive sodium intake, Cushing syndrome, hyperaldosteronism, peritoneal dialysis, vomiting, diarrhea, fistula, diabetes insipidus, osmotic diuresis as seen in alcohol intoxication, burns and others.
4. Hyponatremia – Chronic kidney diseases, cirrhosis, heart failure, diuretic therapy, mineralocorticoid deficiency, SIADH, burns, pancreatitis and others.
5. Hypercalcemia – Primary hyperparathyroidism, multiple myeloma, exogenous vitamin D, bedridden patients, thyrotoxicosis, Paget's disease, vitamin A toxicity, adrenal insufficiency and others.
6. Hypocalcemia – Vitamin D insufficiency, hypoparathyroidism, malabsorption syndromes, insufficient calcium intake and others.
7. Dehydration – Mild, moderate, and severe dehydration. Causes include metabolic acidosis, hypernatremia, gastroenteritis, hyperpyrexia, burns, heatstroke and others.
8. Edema – Congestive heart failure, liver failure, kidney diseases, nephrotic syndrome and others.

Endocrine disorders

A. Adrenal

1. Primary adrenal insufficiency – This is also called Addison's disease.
    A. It is caused by the insufficient secretion of cortisol from the adrenal cortex.
    B. Clinical features are hypotension, adrenal crisis, hyperpigmentation, tiredness, anorexia, vomiting, diarrhea and others. Diagnosis is clinical and confirmed by cortisol and ACTH assay. Treatment is focused on the cause.

2. Cushing syndrome – This is a group of clinical features and abnormalities that are caused by elevated serum levels or corticosteroids/cortisol for a long period.
    A. Cushing syndrome is caused by exogenous intake of corticosteroids, while Cushing's disease is caused by excess secretion of ACTH from a pituitary adenoma.
    B. Clinical features are truncal obesity, moon face, striae, easy bruising, hyperglycemia, thin arms and legs and others.
    C. Diagnosis is clinical and confirmed by assay of serum cortisol.
    D. Treatment is directed at the cause.

B. Glucose-related conditions

1. Type 1 diabetes mellitus – This is insulin-dependent diabetes mellitus.
    A. It is caused by the progressive destruction of B cells in the endocrine pancreas.
    B. Clinical features include hyperglycemia, polyuria, polydipsia, polyphagia, cachexia, glucosuria and ketonuria. The most common complication is diabetic ketoacidosis.
    C. Treatment is the exogenous administration of insulin.
2. Type 2 diabetes mellitus – This is noninsulin-dependent therapy.
    A. It is caused by decreased insulin resistance, decreased insulin sensitivity, hyperinsulinemia and burnout of the endocrine pancreas.
    B. The disease is commonly seen in adults. However, it is becoming common in the younger populations because of obesity.
    C. Treatment modalities include monitoring glucose levels, education, diet modification, exercise and drugs.

C. Thyroid

1. Hyperthyroidism – This is an excess secretion of thyroid hormones due to an intrinsic dysfunction of the thyroid gland (primary hyperthyroidism) or a dysfunction of the hypothalamo-pituitary pathways (secondary hyperthyroidism).
   A. Examples of primary hyperthyroidism are thyroiditis, Graves' disease and multinodular goiter.
   B. Examples of secondary hyperthyroidism are TSH secretory adenoma, choriocarcinoma, hydatidiform moles, stroma ovarii and testicular carcinoma.
   C. The symptoms of hyperthyroidism include weight loss, fatigue, diarrhea, palpitations, tremors and others.
   D. Diagnosis is confirmed with a thyroid function test.
   E. Treatment depends on the cause.
2. Hypothyroidism – This is decreased secretion of thyroid hormone.
   A. Primary causes are Hashimoto's thyroiditis, iodine deficiency and the use of lithium.
   B. Causes of secondary hypothyroidism are insufficient secretion of thyrotropin-releasing hormone and thyroid-stimulating hormone.
   C. Clinical features include dry skin, weight gain, constipation, hoarseness and others.

Immunocompromise

1. Primary immunodeficiency – This is genetically caused and often manifests in infancy and early childhood. It is a result of inborn errors in metabolism affecting cellular immunity, humoral immunity, complement proteins and phagocytes.

2. Secondary immunodeficiency – This is caused by systemic disorders like diabetes, HIV infections, malnutrition, use of immunosuppressants and chronic illness. Other examples may occur as a result of a transplant that has been put in a patient, or if a patient has undergone chemotherapy.

Renal failure

1. Acute kidney injury – Increase in sCr ≥0.3 mg/dL (≥26.5 μmol/L) within 48 hours; or increase in sCr ≥1.5 times baseline, which is confirmed or suspected to have occurred within the prior seven days; or urine volume <0.5 mL/kg/h for 6 hours.
2. Chronic kidney injury – The five stages of kidney disease are:
   A. Stage 1 has normal or high GFR >90 mL/min.
   B. Stage 2 – This is mild CKD, in which GFR 60–89 mL/min.
   C. Stage 3A – This is moderate CKD, in which GFR 45–59 mL/min.
   D. Stage 3B – This is moderate CKD, in which GFR 30–44 mL/min.
   E. Stage 4 – This is severe CKD, in which GFR 15–29 mL/min.
   F. Stage 5 – This is end-stage CKD, in which GFR <15 mL/min.
3. End-stage renal disease – This is stage 5 CKD. The patient will be assessed on the principles of management of a patient with end-stage renal disease. This includes hemodialysis, the filtration of the patient's blood with a dialyzer. It can be continuous or intermittent. Unlike intermittent hemodialysis, continuous hemodialysis reduces the risk of hypotension and is ideal for patients with AKI. Hemodialysis is necessary to correct imbalances of the electrolytes and fluid, remove toxins and wastes, prolong the patient's survival, prevent complications of uremia and improve the patient's blood pressure and comfort.
4. Peritoneal dialysis – Unlike hemodialysis, which requires vascular access, peritoneal dialysis uses the peritoneum as a permeable membrane for

filtration of blood. Unlike hemodialysis, peritoneal dialysis is less stressful on the patient, allows mobility, can be performed at home and does not require intravascular access.

5. Renal transplant – This is used for patients with end-stage renal disease. Survival rates after the first year of transplantation are 98 percent for kidneys from living donors and 95 percent for kidneys from deceased donors. Failure rates for kidney grafts are higher among Black patients compared to White patients.

Sepsis

1. Sepsis is a life-threatening dysfunction of organs that occurs when the body is overwhelmed by infection. It is a clinical syndrome characterized by reduced tissue perfusion and multiple organ failure. Signs of septic shock include fever, oliguria hypotension and altered sensorium.
2. Common causes in immunocompetent patients include infection with gram-negative and gram-positive bacteria.
3. Causes in patients with compromised immunity include atypical bacterial and fungal infections.
4. Septic shock is a consequence of sepsis. It is characterized by persistent hypotension, which is defined as the use of vasopressors to keep the mean arterial pressure above or equal to 65 mm Hg, a serum lactate level > 18 mg/dL even after the patient is resuscitated with intravenous fluids.
5. Treatment involves aggressive resuscitation with antibiotics and fluids, supportive therapy, pus drainage and debridement of infected and dead tissue.

Hypovolemic and distributive shock

Hypovolemic shock occurs when too much blood has been lost and the heart cannot pump enough blood to the body. This is an emergency condition because it can stop the functioning of organs. Distributive shock occurs when the blood flow is not properly distributed throughout the blood vessels, which causes only a small portion of blood to reach the body's organs.

Substance use and abuse

1. Substance-induced disorders – Intoxication, overdose, withdrawal and substance-related psychiatric disorders.
2. Substance abuse disorders – Addiction, tolerance, physical and psychological dependence.

Withdrawal syndrome

Opioid

1. Clinical features – Severe physical dependence. Symptoms are anxiety, tachypnea, diaphoresis, lacrimation, yawning, rhinorrhea, diarrhea, anorexia, tremors, fever, tachycardia, hypertension and stomach cramps. Symptoms are usually not fatal.
2. Treatment – Symptomatic management and treatment with methadone, clonidine and naltrexone.

Alcohol

1. Clinical features – Mild symptoms include headaches, tremors, weakness, diaphoresis, tachycardia, hypertension, seizures, gastrointestinal symptoms and hyperreflexia. Symptoms progress to involve alcoholic hallucinosis characterized by visual and auditory hallucinations and nightmares. Delirium tremens is a late-onset symptom characterized by increasing anxiety, depression, sweating, disorientation, autonomic

features, altered personality, tachycardia and hyperthermia. Alcoholic withdrawal symptoms are fatal.

2. Treatment – Supportive treatment of symptoms, including intravenous fluids, nutrition, treatment of hyperthermia and use of benzodiazepines for sedation.

Anxiolytic

1. Clinical features – Withdrawal symptoms of benzodiazepines are not life-threatening. However, withdrawal from barbiturates can mimic life-threatening symptoms similar to delirium tremens. Features of benzodiazepine withdrawal are tachycardia, tachypnea, hyperpyrexia and seizures. Features of barbiturate withdrawal include restlessness, increasing anxiety, hyperreflexia, muscle weakness, delirium, seizures that can progress to status epilepticus, insomnia, visual and auditory hallucinations and death.
2. Treatment – Supportive management of symptoms in the ICU and use of long-acting benzodiazepines.

Nicotine

1. Clinical features – Nicotine causes strong physical dependence. Features are irritability, difficulty concentrating, anxiety, depression, insomnia, hunger, GI disturbances, headaches and weight gain.
2. Treatment – Bupropion SR, varenicline and nicotine replacement therapy.

Cannabis

1. Withdrawal symptoms of cannabis are generally mild since they do not produce profound physical dependence. Dependence is more psychological.

2. Clinical features – Insomnia, nausea, irritability, anorexia and depression
3. Treatment – Not often needed unless in severe cases, then supportive management is done.

Chapter 7: Musculoskeletal and Wound Emergencies

There are 13 questions in this section of the test. Content areas include:

A. Musculoskeletal Emergencies

Amputation

1. Causes – Include phocomelia and congenital limb deficiency. Acquired causes include vascular causes like diabetes, frostbite, envenomation, peripheral arterial and venous insufficiency, which can cause necrosis and gangrene, infections of the bone, malignant tumors, traumatic amputation, crush injuries, trauma from gunshots, accidents and bites.
2. Treatment – The provision of analgesia, psychological support, rehabilitation and prostheses.

Compartment syndrome

1. Causes – Common causes are crush injuries, fractures, reperfusion injury and severe contusions. Other causes are circumferential devices like casts and bandages, envenomation, severe burns, an overdose of opioids and snakebites.
2. Clinical features – The earliest feature is severe pain, worse than the original injury. This pain is worsened when the muscles in the affected compartment are stretched passively. Late symptoms include paresthesia, pulselessness, paralysis and pallor. Immediate management must commence as soon as compartment syndrome is diagnosed.
3. Treatment
    a) Prompt removal of constricting devices
    b) Analgesia

c) Resuscitation with IV fluids and oxygen
d) Fasciotomy to relieve the pressure
e) Amputation if there is extensive necrosis.

Ligament tendon injuries (strains, sprains and ruptures)

1. Causes – Mostly blunt trauma from sports, falls, domestic accidents and vehicular accidents.
2. Clinical features – Edema, tenderness and erythema of the affected area. Acute complications are bleeding, damage to neurovascular structures and compartment syndrome. Long-term complications are instability, stiffness, reduction of range of motion and osteoarthritis.
3. Treatment
    a) In patients with multiple trauma, severe associated injuries are treated first.
    b) Immobilization, resting of the affected limb, with ice compression and elevation.
    c) Analgesia
    d) Reduction where necessary.

Fractures (open, closed and fat embolus)

1. Fractures – This is a discontinuity in bone.
    A. Causes – Blunt or penetrating trauma from falls, vehicular accidents, home accidents, occupational accidents and abuse.
    B. A fracture can be open or closed. Open fractures are identified when the bone is apparently sticking out of the skin, or if there is a wound that is deep enough to show the bone beneath the skin. A closed fracture occurs when the bone is broken but the skin is not.

C. A fat embolism is a kind of fat that sticks to a blood vessel and impedes the flow of blood. This usually happens when there is a fracture to the bones of the lower body, such as pelvis, shinbone and thighbone.

D. Clinical features – Inability to use the affected joint or bone, pain, redness and edema. In an open fracture, there is bleeding and features of hypovolemic shock. Patients may also present with multiple trauma.

E. Treatment

   a) Acute resuscitation – Immediate complications like hemorrhage, hypovolemic shock and compartment syndrome are treated first.

   b) Open fractures are dressed with sterile dressings, and systemic antibiotics and tetanus prophylaxis are given.

   c) The fracture is reduced under anesthesia.

   d) The fracture is immobilized with splints, casts, or external fixation as indicated.

Dislocations

This is a separation of bones in a joint.

A. Causes – Injuries can occur alone or as part of multisystemic trauma. Most injuries are from blunt trauma from falls, vehicular accidents, home accidents, occupational accidents and abuse.

B. Clinical features – Inability to use the affected joint, pain and joint swelling. Acute complications include pain, damage to neurovascular structures and sepsis. Later complications include instability of the joints, osteoarthritis, osteonecrosis and limited range of motion.

C. Treatment

   a) Acute resuscitation – Immediate complications like hemorrhage, hypovolemic shock, neurapraxia and compartment syndrome are treated first.

b) Open dislocations are dressed with sterile dressings.
c) The joint is immobilized and then reduced using the appropriate methods.

Inflammatory conditions

Costochondritis

1. This is inflammation of the costochondral joints in the ribs.

A. Causes – Trauma to the chest wall, viral infections and some autoimmune diseases like rheumatoid arthritis, systemic lupus erythematosus, inflammatory bowel disease, ankylosing spondylitis, psoriatic arthritis and fibromyalgia.
B. Clinical features – Chest pain, which can be severe enough to disrupt the patient's sleep. Unlike Tietze's syndrome, there is no localized swelling or erythema.
C. Treatment – Analgesia and corticosteroids.

Osteoarthritis

1. Cause – The most common cause is aging, which increases friction between the two bones and increases wearing of cartilage. Obesity is also another cause.
2. Clinical features – Joint pain that is insidious in onset. This pain is aggravated by weight bearing and relieved by rest. Other symptoms include joint stiffness upon rising in the morning, restriction of movement and crepitus.
3. Treatment
    a) Rehabilitation, including weight loss, exercise, physiotherapy and modification of daily activities.

b) Drugs – Including NSAIDs, muscle relaxants, hyaluronic acid formulations and corticosteroids.

Rheumatoid arthritis

1. Cause – Autoimmune reactions to synovial tissues. Risk factors are generics, viral infections and cigarette smoking.
2. Clinical features – Joint stiffness on waking up in the morning, joint pain, erythema, joint swelling and limitation of motion. Patients also experience systemic symptoms like malaise, fatigue, anorexia and low-grade fever. Rheumatoid arthritis affects all joints in the body except the distal interphalangeal joint. As the disease progresses, patients experience flexion contractures, carpal tunnel syndrome and joint instability.
3. Treatment
    a) Rehabilitation, including weight loss, smoking cessation, exercise and rest
    b) Analgesia with NSAIDs
    c) Disease-modifying antirheumatic disease – These drugs reduce the progression of inflammation and tissue remodeling. They include methotrexate, sulfasalazine, hydroxychloroquine and leflunomide.
    d) Corticosteroids therapy.

Gout

1. Deposition of uric acid crystals in the synovial fluid.
    A. Cause – Increased production or decreased excretion of uric acid. Risk factors include male sex, genetics and metabolic syndrome.
    B. Clinical features – Joint pain that is worse at night. The most affected joint is the metatarsophalangeal joint of the big toe. Other features are joint

swelling, erythema and warmth of the affected joint. Patients can experience systemic symptoms like tachycardia, chills, fever and malaise.

C. Treatment
    a) Lifestyle modification – Reduction of alcohol intake and foods high in purines (e.g., beer, beef, poultry and seafood)
    b) Treatment of acute attacks with colchicine, corticosteroids and NSAIDs
    c) Reducing the rate of attacks by reducing serum uric acid by decreasing production of urate with allopurinol, dissolving uric acid deposits with Pegloticase and increasing excretion of uric acid with probenecid.

Osteomyelitis

1. Cause – Infectious spread from infected tissue or prosthetic joint, hematogenous spread, infected open wounds, trauma, pressure ulcers, foreign bodies and ischemia. The most implicated organisms in debilitated and older patients are Staphylococcus aureus and gram-negative bacteria. In intravenous drug abusers, implicated organisms are Pseudomonas aeruginosa, Serratia spp and Staphylococcus aureus. The most implicated organisms in patients with liver disease, sickle cell anemia and immunocompromise are Salmonella spp.
2. Clinical features – In acute cases, clinical features are localized swelling, warmth, erythema and bone tenderness. Systemic features are fever, fatigue and weight loss.
3. Treatment – Antibiotic therapy against gram-negative and gram-positive organism. Surgery to drain sinuses and abscesses and remove the necrotic bone.

B. Wounds

Avulsions and degloving injuries

Avulsions

This includes avulsions of the skin, ear, nail, eyelids, tooth and periosteum.

1. Cause – Animal bites, industrial accidents, missile injuries and motorcycle accidents.
2. Treatment – Control of the bleeding and resuscitation where appropriate, with wound cleaning and debridement.

Degloving injuries

The avulsion of tissues from the muscle, connective tissue and bone. The most often cause is the entrapment of a limb (i.e., in workplace accidents). There is high mortality from hemorrhage. The most affected areas are the lower limbs, fingers, scalp and face.

Wound infections

1. Cause – This is an infection of surgical wounds and surgical sites. Routes of infection include direct contact from the surgical instruments or hands of the surgical team, airborne transmission and self-contamination from the patient's flora in the skin or GI tract. The most implicated organisms are Streptococcus pyogenes, Pseudomonas aeruginosa, Staphylococcus aureus and Enterococci. Risk factors for infection include patient characteristics like obesity, age, malnutrition, metabolic disorders, anemia, tissue hypoxia, immunosuppression and cigarette smoking; and wound characteristics like foreign bodies, ischemia and hematoma.

2. Clinical features – Discharge of purulent material from the wound, pain, edema, erythema, delayed wound healing, offensive odor from the wound, friability of the granulation tissue and lymphangitis.

Injection injuries (eg. Grease gun, paint gun)

1. Causes – These are injuries caused by high-pressure equipment for grease, oil, paint thinner, fuel, paint and other solvents. They cause high-pressure injection wounds with seemingly mild wounds on the surface with extensive injuries in deeper tissues. Risks for amputation are high if the wound is left untreated for about six hours. The severity of injury depends on the type of solvent, including its temperature, thickness and toxicity; the amount of substance injected; the pressure and speed of the equipment; the time between the onset of injury and treatment; the site of injury; and how fast the substance spreads.
2. Clinical features – During early onset, patients present with puncture injuries. Obtaining a history of injection injuries is necessary for appropriate management. Late presentations include edema, erythema and necrosis of the affected area. The risk of amputation is high.
3. Treatment
    a) Immobilization and elevation of the affected area.
    b) Immediate consult to the orthopedic team.
    c) Immediate debridement is required to reduce the risk of amputation.
    d) Antibiotics and tetanus prophylaxis.
    e) Analgesia.

Lacerations

1. Cause – From penetrating injuries to the skin and soft tissues.
2. Treatment – Hemostasis and resuscitation where indicated, wound cleaning and debridement, wound closure and analgesia.

Penetrating injuries (e.g. guns, nail guns)

These are injuries from high-velocity objects like guns. These injuries cause extensive wounds that increase both morbidity and mortality.

Puncture wounds

1. Causes – These wounds are caused by penetration of the skin by sharp and pointed objects. These wounds are narrow and deep. Risk factors are home accidents and occupational accidents. The risk of infections is high.
2. Treatment – Hemostasis and resuscitation where necessary, wound cleaning and debridement, antibiotics and tetanus prophylaxis. HIV postexposure prophylaxis should be given to all patients with puncture wounds from intravenous and blood giving/collecting devices.

Wound Bleeding (e.g. uncontrolled external hemorrhage)

This occurs when blood flows out of the body when there is a wound. If the blood remains in the body after a blood vessel is damaged, it is called internal bleeding. It is possible to treat the bleeding by using bandages and a clean cloth. If nothing is available, the clothing and hands can be used to stop the blood flow in the case of external hemmorhage.

Chapter 8: Maxillofacial and Ocular Emergencies

There are 11 questions in this section of the test. Content areas include:

A. Maxillofacial

Abscess (eg. Peritonsillar, dental)

Peritonsillar abscess/quinsy

1. Cause – A bacterial infection of the pharynx and soft tissues. The most implicated pathogens are Streptococcus, Staphylococcus and Bacteroides.
2. Clinical features – Dysphagia, sore throat, trismus, hot potato voice, fever, ear pain and adenopathy. Patients also present with a toxic appearance, drooling, halitosis and tonsillar erythema.
3. Treatment
   A. Incision and drainage of the abscess under local anesthesia
   B. Systemic antibiotics and supportive management: IV fluids, analgesia and antipyretics
   C. Elective tonsillectomy is indicated for patients with recurrent tonsillitis and obstructive sleep apnea.

Parapharyngeal abscess

1. Cause – Access collection in the parapharyngeal space, which is lateral to the pharyngeal constrictor muscle and medial to the pterygoid muscle. The most implicated organisms are Streptococcus, Staphylococcus and Bacteroides.
2. Clinical features – Fever, odynophagia, sore throat and neck swelling. Abscesses in the anterior space cause induration and trismus with bulging of the tonsils. Abscesses in the posterior space cause swelling in the

posterior part of the pharyngeal wall, with high-grade fever, neurologic deficits and sepsis.

3. Treatment
    A. Airway control
    B. Incision and drainage under local anesthesia
    C. Empirical antibiotic therapy with parenteral antibiotics like clindamycin and ceftriaxone.

Dental conditions (Dental caries)

1. Causes – Caused by bacteria in dental plaques. Risk factors include diets high in carbohydrates and glucose; tooth plaques; dental defects like fissures, grooves and enamel pits that extend to the dentin; reduced salivary secretion from drugs, radiation exposure and systemic disorders; and a low-fluoride, high-acid environment, which can be caused by soft drinks and energy drinks.
2. Clinical features – Asymptomatic if it affects only the enamel. If it affects the dentin, features include dental pain and tooth sensitivity.
3. Treatment – Restorative therapy, root canal and crown as indicated.

Epistaxis

1. Causes – Local trauma is the most common cause of epistaxis. Trauma may be caused by nose blowing, nose picking or drying of the nasal mucosa from very cold weather. Other causes are vestibulitis, coagulopathies, perforation of the nasal septum, foreign bodies, tumors, arteriosclerosis and systemic disorders.
2. Treatment
    A. Measures for anterior epistaxis include pinching the nasal alae, local control with phenylephrine or lidocaine or cauterization with

silver nitrate or electrocauterization. The anterior septum may also be packed with a tampon or a nasal balloon.

B. Control measures of posterior bleeds include the use of commercial nasal balloons, gauze or ligation of the internal maxillary artery and its branches.

Facial nerve disorders

Bell's palsy

1. Causes – Paralysis of the facial nerve. It is mostly idiopathic. Secondary causes include viral infections from herpes simplex, herpes zoster, cytomegalovirus, Epstein-Barr, mumps, rubella, coxsackievirus and influenza B virus.
2. Clinical features – Pain behind the ear is the earliest sign. Other features include paresis of the affected side. The patient complains of a heavy or numb sensation of the face. On examination, the patient is unable to blink, grimace or wrinkle the forehead. In severe cases, the patient is unable to close the eyelids, causing drying of the cornea.
3. Treatment
   A. Antiviral drugs for suspected herpes simplex virus
   B. Prevention of corneal drying by lubrication with isotonic saline, tears or methylcellulose drops
   C. Corticosteroids.

Trigeminal neuralgia

1. Cause – Compression of the fifth cranial nerve by an intracranial artery, a vein, multiple sclerosis plaques or a tumor

2. Clinical features – Excruciating and paroxysmal facial pain that is triggered by brushing the teeth, chewing, smiling or sleeping on the affected side of the face
3. Treatment
   A. Antiseizure drugs like carbamazepine, gabapentin, lamotrigine and phenytoin.
   B. Antidepressants (e.g., amitriptyline).

Maxillofacial infections

1. Otitis – This is an infection of the ear, which may be external, middle or internal ear. Infections may be acute or chronic.
   A. The most implicated organisms are pseudomonas, Proteus, E. coli, Staphylococcus and Aspergillus. In otitis media, implicated organisms are Moraxella, Haemophilus, group A Beta-hemolytic streptococcus and Staphylococcus aureus.
   B. Clinical features include ear pain, ear discharge, deafness and nonspecific features like fever and malaise. In otitis media, patients may present with sore throats and a toxic appearance. Treatment includes analgesics, antipyretics and antibiotics.
2. Ludwig's angina – This is cellulitis of the submandibular space, including the submaxillary and spaces, the suprahyoid soft tissues, and the floor of the mouth. It is not a true abscess, although it is treated as one.
   A. Risk factors include tooth extractions, poor dental hygiene and trauma, including trauma to the mandible.
   B. Clinical features are tenderness in the teeth and affected mandible, with induration of the floor of the mouth and soft tissues of the suprahyoid. Other features include drooling, dysphagia, trismus, stridor, chills, fever and tachycardia.

C. Treatment includes maintenance of the airway, incision and drainage and treatment with empirical antibiotics against aerobic and anaerobic infections.

3. Mastoiditis – This is a bacterial infection of the mastoid air cells. It is often a complication of otitis media.
   A. Clinical features include fever, otalgia, and features of otitis media.
   B. Treatment includes empiric antibiotic therapy with IV ceftriaxone. Incision and drainage are done for a subperiosteal abscess.

Acute vestibular dysfunction

1. Labyrinthitis – This is a bacterial infection of the inner ear.
   A. Clinical features are nystagmus, vertigo, nausea, vomiting, pain, hearing loss, tinnitus and fever.
   B. Treatment includes empirical antibiotic therapy with IV ceftriaxone and myringotomy. Tympanostomy is done to drain the middle ear.
2. Ménière's disease – Risk factors include allergies, autoimmune diseases, family history, trauma, and syphilis.
   A. Clinical features are vertigo, tinnitus, hearing loss, nausea and vomiting. Patients also experience diarrhea, disturbances of gait and diaphoresis.
   B. Treatment includes symptomatic management with antihistamines, antiemetics, diuretics, benzodiazepines and a low-salt diet. In some cases, vestibular ablation is done via surgery or drugs.

Maxillofacial trauma

A. Fractured and avulsed teeth – Patients with fractured teeth that expose the dentin experience tooth sensitivity to cold water and air. Treatment includes analgesia and prompt referral to a dentist. Treatment options include tooth restoration, crowning and root canal. Avulsed primary teeth are not replaced due to the risk of necrosis, infection and ankylosis. Also, these teeth can disrupt the eruption of permanent teeth. Avulsed permanent teeth are rapidly replaced. Rates of retention are high if they are replaced within an hour of the avulsion.

B. Trauma to the external ear – This includes hematoma in the perichondrium, lacerations and avulsions of the external ear.
C. Fracture of the mandible – Patients often present with tenderness and swelling of the affected side. Other features are disruptions of the alveolar ridge, preauricular pain and trismus. Patients with a fracture of the condyle present with a deviation of the jaw to the affected side.
D. Fracture of the nose – Patients present with epistaxis, swelling, tenderness, instability and crepitus. Other features include nasal deformity, ecchymosis, lacerations, nasal obstruction and septal deviation. Some patients may also present with CSF rhinorrhea. Treatment includes immediate control of pain with ice compression and analgesia. Hematomas in the septum are drained, while reduction is done for fractures with nasal obstruction and obvious deformity.

B. Ocular

Abrasions

1. Cause – Contact lens, foreign bodies lodged in the upper eyelid and entropion.
2. Clinical features – Tearing, redness, foreign body sensation and discharge from the eyes.
3. Treatment
    A. Use of ophthalmic ointments like bacitracin. Patients who use contact lenses are given antibiotics that cover pseudomonas infections.
    B. The pupil is dilated with a cycloplegic to reduce eye pain.
    C. Eye patches are not used due to the risk of infections. Also, ophthalmic corticosteroids increase the risk of fungi growth in the eye and reactivation of herpes simplex virus.
    D. Patients are discouraged from wearing contact lenses until the ulcer is completely healed.

Burns

1. Causes – Thermal burns from heat, and chemical burns from alkalis and acids. Ocular burns from acids are less extensive than burns from alkalis because the acids denature and coagulate the proteins in the eye, thereby preventing further absorption of the acids. Alkalis, on the other hand, liquefy the eye proteins and penetrate underlying tissues, thereby causing more extensive burns. Ocular burns from chemicals are usually caused by occupational hazards, assaults and abuse.
2. Treatment
    A. Thermal burns involve more of the eyelids because of the blink reflex. The eyelids are irrigated with copious amounts of normal

saline and then dressed with antimicrobial ointment. Thermal burns to the eye are usually mild. Patients are managed with antimicrobial ointment, cycloplegics and oral analgesia.

B. In chemical burns, the eyeballs and eyelids are irrigated with copious amounts of normal saline or a borate buffer solution under local anesthesia. Irrigation is done until the pH of the cornea is normal.

C. Burns are managed with ocular antibiotics and cycloplegics. Ocular corticosteroids are used only prescribed with an ophthalmologist's discretion. An ophthalmologist should be promptly consulted to reduce the risk of perforation, globe rupture, scarring and deformities of the eyelids.

Foreign bodies

1. Causes and clinical features are the same for corneal abrasions as discussed above

A. Treatment – Surface foreign bodies are managed with irrigation or manual removal under ocular anesthesia by an ophthalmologist.

B. Intraocular foreign bodies are removed surgically by an ophthalmologist. Thereafter, ocular and systemic antibiotics are used. Ointments are not used if there is a rupture of the globe.

Increased intraocular pressure

Increased intraocular pressure is dangerous because it can be an indicator of glaucoma, which can cause blindness. There is high pressure in the eye when different levels of fluids in the eye are being produced as compared to the fluids that are being drained.

Glaucoma

1. Causes – Risk factors for primary open-angle glaucoma are African ethnicity, positive family history, old age, diabetes, myopia and systemic hypertension. Causes of angle-closure glaucoma include inflammatory disorders, contracture of the membranes, lens-induced mechanisms, posterior synechiae and mechanisms that push or pull the iris and block the drainage of the aqueous humor.
2. Clinical features – Primary angle glaucoma is usually asymptomatic until there is marked loss of peripheral vision. However, patients with angle-closure glaucoma experience intense eye pain with conjunctival injection, decreased visual acuity, headache, nausea and vomiting. Some patients complain of colored halos around lights.
3. Treatment – Patients who present to the ER often have angle-closure glaucoma. Treatment must begin quickly after diagnosis to preserve vision. Treatment options include:
    a) Beta-blockers like timolol reduce the secretion of aqueous humor.
    b) Pilocarpine, an acetylcholine agonist, to induce miosis and reduce aqueous humor secretion; Brimonidine, an alpha 2 adrenergic receptor agonist which decreases secretion of aqueous humor and improves uveoscleral drainage; and osmotic agents like mannitol, glycerin and isosorbide to cause movement of fluids from the eye into the intravascular space.
    c) Definite treatment is laser peripheral iridotomy, which is done to create another channel for fluid drainage from the posterior chamber to the anterior chamber.

Ocular infections

Conjunctivitis

1. Conjunctivitis – The most common cause is viral infection from adenovirus, chicken pox, measles, rubella and mumps.
2. Other causes include bacteria, like Streptococcus pneumoniae, Staphylococcus aureus, Haemophilus spp, Chlamydia trachomatis and Neisseria gonorrhoeae; allergens like pollen, dust, hay, mites, dander, airborne spores and pollen; and irritants, like smoke, dust, fumes and ultraviolet light.
3. Clinical features – Eye discharge, which can be thick, copious and cause overnight crusting of the eyes. Other features include tearing, eye pain, conjunctival injection, blurred vision, papillary hyperplasia, chemosis and photophobia.
4. Treatment
   A. Symptomatic treatment.
   B. The patient should be encouraged to wash hands or use hand sanitizer when touching the eye or nose.
   C. Avoid touching the uninfected eye and avoid sharing clothes, pillows, towels and swimming pools.
   D. Health workers must wash their hands after coming in contact with the patient and disinfect all equipment used for examination and treatment. Eye patches are avoided.

Iritis

1. Cause – Infectious: herpes virus, cytomegalovirus, varicella-zoster, tuberculosis, syphilis, Lyme's disease and toxoplasmosis. Other causes are trauma, arthritis, spondyloarthropathies, multiple sclerosis and sarcoidosis.

2. Clinical features – Ocular pain, decreased visual acuity, photophobia and redness. Complications are glaucoma, cataracts, retinal detachment, neovascularization, hypotony and macular edema.
3. Treatment
    a) Topical corticosteroids
    b) Topical mydriatics and cycloplegics
    c) Topical antibiotics for infectious causes
    d) Vitrectomy for severe cases.

Retinal artery occlusion

1. Central retinal artery occlusion – This is caused by embolism from fat, endocarditis, atherosclerotic plaque, atrial myxoma and fat. Thrombosis can occur from systemic vasculitis (e.g., giant cell arteritis and SLE). The risk of stroke is high in the first few weeks of occlusion. It is severe, sudden, unilateral and painless loss of vision.
    A. Treatment includes reduction of intraocular pressure with hypotensive drugs like topical timolol and acetazolamide. High-dose corticosteroids are used for patients with giant cell arteritis.

Retinal detachment

1. Causes – Risk factors for rhegmatogenous detachment are myopia, ocular trauma, cataract surgery, family history of retinal detachment and lattice retinal detachment. Risk factors for traction retinal detachment are sickle cell retinopathy and diabetic retinopathy. Risk factors for serous detachment are cancers, choroid, choroidal hemangiomas and severe uveitis.
2. Clinical features – It is often painless. In the early stage, patients experience vitreous floaters, blurred vision and photopsia. In the late

stage, patients experience grayness in the visual field. If the macula is involved, the central vision is affected. In the ER, patients present with retinal hemorrhage as a result of trauma.

3. Treatment – Treatment options are vitrectomy, scleral buckling, sealing of the retinal breaks and pneumatic retinopexy.

Ocular trauma

1. Hyphema – This is bleeding in the anterior chamber from blunt trauma to the eye. Immediate complications are raised intraocular pressure, glaucoma, recurrent bleeding and permanent blindness in the affected eye. Immediate measures include placing the patient in the semi-Fowler's or high Fowler's position and use of an eye shield to protect the eye. Intraocular pressure is monitored and controlled with the appropriate drugs (e.g., brimonidine and timolol). Corticosteroids are administered to reduce inflammation. Aminocaproic acid or tranexamic acid may be used to control recurrent bleeding.
2. Globe rupture – Immediate interventions for laceration of the globe include using an eye shield to protect the eyes, reduction of intraocular pressure and use of systemic antibiotics to treat infections. Topical antibiotics are avoided. Because vomiting can increase IOP, antiemetics are used. Corticosteroids are not used until the wounds are closed surgically. Tetanus prophylaxis is also given. An ophthalmologist must be consulted immediately.

Ulcerations and keratitis

1. Causes – Infectious (i.e., viruses like herpes simplex, bacteria like pseudomonas, fungi and parasitic infections from acanthamoeba). Risk factors include prolonged wearing of contact lenses, improper disinfection

of contact lenses and reactivation of herpes simplex infections due to immunosuppression (use of topical corticosteroids).

2. Clinical features – Lacrimation, photophobia, feeling of foreign bodies in the eyes, redness and eye pain.
3. Treatment
    A. Empiric antibiotic therapy with topical moxifloxacin, or tobramycin, followed by specific antibiotics after the cause is diagnosed.
    B. Eye patching is contraindicated.
    C. Patients are not to wear contact lenses until the ulcer is completely healed.

Chapter 9: Environment and Toxicology Emergencies and Communicable Diseases

There are 14 questions in this section of the test. Topic areas are:

A. Environment

Burns

1. Thermal burns – From external heat such as hot liquids, steam, hot solid objects, flames and smoke inhalation during fires.
2. Radiation burns – Examples include sunburn from prolonged sun exposure. Also include prolonged exposure to other forms of ultraviolet rays from tanning beds and exposure to nonsolar radiation like X-rays
3. Chemical burns – From acids; alkalis like cement and lye; and exposure to other corrosive agents like mustard gas, cresols, phenols, paint thinner and gasoline. These agents can penetrate deep into the layers of skin and cause extensive burns over hours.
4. Electrical burns – Exposure to live wires and consequent electrocution. Electrical burns extend into deeper tissues even in the face of minimum skin injury. Burns can extend to affect muscles, blood vessels and nerves.

Classification of burns

1. First-degree burns – Burns affect only the epidermis.
2. Second-degree burns – Also called partial-thickness burns. These include superficial partial-thickness burns, which involve the epidermis and the superficial dermis. Healing occurs from the epidermal cells in the hair follicles and sweat glands. Deep partial-thickness burns involve the epidermis and deep dermis. Scarring occurs due to extensive fibrosis. Healing starts only from the hair follicles.

3. Third-degree burns – Also called full-thickness burns. Necrosis involves the epidermis, dermis and subcutaneous fat. Healing starts from the periphery of the skin and requires skin grafting for extensive burns.

A. Acute complications – Smoke inhalation, hypovolemia, hypothermia, sepsis, paralytic ileus, compartment syndrome and metabolic derangements.

B. Late-onset complications – contractures and keloids

C. Management

a) Acute resuscitation

b) Clearing and assessing airway, breathing and circulation

c) Removal of burned clothing, exposure of burned skin, decontamination where necessary

d) IV analgesia as needed

e) Fluid resuscitation with Parkland formula

f) Wound cleaning and dressing with appropriate dressing materials

g) Tetanus toxoid injection where necessary

h) Supportive measures for hypothermia, compartment syndrome, nutritional and others

i) Prompt referral to burns center where appropriate.

Chemical exposure

1. Organophosphates

A. Examples – Chlorpyrifos, malathion, parathion, diazinon, Dursban and fenthion.

B. Clinical features – Acute presentations are a result of stimulation of muscarinic receptors: lacrimation, salivation, diarrhea, emesis, bronchospasm, bradycardia, bronchorrhea, miosis, muscle weakness and muscle fasciculations. Late-onset features include weakness of respiratory muscles and axonal neuropathy.

C. Treatment

   a) Acute resuscitation via ABC of resuscitation
   b) Decontamination when necessary
   c) IV atropine for respiratory symptoms
   d) Pralidoxime for neuromuscular symptoms
   e) Benzodiazepine for seizures.

Electrical injuries

1. Causes – Home accidents are not as serious and can be from exposure to naked wires, frayed cords, faulty electrical sockets and electrical appliances. Severe cases result from exposure to high voltages in factories.
2. Clinical features – Burns that may be more extensive than the cutaneous presentation; ventricular fibrillation; seizures; muscle fasciculation; respiratory arrest; cardiac arrest; damage to the central and/or peripheral nervous system; associated injuries like fractures, dislocations, contusions, lacerations; and blunt injuries to internal organs.
3. Treatment
   A. Acute resuscitation via monitoring of airway, breathing and circulation
   B. Fluid resuscitation for severe cases and patients with rhabdomyolysis, acute kidney injury, or shock
   C. Cardiac monitoring
   D. Wound debridement and wound care
   E. Tetanus prophylaxis
   F. Analgesia
   G. Management of associated complications.

Envenomation emergencies

Causes – Snakes, spiders and aquatic organisms.

Snakebites

1. Causes – Mostly rattlesnakes, cottonmouths and copperheads.
2. Clinical features – Anxiety with autonomic features like nausea, vomiting, diaphoresis, diarrhea and tachycardia. Local signs of envenomation are edema, erythema, ecchymoses, lymph node sweeping, oozing or weeping of the wound and formation of bullae. Systemic features of envenomation are diarrhea, confusion, vomiting, dyspnea hypotension, shock and paresthesia. In rattlesnake bites, patients may complain of a metallic taste in their mouth. Envenomation by pit vipers can cause neuromuscular symptoms like muscle weakness and muscle fasciculations. Patients can also present with anaphylaxis and coagulopathy.
3. Treatment
   A. First-aid measures include reassuring the patient. The bitten area should not be suctioned, incised, or cauterized.
   B. Acute resuscitation via maintaining airway, breathing and circulation
   C. Serial assessment of coagulation profile
   D. Clinical observation
   E. Administration of antivenom
   F. Other supportive measures like tetanus toxoid injection and wound dressing.

Submersion injury

1. Risk factors of drowning – African American, Native American, immigrant children from families with low socioeconomic status, males, people with seizure disorders, people with long QT syndrome, people who are intoxicated with alcohol or other substances and people who participate in dangerous underwater breath-holding activities.
2. Pathophysiology – Includes hypoxia, aspiration of fluid and hypothermia.
3. Clinical features – Patients who survive present to the ER with hypothermia, wheezing, altered consciousness and vomiting.
4. Treatment
    A. Acute resuscitation for apneic patients
    B. Supportive management via assisted ventilation, antibiotics, provision of warmth and control of electrolyte derangement.

Temperature-related emergencies

Frostbite

1. Causes – Extreme cold at high altitudes.
2. Clinical features – Freezing and numbing of affected areas. When these areas are warmed, they present with tenderness, edema, erythema and blisters. In severe cases, affected areas become gangrenous and necrotic. Complications are autoamputation, compartment syndrome and neuropathy.
3. Treatment
    A. Acute resuscitation of the patient. This includes assessment and stabilization of airway breathing and circulation.
    B. Provision of warmth
    C. Rewarming of the affected area
    D. Debriding of the wound and wound care

E. Amputation where appropriate.

Heat exhaustion and heatstroke

1. Risk factors – Young athletes, laborers, children locked in parked vehicles and elderly patients.
2. Clinical features – Patients with heat exhaustion experience headaches, nausea, vomiting and syncope. Patients often have tachycardia and hypotension. In heatstroke, patients have altered sensorium, delirium, confusion and ataxia.
3. Treatment
   A. Nursing the patient in a cool environment
   B. Fluid and electrolyte replacement. Patients with heatstroke are managed with rapid-cooling techniques and supportive measures to treat rhabdomyolysis, DIC and acute kidney injury.

Animal bites

Rabies

1. Cause – Infected saliva transmitted through the bites of dogs, bats, skunks, foxes and raccoons.
2. Clinical features – Pain at the bite area, fever, malaise and headaches. Patients with encephalitis experience hallucinations, insomnia, hydrophobia, bizarre behaviors, agitations, excessive salivation and restlessness. Patients can also present with quadriplegia.
3. Treatment – Once rabies sets in, it is fatal. Mortality rates are as high as 90%. Treatment includes supportive management with fluids and sedatives like ketamine and benzodiazepines.

Lyme disease

1. Parasitic infection.
   A. Cause – A tick that transmits Borrelia spp.
   B. Clinical features – Early localized symptoms include the characteristic rash; and erythema migrans, which are seen in more than 75 percent of patients. Early features of dissemination include fever, neck stiffness, headaches, arthralgias, sore throat, nausea, splenomegaly and lymphadenopathy. Late-stage features include arthritis, neuropathies and disorders of mood, memory and sleep.
   C. Treatment – Antibiotic therapy with ceftriaxone, doxycycline and amoxicillin.

Rocky Mountain spotted fever

1. Rickettsia rickettsii
   A. Cause – Transmitted via the bite of the ixodid ticks in mountainous regions.
   B. Clinical features – Severe headaches, severe myalgia, chills, altered consciousness and hyperpyrexia. Patients also have widespread rashes that extend to the soles and palms. These rashes later coalesce into large ecchymosis and then ulcerate.
   C. Treatment – Antibiotic therapy with doxycycline.

B. Toxicology

Acids and alkalis

1. Sources – Toilet cleaners and liquid or solid drain cleaners. Caustic poisoning in children is often accidental ingestion, while in adults it is often intentional.
2. Clinical features – Symptoms of initial poisoning are dysphagia and drooling. In severe poisoning, patients experience vomiting and upper GI bleeding. If the airway is burned, patients present with stridor and cough. Complications like esophageal and gastric perforation are very likely. Esophageal strictures are late-onset complications.
3. Treatment – Treatment is supportive with intravenous fluids and monitoring of metabolic and hematologic profiles. Patients with perforation are managed with IV antibiotics and surgery. Gastric emptying is contraindicated due to the risk of re-exposing the upper GI tract to the agent. The use of activated charcoal is contraindicated due to the risk of disrupting endoscopy. Insertion of gastrointestinal tubes is contraindicated, and so is the use of acids or alkalis to neutralize the agent.

Carbon monoxide

1. Sources – Fumes from automobiles, kerosene heaters, charcoal or wood stoves, water heaters, furnaces and gas heaters.
2. Clinical features – As a result of hypoxia, features include nausea, headaches, dizziness, impaired judgment, inability to concentrate, chest pain and difficulty breathing. In severe poisoning, patients experience seizures and syncope. Death ensues from severe hypoxia.
3. Treatment – Supplemental 100 percent oxygen, or hyperbaric oxygen that displace carbon dioxide from the red blood cells.

Cyanide

1. Sources – Bitter almond oil, poorly processed cassava products, sodium nitroprusside, wild cherry syrup, prussic acid, hydrocyanic acid and potassium cyanide.
2. Clinical features – Drowsiness, headaches, disorientation, dizziness and tachycardia. In severe cases, patients experience hypotension, seizures and coma. The presence of bright red mucosal surfaces requires rapid intervention due to the high risk of mortality. Cyanide is very lethal.
3. Treatment – Supplemental 100% oxygen, use of inhalational amyl nitrate and sodium thiosulfate.

C. Communicable diseases

Clostridium difficile (*C. difficile*)

1. Cause – The most common cause of antibiotic-induced colitis; it is a nosocomial infection of the anaerobe, Clostridium difficile. It is the most common cause of hospital-acquired diarrhea. Risk factors include prolonged hospital admission, elderly patients, neonates and infants, debilitating disease, chronic use of proton pump inhibitors and H2 receptor antagonists and cross infection from health workers. Disruption of the normal microbiota in the gut causes unchecked proliferation of this organism.
2. Clinical features – Gastroenteritis characterized by diarrhea and abdominal cramps. Nausea and vomiting are not common features. The stool may be watery or bloody. Complications are toxic colitis and perforation of the colon.
3. Treatment – Supportive, oral vancomycin, a nonabsorbable antibiotic that exerts direct antibacterial action on the gut. Oral metronidazole is no longer a first-line drug.

Vaccine-preventable diseases

Measles

1. Source – Respiratory droplets infected by a paramyxovirus.
2. Clinical features – Prodromal phase characterized by fever, conjunctivitis, coryza, cough, Koplik's spots and sore throat. The rash appears three to five days after symptom onset, usually one to two days after Koplik's spots appear. It begins on the face in front of and below the ears and on the side of the neck as irregular macules, soon mixed with papules. Within 24 to 48 hours, lesions spread to the trunk and extremities (including the palms and soles) as they begin to fade on the face. Petechiae or ecchymoses may

occur with severe rashes. At the peak stage, the patient experiences hyperpyrexia, photophobia, cough and an extensive rash. Complications include pneumonia, viral encephalitis, hepatitis and acute thrombocytopenic purpura.

3. Treatment – Supportive management of symptoms, which includes antipyretics, intravenous fluids and nutrition. Antibiotics may be used in superimposing bacterial infections.

Mumps

1. Source – Respiratory and aerosolized droplets infected by a paramyxovirus.
2. Clinical features – Headaches, malaise, hyperpyrexia, headaches and bilateral parotitis. Pain is worsened when the patient chews food or takes acidic substances like citrus. The submandibular and submaxillary glands may also be inflamed. Complications include meningitis, pancreatitis, orchitis, or oophoritis.
3. Treatment – Supportive management of symptoms. The child is fed soft semisolid foods. Very hot foods and acidic foods are avoided.

Pertussis

1. Cause – Respiratory droplets and aerosol infected by Bordetella pertussis.
2. Clinical features – Otitis media, pharyngitis, bronchopneumonia, febrile seizures, encephalitis, DIC and spastic paralysis in severe cases.
3. Treatment – Supportive management of symptoms. Antibiotic therapy with erythromycin and azithromycin.

Chicken pox

1. Cause – Via respiratory droplets and aerosols infected with varicella-zoster virus; also via direct contact with skin lesions.
2. Clinical features – Chicken pox is not severe in healthy children. It is, however, severe in adults and immunocompromised children. Symptoms include fever, malaise, headaches in the prodromal phase. It is then followed by macular rashes that erupt in crops. These rashes change from macules to papules and are very pruritic. Papules eventually form crusts. The patient can present with ulcers on the mouth, rectal and vaginal mucosa, conjunctiva and throat. Complications are superseding bacterial infection, pneumonia, hepatitis, myocarditis, encephalitis and coagulopathies. These complications are more likely to occur in immunocompetent adults and immunocompromised children. Reye's syndrome is a fulminant hepatic failure caused by the use of aspirin in children with varicella-zoster.
3. Treatment – Treatment of symptoms, use of antiviral in patients older than 12 years and immunocompromised patients (i.e., symptomatic treatment) and antibiotics for bacterial infections.

Influenza

Influenza is a viral infection that affects the respiratory system. It is known as the flu and there are vaccines available to help prevent one from catching the flu. Symptoms include runny nose, coughing, sneezing, muscle pain, chills and headaches.

Multidrug-resistant organisms

1. Methicillin-resistant Staphylococcus aureus (MRSA) – Becoming increasingly common in hospitals due to antibiotic therapy. These strains

are resistant to beta-lactamase because they secrete penicillinase. MRSA infections are treated with vancomycin, aminoglycosides and rifampin. Other drugs include daptomycin, linezolid, tigecycline and telavancin.

2. Vancomycin-resistant enteritis (VRE) – Caused by Staphylococcus aureus that is resistant to vancomycin. These strains are treated with daptomycin, trimethoprim-sulfamethoxazole, linezolid, tedizolid and others.

Tuberculosis

1. Cause – Aerosols and droplets infected with Mycobacterium tuberculosis, slow-growing aerobic bacilli.
2. Clinical features – Initial symptoms are chronic cough productive of sputum, night sweats and low-grade fever. Other symptoms include anorexia, chest pain, weight loss, fatigue and lymph node swelling. Hemoptysis occurs when cavities extend to the blood vessels.
3. Treatment – Directly observed therapy of two months of induction phase with first-line drugs (rifampicin, isoniazid, pyrazinamide and ethambutol), followed by six months of consolidation phase with second-line drugs (fluoroquinolones and aminoglycosides). Contact tracing.

Hemorrhagic fevers

These fevers can cause serious illness that can result in death. They can break the walls of blood vessels leading to leakages and can also prevent blood from clotting. Even if the bleeding does not cause death, the disease can cause death instead. Examples of such diseases include dengue, lassa, yellow fever and ebola. Symptoms include diarrhea, fever, tiredness, and dizziness. Life-threatning symptoms include coma, liver failure, respiratory failure and kidney failure.

Chapter 10: Professional Issues

There are 14 questions in this section of the exam. Topic areas are:

A. Nurse

Ethical dilemmas

The principles of ethics in clinical practice include:

1. Fidelity – This means confidentiality. In clinical practice, the ethical principle of fidelity means that health workers are expected to keep all health information about their patients private and confidential. This ethical principle is breached when health workers discuss their patients' information with third parties. Events as casual as discussing the health conditions of patients with spouses who are not involved are still a breach of fidelity.
2. Veracity – This means truthfulness. In ethical practice, emergency nurses are expected to provide their patients with all the information needed to give informed consent.
3. Autonomy – This means patients have the final say in the way they receive treatment. The principle of autonomy works with informed consent. Patients must be educated on their condition, as well as the indications of the treatment provided, including side effects and complications. After this information is given, the patients then decide if they want to go on with treatment.
4. Beneficence – This principle means that the health worker is expected to act in the patient's best interest.
5. Nonmaleficence – In this principle, the health worker is expected to not harm a patient, either intentionally or unintentionally. This principle

addresses the issues of negligence, malpractice and other breaches of civil law in medicolegal practice.

6. Justice – This principle means that the health worker is to be fair, impartial and unbiased in the treatment of all patients regardless of their race, religion, tribe, sexual orientation and sex.

Evidence-based practice

This is the use of clinical practices that are based on research evidence, patient values and clinical expertise. Evidence-based practice aims to improve patient outcomes. The steps involved in evidence-based practice include asking valid clinical questions, performing clinical research, evaluating the evidence, incorporating the evidence into clinical practice and evaluating patient outcomes.

Lifelong learning

Continuing education is a requirement for professional practice in emergency nursing. The requirements of continuing education for CEN recertification are discussed in chapter two of this book.

Impaired nurse and drug diversion

Impaired nurses cannot carry out their duties properly. They may become impaired due to substance abuse. Impaired nurses should seek treatment before continuing work. Moreover, if a nurse is found to be diverting drugs or misusing drugs, the regulating bodies of the jurisdiction can take action against the nurse. The nurse may face criminal charges and lose the nursing license that was originally granted by that jurisdiction.

Workplace violence

Workplace violence is defined as violence of any nature that occurs at the workplace including physical, verbal, emotional, psychological or sexual abuse. Workplace environments should be designed to ensure the safety of all healthcare workers. Courses from univerisites and colleges should be taught that provide resources on how to prevent and resolve issues among staff. There can also be technological tools such as panic buttons and alarms that help to keep the workplace safe.

Stress management (burnout, compassion fatigue, PTSD)

Burnout

Nurse burnout occurs when nurses are exhausted from working long hours in a sustained fashion. The pressure from continuous and spontaneous decision making along with the toll that comes from caring for patients can cause burnout. This is a physical, emotional and mental state. The most common causes are lack of sleep and high stress. Treatment requires time off work as there is no other quick solution to burnout.

Compassion fatigue

In nursing, compassion fatigue refers to the fact that a nurse slowly become less compassionate about a patient's medical issues as time goes by. Compassion fatigue occurs because of high stress, low resources and a risk of being abused by patients. The best way to deal with compassion fatigue is to provide yourself with self-care including a healthy diet, exercise and enjoyable hobbies.

PTSD

Critical incident stress management provides psychological help to people who have experienced unexpected and sudden traumatic events. This is done by providing the resources and environment that can facilitate the recovery process of affected individuals, evaluating those who need further therapy, helping affected individuals return to their normal routine and work activities and allowing them to talk about their experiences and explore the feelings that surround the event. Components of CISM include precrisis intervention, community support programs, defusing and critical incident stress debriefing.

Just Culture

Just culture refers to a system in which all staff share accountability for mishaps and mistakes that occur in the workplace. It is a workplace environment that places the onus of accountability on organizations for the systems that are in place for healthcare workers. Organizations are meant to treat employees fairly and justly. Along with this, staff are accountable for the choices they make and for reporting their mistakes. A fair culture ensures that staff are not held accountable for failures over which they had no control to begin with.

B. Patient

Discharge planning

Discharge planning is required to initiate the transition of patient care. Discharge plans are authorized by a physician. It can, however, be created by a nurse, social worker, or caseworker. The components of discharge planning are:

1. Identification – Here, the nurse identifies the patient who is fit for discharge. Identification is done after the physician assesses a patient's clinical state, including vital sign data and response to treatment compared to the goal of treatment.
2. Assessment – In this stage the nurse assesses the patient to identify their needs, which may be simple or complex. These needs can be physical, psychological, financial and psychological. Identifying needs helps the nurse determine the depth of collaboration needed with other health workers inside and outside the ER.
3. Collaboration – The nurse initiates collaboration with the patient, caregivers and other members of the health team and incorporates their recommendations for discharge into the discharge plan.
4. Planning – A discharge plan and summary are written to formally initiate the transition of the patient's care. The discharge plan contains instructions for the patient's care and the discharge summary contains information on the patient's clinical condition during admission, current clinical state (including current vital sign data), current drug prescription, drug and food allergies and other aspects of their clinical history.
5. Patient education – Before the patient is discharged, the nurse must educate them on important information concerning the treatment plan. This includes side effects of drugs, drug interactions, postoperative care instructions, follow-up and more.

End-of-life and Palliative Care

1. Organ and tissue donation – Organ donation is incorporated into end-of-life care. However, emergency nurses and other health workers in the ERs must be trained on how to identify candidates suitable for organ donation and know the different cultural and religious beliefs that influence organ donation.
2. Advance directives – In advance care planning, patients are allowed to make decisions about their health-care management plans in the case of crises. These decisions are often based on the patient's values and discussions with loved ones and caregivers.
   The principles of advanced care planning include education on life-sustaining treatments available, making decisions on the forms of preferential treatment in the event of a life-limiting illness, discussing such plans with loved ones and caregivers and filling out the advanced directives forms. An advanced directive is a written statement of a patient's preferential medical treatment at the end of life.
   It includes a living will, which is a legal document that states the forms of treatment a patient prefers if he or she is no longer able to give consent. These treatment options include resuscitation and other end-of-life treatment. A healthcare proxy or durable power of attorney for healthcare is a document that states the patient's appointed attorney in cases when he or she is unable to give consent. A durable power of attorney doesn't nullify a living will. Medical orders for life-sustaining treatment (MOLST) or Provider Orders for Life-Sustaining Treatment (POLST) are documents that contain the patient's medical orders for end-of-life treatment.
3. Family presence – The nurse should know the importance of family dynamics in patient recovery and must have the ability to cope with stressful conditions. The nurse is also expected to know the religious and

ethnic factors that affect family dynamics. The emergency nurse should also be able to recognize features of caregiver burden.

4. Palliative care – This care is given to end-of-life patients to provide comfort and relieve symptoms and distress in end-of-life patients or patients with an incurable and terminal illness. Relief is offered for physical symptoms (pain, nausea, vomiting, pressure ulcers, constipation and delirium) and psychological symptoms (guilt, depression and suicide). Also, solutions are offered for religious, social and emotional needs.
5. Withholding or withdrawal of life-sustaining care – This is a process in which medical interventions that prolong a patient's life are either removed or withheld with the full knowledge that the patient may die. This directive is always given by a competent patient, advance directives or a surrogate decision-maker. These scenarios are often seen in ICUs where patients are sustained on interventions like ventilators, vasopressors and cardiopulmonary resuscitation.

Forensic evidence collection

1. Chain of custody – A chain of custody ensures that forensic samples are authentic and untampered with during collection, transportation and processing.
2. Chain of custody requires that forensic samples be in the possession of identified and designated individuals at all times. This is made possible by maintaining a chain of documentation.
3. When the sample is passed on to a designated individual, both the sender and recipient of the sample are required to document the exchange.
   A. Important data required include date and time of collection, name of the investigator, location of collection, reason for collection, name of

the owner of the sample, type of sample, identification number of the sample and signatures of both the sender and recipient of the sample.

Pain management and procedural sedation

The severity of pain should be assessed in all patients. Assessment is done by evaluating the patient's feedback, evaluating vital sign data and physiologic features and using pain scales. Some of these pain scales include visual analog, numeric and verbal category. The use of pain scales is based on the patient's cognition and comprehension. Types of drugs used in controlling pain are:

1. Nonopioid analgesics – These include nonsteroidal anti-inflammatory drugs like selective and nonselective COX1 and COX2 inhibitors and acetaminophen. NSAIDs are used for first-line pain relief due to their low risk of addiction. They are, however, unsuitable for controlling severe pain.
2. Opioid analgesics – These drugs bind to opioid receptors in the CNS to produce both analgesia and sedation. These drugs have a high risk for abuse due to tolerance and desensitization. The risk for abuse is higher in pure agonists than in agonist-antagonists. Opioid analgesics are useful in managing severe pain, cancer pain and end-of-life pain. To reduce the risk of addiction and abuse, acute pain is managed with pure agonists with a short duration of action. These drugs are used for a short period. In patients under end-of-life care and palliative care, the risk for addiction is not an immediate concern. Longer-acting opioids are used in combination with adjuvant therapies.
3. Adjuvant drugs – These include antiseizure drugs like gabapentin, carbamazepine and pregabalin; antidepressants like antitricyclic agents and selective serotonin reuptake inhibitors; corticosteroids like dexamethasone; alpha 2 adrenergic agonists like clonidine; muscle

relaxants like baclofen and oral sodium channel blockers; and NMDA receptor antagonists.

4. Neural blockade – This is the process of blocking the transmission of pain signals to the CNS via the use of physical methods or drugs. Local anesthetics like lidocaine are injected intrathecally, epidurally, subcutaneously or intrapleurally. This method is used for patients with postoperative pain and patients with localized pain and short life expectancy. Neuro ablation, which is the physical and permanent destruction of pain fibers, is rarely used.
5. Neuromodulation – This is the electrical stimulation of nerves to stimulate endogenous pain modulation. This method is used in patients with neuropathic pain.

Patient safety

The emergency nurse is expected to uphold the ethical principles of beneficence and nonmaleficence to ensure the patient's safety. This is done by following best practices in providing nursing care.

Patient satisfaction

Communication promotes patient satisfaction. The principles of ethics in clinical practice ensure that patients are satisfied with the clinical care they receive.

Transfer and stabilization

The following are required in order to safely transfer patients from one point to the other:

1. Proper communication and collaboration with all members of the managing team. This also includes corroboration with the team about to receive the patient.

2. Proper documentation of the patient's clinical condition.
3. Stabilization of patients before they are transferred. This is done by monitoring and stabilizing a patient's vital signs before and during the transfer.
4. Proper mode of transfer. This is often the fastest and safest mode of transferring the patient inside or outside the hospital.

Transition of care

1. Handoff – This includes both internal handoffs within a facility and external handoffs from one facility to the other. Handoffs are required to transmit a patient's health information, transfer the responsibility of caring for a patient and provide patient safety and continuity of care.
2. Patient boarding – This is the practice of keeping patients on stretchers and boards in the ER for hours or days due to lack of bed space in the ER. A primary cause of this phenomenon in ERs is the presentation of subacute cases to the ER due to an insufficient number of primary health-care providers and long waiting times in consulting with PCPs. Because the law requires that all patients who present to the ER be attended to and stabilized, patient boarding persists.

   The effects of patient boarding

   A. Increased traffic also increases the risk of sepsis via aerosolized, respiratory and contact routes of spread
   B. Delayed attention to emergent and urgent patients
   C. Burnout of health workers
   D. Increased risk of assault of health workers
   E. Delayed turnover of radiological reports
   F. Reduced patient satisfaction

G. Increased risk of medication errors
H. Reduced profits for hospitals that must care for all patients who present to the ER.

3. Shift reporting – This involves educating nurses and medical staff who have taken over management of a patient on the patient's health information and previous management plan. This is necessary for continuity of care.

Cultural considerations

The emergency nurse must be aware of the cultural values that affect the patient's acceptance or refusal of care. Some cultural considerations in health care include:

A. Cultural imposition – This occurs when a health worker imposes his or her cultural values on a patient.
B. Cultural stereotyping – This occurs when a health worker generalizes patients based on their cultural background. This may seem similar to cultural awareness, but cultural stereotyping often operates on bias and prejudice.
C. Cultural blindness – This occurs when a health worker treats all patients the same way regardless of their cultural differences.
D. Cultural awareness – This is sensitivity and acceptance of the cultures of all patients.

Abuse and neglect

1. Abuse – This can be physical, emotional, sexual or medical (Munchausen by proxy).
2. Neglect – This is the failure to meet the basic physical, emotional, educational and medical needs of a dependent. Neglect can be physical, emotional, medical or educational.

3. Self-harm – This is an intentional injury of one's own body, without the intention of causing suicide. Risk factors for self-harm include substance abuse, psychotic illness, bipolar disorder, anxiety disorder and others.

Human Trafficking

Human trafficking affects the healthcare sector in a variety of ways. Most victims of human trafficking are women and children. They may present to the hospital with infections or diseases. Most common diseases include STIs, anxiety, physical injuries, PTSD, suicidal ideation, malnutiriton, depression and various other illnesses.

Victims of human trafficking usually fear authorities and are scared to disclose their situation. Since many of the victims may not speak English well, there may be a need to get an interpreter. The nurse should pay attention to subtle clues since the victims will most likely hide the fact that they are victims.

Gender equity (e.g. inclusion, gender transition)

Gender inclusion

Gender inclusion means using language that does not discriminate against any specific sex, gender identity or social gender. Using gender-inclusive language is a powerful way to promote gender equality amongst patients and staff.

Gender transition

Gender transition refers to the process of altering appearance and how one sees their own gender internally. The goal is to become the gender one feels on the inside.

C. System

Delegation of tasks to assistive personnel

As a registered nurse, the CEN is expected to delegate duties to the nursing assistant and licensed practical nurse based on their scope of practice.

Duties of a nursing assistant

A. Take patients' vital signs
B. Assist patients in feeding, bathing, dressing and positioning
C. Set up medical equipment
D. Assist in nursing procedures
E. Answer patients' calls for help
F. Keep patients' environment clean.

Duties of a licensed practical nurse

A. Measure, record and report patients' vital signs data to the registered nurse
B. Document patients' medical history
C. Assist in giving certain oral medications under supervision
D. Collect samples under supervision
E. Assist patients in dressing, feeding and positioning
F. Monitor and report patients' condition to the registered nurse.

Disaster management

This includes employing the principles of preparedness, mitigation, response and recovery from natural and man-made disasters.

Mass Casualty

Mass casualty refers to an incident or affliction (such as a pandemic or natural disaster) that limits the capacity of a healthcare facility to provide adequate care to its patients. Normal operations may be disrupted and nurses may have to make critical decisions that they would not normally make. Patients may have to be selected and organized based on the seriousness of illness and urgency of care that would be needed per patient.

Federal regulations

1. HIPAA – The Health Insurance Portability Accountability Act regulates the use and transmission of a patient's health information used by covered entities. These covered entities are:

A. Health plans, like HMOs, company health plans, health insurance companies and government insurance plans like Medicare and Medicaid.
B. Health care providers – All health workers and health facilities.
C. Health care clearinghouses – These are organizations that process health information from nonstandardized formats to standardized formats.
D. Business associates of covered entities – Billing companies, companies that provide health care plans, companies that store health information, accountants, lawyers and IT personnel dealing with health care.

Organizations that have a right to an individual's health information are employers, life insurers, law enforcement agencies, schools, state agencies and municipal offices. The forms of health information that are protected include medical records, medical conversations, health billing information and health information given to insurance companies.

2. EMTALA – The Emergency Medical Treatment and Labor Act requires that all patients who present to the ER be treated, stabilized and referred regardless of their insurance or ability to pay. The three obligations of EMTALA are:

A. Medical screening for all individuals who present to the ER. This screening is done to determine if the individual has an emergency condition. Screening must not be delayed to assess the individual's insurance or ability to pay for treatment. Emergency rooms are mandated to post signs that inform patients of their right to medical screening.
B. Provision of resuscitation and stabilization to patients who are diagnosed with an emergency. Hospitals that do not have the needed resources to attend to the emergency must transfer the patient to the appropriate facility according to the provisions set by EMTALA.
C. Hospitals with emergency provisions must receive patient transfers from hospitals without the resources to attend to patients with emergencies.

Patient consent for treatment

1. Disclosure of information – The patient must be educated on the facts of the procedures, the implication of accepting/declining, the possible alternatives and the implication and consequences of these alternatives. After education, the CEN must make sure that the patient demonstrates a full understanding of the disclosure by asking questions to test recall and understanding.
2. Competency of the patient or surrogate to make a decision – Competency means the patient's ability to make decisions. For patients to be competent, they must understand the disclosed information, including its processes, implications and side effects. The patient must also be able to demonstrate an understanding of the implications of refusal of treatment and the process, including the implications and side effects of other available options.

3. Voluntariness – Patients must be able to decide on medical treatment without duress and should also be made aware of their right to refuse or accept treatment.
4. Documentation – Informed consent is obtained in a written form for medical and legal reasons. The written document must contain an explanation of the medical condition that justifies the medical treatment; an explanation of the benefits of the medical treatment, including its complication and adverse effects; an explanation of the available alternative treatments and an explanation of the consequences of not accepting the test. The consent form should be signed by both the health worker and the patient/surrogate.

Performance and process improvement

Performance improvement

This is the act of improving patient outcomes and ensuring patient safety to reduce the cost of providing care and risks of liability. Performance improvement activities are regulated by bodies like the Joint Commission on the Accreditation of Healthcare Organizations (JCAHO), the state department of health and the Centers for Medicare & Medicaid Services. Activities include identifying opportunities for improvement, organizing groups for assessing current practices, collecting and analysis of empirical data and implementation of evidence-based practices.

Process improvement

Processes are continuosly revised to enhance the quality of healthcare while reducing costs. Some of the processes include hospital admissions, billing, patient transfers and patient discharges. The goal is to save time and also to reduce costs while providing optimal healthcare.

Risk management

There are three types of transmission-based precautions: contact precaution, droplet precaution and airborne precaution.

Symptom surveillance

1. Recognizing symptom clusters – This is required for the prompt report of diseases that ought to be reported to the authorized bodies. Symptom surveillance is required for reporting infectious diseases that can lead to outbreaks and epidemics, chronic diseases and their complications, mass casualties from natural or man-made disasters and environmental conditions. Symptoms clusters are used to alert the authorized bodies before a diagnosis is confirmed.
2. Mandatory reporting of diseases – This includes mandatory reporting of diseases classified as notifiable diseases that have an impact on public health. This report allows health authorities to identify disease trends and outbreaks and help prevent them in the future.
3. Triage – This is the evaluation and categorization of patients involved in mass casualties. Triage is used to prioritize care to patients who have the most need for it and to use limited resources in attending to such patients. The Simple Triage and Rapid Treatment (START) form of triage quickly assesses patients based on consciousness, respiration and circulation into four categories:
    A. Red labels (immediate) – These patients require immediate treatment for survival. They are prioritized above other patients.

B. Yellow labels (urgent) – These patients' treatment can be delayed for observation because their conditions do not put them at immediate mortality risk. In normal circumstances, these patients ought to be quickly treated.
C. Green labels (delayed) – These patients have minor injuries that do not require urgent interventions. Management of these patients can be delayed until patients in the above categories are stabilized.
D. Blue labels (expectant) – These patients require interventions that are beyond the provision of the hospital for survival. In these patients, life support is of no benefit.
E. Black labels (dead) – Patients in cardiopulmonary failure for which resuscitation will not be given.

Test 1: Questions

1. A patient with a peritonsillar abscess is likely to have which of these?

   A. Stridor
   B. Wheezing
   C. Whooping cough
   D. Hot potato voice

2. A patient who presents to the ER with anterior epistaxis secondary to drying of the mucosa from extreme weather is being managed with silver nitrate. Which of these best describes the action of silver nitrate?

   A. Anesthesia
   B. Vasoconstriction
   C. Lubrication
   D. Cauterization

3. A patient who presents to the ER with acute kidney injury is placed on a low-potassium diet. Which of these is most appropriate?

   A. Bone broth
   B. A cup of bananas
   C. Baked potatoes
   D. Pasta

4. A patient is being managed with streptokinase for deep vein thrombosis. The nurse is expected to monitor which of the following?

A. Urine volume
B. Urine color
C. Blood pressure
D. Skin turgidity

5. Which of the following is a discrete variable?

A. Number of neonates in the NICU
B. Occipitofrontal circumference
C. Height
D. Weight

6. Which of the following is not a risk factor for epistaxis?

A. Hypertension
B. Drug abuse
C. Foreign bodies
D. Autoimmune response

7. A 55-year-old hypertensive male is being managed in the ER for NSTEMI. Which of the following treatment modalities is inappropriate for this patient?

A. Angiography
B. Fibrinolytic therapy
C. ACE inhibitors
D. Morphine

8. A 56-year-old hypertensive male is being managed for STEMI secondary to atherosclerosis. Which of the following eliminates the need for thrombolytic therapy?

A. Previous history of myocardial infarction
B. Available PCI
C. Recent aspirin use
D. The onset of symptoms 12 hours before arrival

9. A 57-year-old female presents to the ER with diaphoresis, shortness of breath and crushing chest pain. A diagnosis of acute coronary syndrome is made. Which of the following is not a component of care given before diagnosis is confirmed?

A. Oxygen therapy
B. Nitrates
C. Beta-blockers
D. Angiography

10. Which of the following is most appropriate for a 46-year-old male who is being managed for uncomplicated NSTEMI?

A. Emergency angiography
B. Fibrinolytic therapy
C. Beta-blockers
D. CABG

11. A 57-year-old male is being managed in the ER for unstable angina. Which of the following is not a presentation of this condition?

A. Angina at rest
B. New-onset angina
C. Progressive angina
D. ST elevation

12. Which of the following patients is least at risk of aspiration?

A. A 56-year-old male with status epilepticus
B. A 36-year-old female with myasthenia gravis
C. A 23-year-old male with upper GI bleeding
D. A 45-year-old male with chronic bronchitis

13. Which of the following modalities is not useful in reducing the risk of aspiration in a 45-year-old male who presents to the ER with altered consciousness secondary to opioid overdose?

A. Semi-Fowler's position
B. Parenteral nutrition
C. IV drugs and fluids
D. Endotracheal tube

14. Which of the following antibiotics is most suitable for use in treating a 45-year-old male who is being managed in the ER for aspiration pneumonitis secondary to opioid overdose?

A. Clindamycin
B. Doxycycline
C. Erythromycin
D. Streptomycin

15. Which of the following treatment modalities is not indicated in managing a four-year-old male who ingested paint thinner an hour before presentation?

A. Gastric lavage
B. Oxygen supplementation
C. IV fluids
D. Vital sign monitoring

16. Which of the following investigations is not required in diagnosing myasthenia gravis in a 35-year-old female who presents to the ER with diplopia, ptosis and weakness of the distal muscles?

A. Electromyography
B. CT of the thorax
C. Serum AchR antibodies
D. Ice pack test

17. A patient who presents to the ER with ptosis, dysphagia and diplopia is being managed with pyridostigmine for myasthenia gravis. The patient should be informed of which of the following side effects?

A. Diarrhea
B. Tachycardia
C. Urinary retention
D. Conjunctivitis

18. Which of the following investigations is most appropriate in diagnosing multiple sclerosis?

A. Electromyography
B. MRI
C. CT scan
D. CSF analysis

19. A 15-year-old male with multiple sclerosis is being managed in the ER with Baclofen. This drug provides relief from which of the following symptoms?

A. Paresthesia
B. Confusion
C. Spasticity
D. Urinary incontinence

20. Which of the following is used in assessing the facial nerve in a 56-year-old male who presents to the ER with Bell's palsy?

A. Blowing of the cheeks
B. Raising of the shoulders
C. Jaw jerk
D. Grinding the teeth

21. A patient who presents to the ER with a cerebrovascular accident has a positive Romberg's test. Which of the following is not assessed by Romberg's test?

A. Proprioception
B. Coordination
C. Vestibular function
D. Attention

22. Which of the following is not a cause of flaccid paralysis?

A. Myasthenia gravis
B. Poliomyelitis
C. Guillain-Barré
D. Multiple sclerosis

23. A five-year-old male presents to the ER with a history of salicylate poisoning. To alkalinize the urine, the nurse is expected to do which of the following?

A. Give 1 L of sodium chloride in 30 minutes.
B. Give IV $NaHCO_3$ 1–2 mEq/kg as a bolus injection.
C. Give dextrose potassium insulin infusion.
D. Give IV furosemide.

24. Which of the following clinical features excludes delirium from dementia?

A. Sudden onset
B. Age
C. Sex
D. Orientation

25. Which of the following describes an inability to identify objects despite having normal sensory function?

A. Agnosia
B. Apraxia
C. Aphasia
D. Akinesia

26. A 56-year-old male with Parkinson's disease is unable to move his lower limbs against gravity. What grade of power is this?

A. Grade 1
B. Grade 2
C. Grade 3
D. Grade 4

27. A 55-year-old female with Alzheimer's disease is being managed in the ER with acute pyelonephritis. Part of her treatment plan includes donepezil. Which of the following best describes the mechanism of action of this drug?

A. NMDA antagonist
B. Selective serotonin reuptake inhibitor
C. Acetylcholine receptor blocker
D. Cholinesterase inhibitor

28. A 65-year-old female who presents to the ER with Parkinson's disease is being managed with amantadine. Which of the following best describes the mechanism of action of this drug?

A. Dopamine receptor agonist
B. Acetylcholinesterase inhibitor
C. NMDA receptor antagonist
D. MAO-B inhibitor

29. Which of the following is not seen in acute appendicitis?

A. Rebound tenderness
B. Rovsing's sign
C. Cullen's sign
D. Obturator sign

30. Which of the following is most necessary in making a diagnosis of acute appendicitis?

A. Abdominal ultrasound scan
B. Clinical evaluation
C. CT scan of the abdomen
D. Abdominal X-ray

31. Which of the following is not a cause of lower GI bleeding?

A. Peptic ulcer disease
B. Colorectal cancer
C. Anorectal fistula
D. Hemorrhoids

32. Which of the following is not a stigmata of chronic liver disease?

A. Testicular atrophy
B. Finger clubbing
C. Lanugo hair
D. Acanthosis nigricans

33. A 25-year-old female who presents to the ER with abdominal pain, fever, chills and vomiting demonstrates a positive Murphy's sign. Which of the following maneuvers best elicit this sign?

A. Palpation of the epigastric region on deep inspiration
B. Palpation of the right hypochondrium on deep inspiration
C. Auscultation of the right hypochondrium
D. Percussion of the right hypochondrium

34. Which of the following is not a therapeutic function of IV theophylline administered to a 22-year-old female being managed for severe acute asthma?

A. Bronchodilation
B. Leukotriene inhibitor
C. Increased heart rate
D. Immunosuppression

35. A 16-year-old female who is being managed for severe acute asthma has worsened symptoms despite management with supplemental oxygen, IV epinephrine, corticosteroids and nebulized albuterol. Arterial blood gases show PaCo2 62 mmHg. Which of the following interventions is most appropriate?

A. IV theophylline
B. NIPPV
C. Mechanical ventilation
D. IV diazepam

36. Which of the following treatments is inappropriate in a five-year-old asthmatic male who presents to the ER with cough, wheezing, breathlessness and chest pain?

A. Nebulized albuterol
B. Subcutaneous epinephrine
C. IV hydrocortisone
D. IV amoxicillin

37. Which of the following is not a differential of wheezing in a two-year-old child?

A. Asthma
B. Foreign body aspiration
C. Heart failure
D. Bronchitis

38. As part of the discharge requirements for a six-year-old female admitted 24 hours ago with acute asthma, the attending physician prescribes omalizumab. Which of the following best describes the mechanism of action of this drug?

A. Leukotriene receptor antagonist
B. Mast cell stabilizer
C. Cyclooxygenase inhibitor
D. Mucus plug degradation

39. Which of the following histories is most important to obtain from a 45-year-old female who presents to the ER with a history of chronic productive cough of three months duration, pedal edema and hypertension?

A. Family history of hypertension
B. Contact with someone with a recent cough
C. Cigarette smoking
D. IV drug abuse

40. Which of the following drugs should be administered first to a patient who presents to the ER with diarrhea, wheezing, shortness of breath and hypotension following ingestion of seafood?

A. Diphenhydramine
B. Epinephrine
C. Albuterol
D. Hydrocortisone

41. Which of the following features is most appropriate in distinguishing diverticulitis from appendicitis?

A. Right suprapubic pain
B. Rebound tenderness
C. Vomiting
D. Palpable sigmoid

42. A 46-year-old male who is being managed for renal calculi is treated with hydrochlorothiazide. Which of the following best explains the mechanism of action of this drug in this patient's condition?

A. Dissolution of calculi
B. Alkalinization of urine
C. Lowers excretion of calcium
D. Muscle relaxant

43. A 35-year-old male who presents to the ER with upper GI bleeding secondary to GERD is set to be discharged to his primary care physician. Part of his discharge requirements include aluminum hydroxide. The patient should be warned of which of the following potential side effects?

A. Diarrhea
B. Constipation
C. Drowsiness
D. Rashes

44. Which of the following best describes Barrett's esophagus?

A. Hypertrophy of the esophageal mucosa
B. Atrophy of the esophageal mucosa
C. Metaplasia of the esophageal mucosa
D. Atrophy of the gastric mucosa

45. Which of the following is not a cause of erosive gastritis?

A. NSAID
B. H. pylori
C. Cytomegalovirus
D. Alcohol

46. A nurse is monitoring the vital signs of a gravid patient being managed with magnesium sulfate for severe eclampsia. The nurse assesses the patient's patellar reflex and records it as 2+. Which of the following best describes this grade?

A. Diminished reflex
B. Normal reflex
C. Brisk reflex
D. Hyperactive reflex

47. Which of the following is not an expected presentation in a 55-year-old male who is being managed for aortic dissection?

A. Chest pain
B. Syncope
C. Heart murmurs
D. Collapsing pulse

48. A 56-year-old male who presents to the ER with tearing chest pain, hypertension and aortic regurgitation is being managed for aortic dissection. Which of the following drugs is the first-line treatment of hypertension in this patient?

A. Beta-blockers
B. Calcium channel blockers
C. ACEI inhibitors
D. Nitrates

49. A 55-year-old male who is being managed for aortic dissection has an underlying pathology in which of the following parts of the blood vessel?

A. Tunica intima
B. Tunica media
C. Tunica adventitia
D. Tunica serosa

50. You are to commence CPR on a 45-year-old female who is being managed for an opioid overdose. Which of the following is most useful in signaling an appropriate positioning of the patient's airway?

A. External auditory meatus in the same plane as the sternum
B. Head flat on the stretcher
C. Head tilt position
D. The rami of the mandible pointing downward

51. A patient who was managed for trichomoniasis is about to be discharged on oral metronidazole. Which of the following statements is accurate when educating the patient on the use of the medication?

A. It should be taken with orange juice to increase absorption.
B. It should not be taken with alcohol.
C. It should be taken on an empty stomach.
D. It should be taken with fatty foods.

52. A patient with cystic fibrosis is treated in the ER with nebulized hypertonic saline. Which of the following best describes the rationale behind this treatment?

A. Bronchodilation
B. Mucus thinner
C. Cough suppressant
D. Vasodilation

53. A patient is being managed with a continuous infusion of epinephrine for anaphylaxis and angioedema. The attending nurse is expected to monitor the patient for all of the following side effects except?

A. Pulmonary edema
B. Hypertension
C. Tachycardia
D. Hypoglycemia

54. Which of the following is not an immediate concern in a patient who presents to the ER with full-thickness burns secondary to a fire incident?

A. Dehydration
B. Eschar
C. Contractures
D. Hypothermia

55. Part of the initial management of a patient with third-degree burns is IV cimetidine. This drug is useful in preventing which of the following?

A. Nausea
B. Stress ulcers
C. Diarrhea
D. Anxiety

56. Which of the following is not a clinical feature of organophosphate poisoning?

A. Lacrimation
B. Diarrhea
C. Mydriasis
D. Urinary frequency

57. A patient with organophosphate poisoning is being managed with IV pralidoxime. Which of the following symptoms is best treated with pralidoxime?

A. Seizures
B. Muscle fasciculations
C. Nausea
D. Lacrimation

58. Which of the following is not a complication of electrical injury?

A. Hemolysis
B. Burns
C. Compartment syndrome
D. Distal leg paresis

59. Which of the following is not a component of critical incident stress management?

A. Defusing
B. Debriefing
C. Psychoanalysis
D. Follow-up

60. Which of the following is not a purpose of critical incident stress management?

A. Helping patients cope with depressive disorders
B. Reducing the risk of post-traumatic stress disorder
C. Offering psychological first aid
D. Helping patients cope with trauma

61. Which of the following is not an example of a critical incident?

A. Work-related death
B. Suicide of a coworker
C. Assault
D. Stage IV colorectal cancer

62. Critical incident stress management should be managed by which of the following?

A. Physician
B. Emergency nurse
C. Psychologist
D. None of the above

63. A patient's right to refuse treatment is supported by which of the following principles of ethics?

A. Beneficence
B. Veracity
C. Autonomy
D. Privacy

64. Which of the following is necessary for confirming a diagnosis of variant angina in a 45-year-old female with a history of nocturnal chest pain?

A. Exercise test
B. Provocative test
C. Chest X-ray
D. Echocardiography

65. A 56-year-old female who presents with diaphoresis, crushing chest pain and breathlessness was given sublingual nitroglycerin for acute myocardial infarction. Which of the following is not a mechanism of action of nitroglycerin in this patient?

A. Reduces preload
B. Reduces afterload
C. Arterial dilatation
D. Reduces heart rate

66. Which of the following is not an immediate concern in a 56-year-old male currently being managed for an abdominal aortic aneurysm?

A. Hypovolemic shock
B. Disseminated intravascular coagulation
C. Acute peripheral arterial occlusion
D. Pulmonary embolism

67. Which of the following radiologic investigations is most suitable in a 75-year-old female with a suspected rupture of an abdominal aortic aneurysm?

A. CT angiography
B. Magnetic resonance angiography
C. Abdominal ultrasonography
D. Plain abdominal X-rays

68. A 65-year-old male is being booked for an emergency repair of an abdominal aortic aneurysm. Which of the following is the patient most at risk of having in the early postoperative phase?

A. Hemorrhagic shock
B. Myocardial infarction
C. Acute kidney injury
D. Erectile dysfunction

69. Which of the following is not a risk factor of aortic dissection?

A. Hypertension
B. Black race
C. Female sex
D. Elderly age

70. Which of the following is an indication of gastric lavage?

A. Ingested hydrocarbons
B. Drugs that are absorbed by activated charcoal
C. Heavy metal poisoning
D. Short duration of ingestion of toxic material

71. Which of the following is not a cause of deviation of the QRS complex to an angle that is more than +90°?

A. Right ventricular hypertrophy
B. Hyperkalemia
C. Left ventricular hypertrophy
D. Chronic bronchitis

72. A six-year-old male who presents to the ER with cough, wheezing and chest tightness is being managed for an acute asthmatic attack. Which of the following clinical signs will alert the attending nurse to worsening symptoms?

A. Crackles
B. Silent chest
C. Tachypnea
D. Fever

73. A 56-year-old female who presents to the ER with severe anemia is being managed for atrophic gastritis. Her management plan will include foods rich in which of the following?

A. Legumes
B. Cabbage
C. Red meat
D. Fat

74. A 15-year-old male who presents to the ER with sickle cell crisis is being managed with hydroxyurea. Which of the following best explains the mechanism of action of this drug?

A. Stimulates vasodilation
B. Controls pain
C. Increases HbF
D. Increases oxidation

75. Which of the following clinical features is unlikely to be seen in a 25-year-old sickle cell patient with vaso occlusive crisis?

A. Jaundice

B. Hepatosplenomegaly

C. Pallor

D. Fever

76. A 68-year-old male presents with widespread petechiae rashes and decompensated liver failure. Which of the following is not a pathophysiology of this patient's bleeding condition?

A. Vitamin K deficiency

B. Thrombocytopenia

C. Elevated liver enzymes

D. Hypofibrinogenemia

77. A patient with DIC is being managed with cryoprecipitate. Which of the following substrates is provided by cryoprecipitate?

A. Fibrinogen

B. Thrombin

C. Plasminogen

D. Platelets

78. Which of the following is responsible for initiating the clotting cascade in DIC?

A. Thrombin

B. Tissue factor

C. Calcium

D. Vitamin K

79. A five-year-old male who presents to the ER with an acute exacerbation of asthma is being managed with nebulized ipratropium. Which of the following best describes the mechanism of action of this drug?

A. Muscarinic receptor blocker
B. Nicotinic receptor blocker
C. Beta receptor agonist
D. Beta receptor blocker

80. Which of the following is not a pathophysiologic process involved in Alzheimer's disease?

A. Short-term memory loss
B. Visuospatial dysfunction
C. Impaired consciousness
D. Poor judgment

81. Which of the following drugs is not useful in the management of trigeminal neuralgia?

A. Carbamazepine
B. Gabapentin
C. Baclofen
D. Acetaminophen

82. Which of the following treatments is contraindicated in a patient with traumatic rupture of the eardrums?

A. Aural irrigation
B. Oral antibiotics
C. Topical antibiotics
D. Oral analgesia

83. Which of the following is not a clinical feature of Ludwig's angina?

A. Tenderness
B. Abscess
C. Induration
D. Drooling

84. A patient with Ménière's disease will benefit from a diet low in which of the following?

A. Sodium
B. Potassium
C. Protein
D. Calcium

85. Which of the following is not a clinical feature of Ménière's disease?

A. Tinnitus
B. Vertigo
C. Sensorineural deafness
D. Nystagmus

86. Which of the following drugs is not implicated in ototoxicity?

A. Gentamicin
B. Furosemide
C. Vancomycin
D. Tetracycline

87. The pain in trigeminal neuralgia is often described as:

A. Persistent
B. Paroxysmal
C. Nocturnal
D. Throbbing

88. A patient who has just had a reduction of his dislocated mandible will be counseled on doing which of the following?

A. Avoiding hot foods
B. Eating only semisolids for three weeks
C. Cutting food into smaller pieces before chewing
D. Gargling with warm saline water

89. Which of the following measures is not useful in managing myoglobinuria in a patient with electrical injuries?

A. Alkalinization of urine
B. Surgical debridement
C. IV fluids
D. Allopurinol

90. Which of the following first aid interventions is inappropriate in a patient who is suffering from a snakebite?

A. Establishing IV access
B. Securing the airway
C. Applying a tourniquet
D. Reassuring the patient

91. Which of the following ethnic groups in the United States is least at risk of drowning?

A. African American
B. Asian American
C. Native American
D. North American

92. Which of the following measures is not appropriate in providing a safe and secure environment for a patient with Alzheimer's disease?

A. A bright, familiar environment
B. New stimulation
C. Regular exercise
D. Frequent orientation

93. Which of the following is not a feature of myasthenic crisis?

A. Lacrimation
B. Tachypnea
C. Muscle weakness
D. Diplopia

94. Which of the following is the most common cause of cholecystitis?

A. Septicemia
B. Cholelithiasis
C. Drugs
D. Liver flukes

95. A 56-year-old male who presents to the ER with altered consciousness, jaundice and ascites is managed for hepatic encephalopathy secondary to alcoholic liver disease. His treatment management includes lactulose. The therapeutic action of lactulose is seen in which of the following organs?

A. Liver

B. Colon

C. Brain

D. Gallbladder

96. Which of the following treatment modalities is contraindicated in a patient with hepatic encephalopathy?

A. Low-protein diet

B. Motility agents

C. Sedatives

D. Antibiotics

97. A 56-year-old male who presents to the ER with upper GI bleeding secondary to ruptured esophageal varices is administered octreotide. Which of the following best describes the mechanism of action of this drug?

A. Inhibition of glucagon

B. Vasoconstriction

C. Platelet aggregation

D. Antimotility agent

98. Which of the following procedures is most suitable for use in a 56-year-old male with ruptured esophageal varices and persistent upper GI bleeding despite interventions with IV octreotide and endoscopic banding?

A. Liver transplantation
B. TIPS procedure
C. Sengstaken-Blakemore tube
D. IV vasopressin

99. A patient is being managed in the ER for acute watery diarrhea secondary to norovirus infection. Which of the following measures is not useful in reducing the risk of spread?

A. Handwashing
B. Sterile gloves
C. Isolation
D. Disinfection of surfaces

100. Nurse E tells a patient that she cannot return if she is discharged against medical advice. Nurse E has demonstrated which of the following?

A. Fraud
B. Battery
C. Malpractice
D. False imprisonment

101. Which of the following is not a component of malpractice?

A. Breach of duty
B. Effect
C. Causation
D. Damages

102. Which of the following is not a characteristic of a qualitative research method?

A. Use of open-ended questions
B. Use of structured questionnaires
C. Aims to describe data
D. Use of a small sample size

103. Which of the following is not an objective of quantitative research?

A. Testing cause and effect
B. Testing a hypothesis
C. Interpreting social interactions
D. Explaining a phenomenon

104. Nurse M believes that taking out alternate stitches on the first day of the postoperative period encourages rapid wound healing. To prove this to the team, Nurse E will obtain information from which of the following?

A. Case notes
B. Patients' reports
C. Clinical journals
D. Nurses' reports

105. A four-year-old male who is being managed in the ER with prolonged bleeding secondary to hemophilia will be managed with which of the following blood products?

A. Red blood cells
B. Platelets
C. Fresh frozen plasma
D. Whole blood

106. A patient is being managed with heparin. The nurse has the antidote, protamine sulfate, in the drug tray in case of emergencies. Which of the following best describes the mechanism of action of this drug?

A. Receptor blocker
B. Heparin degradation
C. Heparin binder
D. Heparin excretion

107. A 56-year-old female with atrial fibrillation is being managed with warfarin. Her INR is 4.5. Which of the following responses is most appropriate?

A. Withhold the next dose of warfarin
B. Reduce the next dose of warfarin by half
C. Continue with the next dose of warfarin
D. Give protamine sulfate

108. Which of the following methods is most effective in controlling posterior epistaxis?

A. Nasal balloons
B. Pinching the alae of the nose together
C. Electrocauterization
D. Topical lidocaine

109. A patient with trigeminal neuralgia is unlikely to experience increased pain when performing which of the following activities?

A. Chewing
B. Brushing teeth
C. Smiling
D. Swallowing

110. Which of the following is a side effect expected to be seen in a patient given Fab antivenom?

A. Anorexia
B. Serum sickness
C. Redman syndrome
D. Postural hypotension

111. Which of the following organisms is most implicated in food poisoning?

A. Staphylococcus aureus
B. Escherichia coli
C. Clostridium perfringens
D. Vibrio cholera

112. Which of the following treatment modalities is not useful in managing acute food poisoning caused by Clostridium perfringens?

A. IV fluids
B. Antiemetics
C. Oral metronidazole
D. Bed rest

113. A patient with intense pruritus secondary to obstructive jaundice is being managed with cholestyramine. Which of the following best explains the mechanism of action of this drug?

A. Histamine receptor blocker
B. Relaxation of the neck of the gallbladder
C. Bile acid sequestrant
D. HMG CoA reductase inhibitor

114. Which of the following treatment modalities is unnecessary in a patient being managed for acute hepatitis A infection?

A. Ribavirin
B. IV fluids
C. Cholestyramine
D. Antipyretics

115. Which of the following microorganisms is implicated in hemolytic uremic syndrome?

A. Campylobacter jejuni
B. Vibrio cholerae
C. Escherichia coli
D. Entamoeba histolytica

116. Which of the following treatment modalities is contraindicated in managing a 15-month-old female who presents to the ER with acute watery diarrhea secondary to rotavirus infection?

A. IV crystalloids
B. Loperamide
C. Ondansetron
D. Zinc

117. Which of the following statements is false about a direct inguinal hernia?

A. It does not pass through the inguinal canal.
B. It is more likely to herniate into the scrotum.
C. It can be manually reduced.
D. It can be elicited by a cough impulse.

118. A 56-year-old male with a strangulated inguinal hernia is at risk of all of the following except:

A. Intestinal obstruction
B. Peritonitis
C. Hemorrhage
D. Shock

119. Which of the following is not used in differentiating Crohn's disease from ulcerative colitis?

A. The small bowel is mostly affected.
B. Rectal bleeding is present.
C. The right colon is most affected.
D. A fistula is a common complication.

120. Which of the following is not a route of transmission of giardiasis?

A. Waterborne
B. Sexual contact
C. Foodborne
D. Respiratory droplet

121. You are inserting a nasopharyngeal airway in a 45-year-old being managed for ventilatory failure. Which of the following is used in measuring the appropriate length of tubing to be used in this patient?

A. Distance from the tip of the nose to the tragus of the ear
B. Distance from the tip of the nose to the ramus of the mandible
C. Distance from the tip of the nose to the sternal notch
D. Distance from the tip of the nose to the xiphisternum

122. You are inserting an oropharyngeal airway in a conscious 19-year-old male. Which of the following steps is incorrect?

A. Clearing the oropharynx of secretions and vomitus
B. Collecting the appropriate measurement of the tube
C. Inserting the airway with its tip pointing to the floor of the mouth
D. Turning the airway about 180 degrees as you approach the posterior oropharynx

123. Which of the following is an absolute contraindication to the Heimlich maneuver?

A. Infants
B. Obesity
C. Pregnancy
D. Cyanosis

124. You are to commence a bag valve mask ventilation in a conscious 27-year-old male with apnea. Which of the following statements is incorrect?

A. You should insert an oropharyngeal airway.
B. You should use your hand to hold the mask over the patient's mouth, with your thumb and index finger anchoring the connector stem of the mask.
C. You should avoid covering the patient's eyes.
D. To achieve a proper seal, you should ensure the mask covers the bridge of the nose, mandibular alveolar ridge and malar eminences.

125. A 47-year-old female presents to the ER with palpitations, dizziness and dyspnea in exertion. Emergency ECG reveals a sawtooth pattern in leads II, III and aVF. Which of the following diagnoses is most appropriate?

A. Atrial fibrillation
B. Atrial flutter
C. Ventricular tachycardia
D. Ventricular fibrillation

126. Which of the following drugs is not a scabicide?

A. Permethrin
B. Lindane
C. Sulfur
D. Praziquantel

127. In a patient who presents to the ER with radiologic exposure, which of the following is not a principle of decontamination?

A. Removing clothing and all external material
B. Using a monitor to measure decontamination
C. Decontaminating intact skin before wounds
D. Irrigating exposed eyes with normal saline

128. Which of the following cells is most susceptible to radiation?

A. Bone cells
B. Hepatic cells
C. Lymphoid cells
D. Brain cells

129. A health worker is expected to divulge all the information necessary in helping a patient make an informed decision, even if such information can affect the patient's coping mechanisms. This is in accordance with which health-care principle?

A. Beneficence
B. Veracity
C. Fidelity
D. Autonomy

130. You are attending to a 17-year-old female who presents to the ER with acute PID. You suspect that she has an STI. She is unwilling to divulge this information to her parents, who are also present in the ER. The results of the STI screening reveal that the patient has a chlamydial infection. Which of the following responses is most appropriate?

A. Discuss the results of the test with the parents first.
B. Obtain permission from your patient to discuss the results with her parents.
C. Send a consult to the psychologist.
D. Discuss the results of the test with your patient first.

131. Which of the following is the most appropriate way to obtain a sexual history from a patient who presents to the ER with foul-smelling vaginal discharge and fever?

A. Are you married?
B. Do you have a boyfriend?
C. When was the last time you had sex?
D. Are you sexually active?

132. Which of the following is an example of battery?

A. Use of physical restraints on a patient with psychosis
B. Attempting a venipuncture without permission
C. Forgetting to take off a tourniquet after venipuncture
D. Punching a patient in the face

133. Which of the following is an example of negligence?

A. Giving a vesicant drug intramuscularly
B. Attempting a venipuncture without permission
C. Applying physical restraints on a patient with delirium
D. Refusing flowers for a patient with third-degree burns

134. Which of the following statements is false about a laryngeal mask airway?

A. It reduces the risk of jaw and tongue displacement.
B. It reduces the risk of gastric inflation.
C. It can be used as a bridging device.
D. It reduces the risk of regurgitation in conscious patients.

135. Which of the following positions is unsuitable for use in an unconscious 17-year-old who presents with a road traffic accident and suspected cervical spine injury?

A. Sniff position
B. Jaw thrust
C. Chin lift
D. Supine position

136. A patient who is being managed with digoxin for arrhythmia presents to the ER with palpitations and dizziness. Emergency ECG reveals irregular and rapid QRS complexes that twist around the baseline. Which of the following treatment modalities is most appropriate?

A. Amiodarone
B. Procainamide
C. Magnesium sulfate
D. Calcium gluconate

137. Which of the following arrhythmias is amenable to direct-current defibrillation?

A. Pulseless ventricular tachycardia
B. Supraventricular tachycardia
C. Atrial fibrillation
D. Atrial flutter

138. Which of the following electrolytes must be monitored in a 58-year-old male who is being managed with digoxin and verapamil for congestive heart failure?

A. Potassium
B. Bicarbonate
C. Sodium
D. Calcium

139. Which of the following is not a clinical presentation of emphysema?

A. Cachexia
B. Cyanosis
C. Dyspnea
D. Dome-shaped chest

140. Blue bloater is used to describe a patient with which of the following diseases?

A. Emphysema
B. Asthma
C. Chronic bronchitis
D. Cystic fibrosis

141. A patient with severe anemia is being evaluated with the Schilling test. The patient is likely to have any of the following diseases except:

A. Atrophic gastritis
B. Gastric bypass surgery
C. Inflammatory bowel disease
D. Hemorrhoids

142. Which of the following methods is not useful in correcting hyperkalemia?

A. Polystyrene sulfate
B. Salbutamol
C. Calcium gluconate
D. Dextrose insulin infusion

143. You are to assess the hydration status of a four-year-old male who presents with acute watery diarrhea. Which of the following is not suitable in assessing hydration?

A. Conjunctiva
B. Buccal mucosa
C. Capillary refill
D. Skin turgidity

144. Which of the following drugs is unlikely to cause hypokalemia?

A. Furosemide
B. Amiloride
C. Hydrochlorothiazide
D. Albuterol

145. Which of the following is required in eliciting the Chvostek sign?

A. Inflating the midarm with the cuff of a sphygmomanometer
B. Tapping the skin 2 cm in front of the tragus
C. Asking the patient to blow out his or her cheeks
D. Tapping the patient's chin while the patient holds his or her mouth open

146. Which of the following is not a cause of hypovolemic hypernatremia?

A. Iatrogenic sodium chloride overload
B. Diabetes mellitus
C. IV furosemide
D. Heatstroke

147. Which of the following is not a clinical presentation of diabetes insipidus?

A. Polyuria
B. Polydipsia
C. Hyponatremia
D. Dehydration

148. A 56-year-old female who presents to the ER with diabetic ketoacidosis will require initial resuscitation with which minimum amount of normal saline?

A. 2 L
B. 4 L
C. 5 L
D. 3 L

149. A 56-year-old female who was admitted with chronic cough, pedal edema and hypertension is prepared to be discharged to the clinic on a long-acting beta-agonist. Which of the following fit this criteria?

A. Salbutamol
B. Albuterol
C. Salmeterol
D. Ipratropium

150. A 56-year-old male who was admitted into the ER with opioid overdose has been relatively stable in the last six hours. However, the nurse notices that the patient develops an abnormal breathing pattern in which there are regular deep inspirations that are followed by regular apnea. Which of the following abnormal respiratory patterns is being demonstrated?

A. Cheyne-Stokes respiration
B. Biot's respiration
C. Kussmaul breathing
D. Orthopnea

151. A 56-year-old male presents to the ER with difficulty breathing, cachexia and restlessness. A differential diagnosis of chronic obstructive disease is made after obtaining a significant cigarette smoking history of 45 pack-years. The nurse counsels the patient to practice pursed-lip breathing. Which of the following best explains the purpose of this method?

A. Increased oxygenation
B. Increased lung expansion
C. Increased carbon dioxide excretion
D. Strengthening of accessory muscles

152. A 25-year-old female with Guillain-Barré syndrome is being managed in the ER. Which of the following is not a danger sign indicating worsening respiratory function?

A. Respiratory rate – 12 cpm
B. Vital capacity – 15 mL/kg
C. Inability to lift the head from the pillow
D. Cyanosis

153. Which of the following treatments is definitive in managing Guillain-Barré syndrome?

A. IV corticosteroid
B. Plasma exchange
C. Heat therapy
D. Baclofen

154. Which of the following treatment modalities is contraindicated in the management of Guillain-Barré?

A. IV immunoglobulin
B. Heat therapy
C. IV corticosteroids
D. Low-weight molecular heparin

155. Which of the following initial interventions is most appropriate in a 56-year-old female who presents to the ER with weakness of the left arm and aphasia?

A. Emergency CT of the brain
B. IV rt-PA
C. Oral aspirin
D. Sublingual nitroglycerin

156. Which of the following complications is most likely to increase morbidity in a patient who presents with Parkinsonian crisis?

A. Hyperthermia
B. Acute urinary retention
C. Delirium
D. Spastic paralysis

157. A 35-year-old male presents to the ER with upper GI bleeding secondary to erosive gastritis from chronic use of NSAIDs. Which of the following treatment modalities is inappropriate in managing this patient?

A. IV crystalloids
B. Endoscopic banding
C. Angiography
D. Proton pump inhibitors

158. Which of the following medications is unsuitable for use in a 35-year-old known depressive disorder patient recently diagnosed with GERD?

A. Omeprazole
B. Cimetidine
C. Aluminum hydroxide
D. Magnesium hydroxide

159. Which of the following is not a clinical feature of hepatocellular jaundice?

A. Jaundice
B. Pruritus
C. Pale stools
D. Dark-colored urine

160. A patient who is being managed for DIC secondary to a snakebite is being managed with aminocaproic acid. Which of the following best describes the mechanism of action of this drug?

A. Converts plasminogen to plasmin
B. Inhibits formation of thrombin
C. Inhibits formation of plasmin
D. Converts fibrinogen to fibrin

161. You are about to discharge a four-year-old male who was managed with iron deficiency anemia. You counsel the mother to serve him foods rich in iron. Which of the following is not a good example of this kind of food?

A. Dairy
B. Broccoli
C. Offal
D. Rice

162. Which of the following is the most common form of dislocation of the temporomandibular joint?

A. Anterior
B. Posterior
C. Medial
D. Lateral

163. A patient who presents to the ER with GERD is being discharged on antacids containing calcium hydroxide. The patient is most likely to experience which of the following?

A. Tetany
B. Paresthesia
C. Flatulence
D. Constipation

164. Nurse P, who is ready to discharge a patient, counsels the patient on drug supplements that should not be taken with oral warfarin. Which of the following drugs is not implicated?

A. Ginkgo biloba
B. Vitamin E
C. Ginseng
D. Cod liver oil

165. An elderly patient who presents to the ER with hemorrhagic stroke has hyperpyrexia. Which of the following best describes the mechanism of this pathophysiology?

A. Microbial infection
B. Hyperventilation
C. Damage to the hypothalamus
D. DIC

166. A patient who is being managed with IV Lasix is noted to have recent serum potassium of 3 mmol/L. Which of the following ought to be the initial response?

A. Administer IV potassium chloride
B. Administer oral slow K
C. Check ECG function
D. Stop Lasix

167. Which of the following is not a pathophysiologic process of drowning?

A. Hypoxia
B. Aspiration
C. Hypothermia
D. Hyperventilation

168. Which of the following is not a factor contributing to the risk of hypothermia in the elderly?

A. Diminished subcutaneous fat
B. Diminished sensation of temperature
C. High surface area/mass ratio
D. Impaired mobility

169. Which of the following is unlikely to be seen in a patient who presents to the ER with hypothermia following a near-drowning accident?

A. Hypotension
B. Lethargy
C. Tachypnea
D. Bradycardia

170. Which of the following is the typical rash seen in infection with borrelia?

A. Erythema migrans
B. Erythema nodosum
C. Erythema marginatum
D. Erythema capsulatum

171. What is the drug of choice in a patient who presents to the ER with Rocky Mountain spotted fever?

A. Vancomycin
B. Doxycycline
C. Penicillin G
D. Ceftriaxone

172. Which of the following is not a method of data collection for qualitative research?

A. Interviews
B. Focus groups
C. Surveys
D. Probability sampling

173. Which of the following is not a model of quantitative research?

A. Experimental studies
B. Correlational studies
C. Ethnographic studies
D. Survey studies

174. Which of the following is a nominal variable?

A. Hair color
B. Age
C. Blood pressure
D. Height

175. Which of the following is an example of an interval variable?

A. Temperature
B. Age
C. Weight
D. Eye color

Test 1: Answers and Explanations

1. (D) Hot potato voice.

A patient with a peritonsillar abscess is likely to have a hot potato voice. In this condition, patients speak as if they have hot food in the mouth. Stridor is a high-pitched sound heard on inspiration. Causes include epiglottitis, croup and foreign body aspiration. Whooping cough is a paroxysmal cough seen in children with pertussis. Wheezing is a high-pitched sound heard as a result of obstruction of small to medium airways. Causes of wheezing include bronchitis, foreign body aspiration and asthma.

2. (D) Cauterization.

Silver nitrate is an anti-infective agent used to cauterize open wounds and tissues. It is applied to bleeding sites with an applicator stick. Electrocauterization can be used in place of silver nitrate.

3. (D) Pasta.

Foods that are rich in potassium include bone, chicken, poultry, oranges, spinach, broccoli, bananas, raisins, prunes, mushrooms, cucumbers, sweet potatoes and cantaloupe. Therefore, pasta, which is not rich in potassium, is the best option for this patient.

4. (B) Urine color.

This patient has a risk of bleeding. The nurse should assess the patient's urine for hematuria, which can manifest as rust-colored, dark-brown or Coke-colored urine.

5. (A) Number of neonates in the NICU.

A discrete variable is counted, while a continuous variable is measured. This is because discrete variables are finite, while continuous variables are infinite. For example, a discrete variable includes counting the number of beds in a ward, the number of neonates in the NICU or the number of patients who present to the ER with burns injuries. A discrete variable often involves a particular place and time.

6. (D) Autoimmune response.

Local trauma is the most common cause of epistaxis. Trauma may be caused by nose blowing, nose picking or drying of the nasal mucosa from very cold weather. Other causes are vestibulitis, coagulopathies, perforation of the nasal septum, foreign bodies, tumors, arteriosclerosis and systemic disorders. Autoimmune response is not a risk factor for epistaxis.

7. (B) Fibrinolytic therapy.

Fibrinolytic therapy is contraindicated in patients with NSTEMI and unstable angina. The preferable mode of treatment is emergency angiography to diagnose patients with a need for PCI or CABG. Fibrinolytic therapy is used for patients with STEMI who do not have access to immediate PCI.

8. (B) Available PCI.

PCI (percutaneous coronary intervention) should be done within 90 minutes for all patients who present with STEMI. If PCI is not available, thrombolytic therapy must be commenced. Thrombolytic therapy is contraindicated for patients who present with symptoms of STEMI that are more than 24 hours. Aspirin is used as part of supportive therapy for all patients who present with myocardial infarction.

9. (D) Angiography.
Angiography is not a component of care given before diagnosis is confirmed. It is a component of treatment for patients with NSTEMI. Components of prehospital care are oxygen therapy, nitrates, morphine, beta-blockers (where indicated), aspirin and anticoagulant therapy.

10. (C) Beta-blockers.
Treatment modalities for patients with stable NSTEMI are supportive management with oxygen, beta-blockers, aspirin, diuretics and anticoagulants. Angiography is done about 24 to 48 hours after hospitalization. This is because the risk of a completely blocked coronary artery has been ruled out. Angiography is done to identify the need for a PCI or a CABG. Fibrinolytic therapy is contraindicated in all patients with NSTEMI.

11. (D) ST elevation.
Clinical features of unstable angina are angina that occurs at rest and lasts more than 20 minutes and new-onset angina that increases in intensity, duration and frequency. These anginas also have a low threshold. However, unlike acute myocardial infarction, the levels of the cardiac biomarkers are much lower. ECG findings during presentation include elevation/depression of the ST segment and inversion of the T waves. These findings are short-lived.

12. (D) A 45-year-old male with chronic bronchitis.
The risk factors for aspiration are impaired consciousness, gastrointestinal procedures, impaired swallowing, vomiting, GERD, respiratory and dental procedures. Therefore, the patient in Option D is least at risk of aspiration.

13. (D) Endotracheal tube.
An endotracheal tube will assist this patient in ventilation but is not used to reduce the risk of aspiration. Respiratory procedures, like the passage of an endotracheal tube, can increase a patient's risk of aspirating gastric contents and gastric secretions.

14. (A) Clindamycin.
According to the Infectious Diseases Society of America, antibiotics used for treating aspiration pneumonia are clindamycin, a beta-lactamase inhibitor like tazobactam, clavulanic acid, sulbactam or a carbapenem.

15. (A) Gastric lavage.
Gastric emptying is contraindicated in this patient, who has hydrocarbon poisoning, in order to avoid the risk of aspiration pneumonia. Treatment modalities in this patient are largely supportive. Patients who do not show signs of pneumonitis are discharged about six hours after admission.

16. (B) CT of the thorax.
Myasthenia gravis is confirmed with electromyography and measuring serum levels of AchR antibodies. Electromyography is sensitive in about 60 percent of patients, while serum AchR antibodies are sensitive in about 95 percent of patients with generalized myasthenia gravis. The ice pack test is a bedside test used for screening. CT of the thorax is only done after confirmation of the diagnosis to exclude or confirm hyperplasia of the thymus or thymoma.

17. (A) Diarrhea.
Pyridostigmine is an anticholinesterase inhibitor that prolongs the action of acetylcholine in the neuromuscular junction. Side effects are from stimulation of the muscarinic and nicotinic receptors in the parasympathetic nervous system. These side effects include bradycardia, hypermotility of the GI tract, hypertonia of the lower esophageal sphincter, nausea, vomiting, bronchoconstriction, diarrhea, abdominal cramp, low blood pressure, frequent urination, insomnia, headaches and allergic reactions.

18. (B) MRI.
Diagnostic investigations for multiple sclerosis include clinical evaluation, MRI and analysis of CSF. However, the most sensitive test is an MRI, which can differentiate multiple sclerosis from other disorders that may mimic it. An MRI is also used to differentiate new plaques from old ones.

19. (C) Spasticity.
Baclofen is a GABA derivative used to treat spasticity in patients with multiple sclerosis. About 10 to 20 mg of oral Baclofen is given three to four times a day. Other treatment options for spasticity are gait training and physiotherapy.

20. (A) Blowing of the cheeks.
Clinical examination of the facial nerve includes asking the patient to raise his eyebrows, close his eyes against resistance, show his teeth or blow out his cheeks. The facial nerve innervates the muscle of facial expressions. Option B is used to assess the trapezius muscle. Options C and D are used to assess the mandibular branch of the trigeminal nerve.

21. (D) Attention.
Attention, which is a function of cognition, is tested with the mini-mental state exam. Romberg's test is used to test for proprioception, motor coordination, joint position and vestibular function. It is also used to test the dorsal column of the spinal cord. In this test, patients are asked to stand straight with the eyes closed and feet together. Patients with a positive Romberg's test will be unable to stand straight with eyes closed. Instead, they will sway. Examiners should stand at the back of patients to catch them if they fall.

22. (D) Multiple sclerosis.
Multiple sclerosis causes muscle spasticity, not flaccid paralysis. Some causes of flaccid paralysis are metabolic neuropathies, West Nile virus, botulism and tick paralysis. Flaccid paralysis is attributed to lower motor neuron lesions that affect the neurons in the motor nuclei of cranial nerves, anterior horn of the spinal cord and motor nuclei in muscles.

23. (B) Give IV $NaHCO_3$ 1–2 mEq/kg as a bolus injection.
In the treatment of salicylate poisoning, urine and plasma are ionized to increase the excretion of salicylic acid and reduce the risk of its absorption through the blood-brain barrier. Alkalizing the urine keeps the drug in its ionized form, making it easy for excretion by the renal tubules. The pH of the urine should be about 7.5 to 8.

24. (A) Sudden onset.
Delirium is often sudden in onset because it is mostly caused by acute illness or drug toxicity. Dementia, on the other hand, is insidious because it is caused by pathologic changes in the brain. Options B and C are incorrect. Patients with delirium have varying degrees of impairment of their orientation. Patients with

dementia have an impaired orientation. Therefore, Option D is not as clear-cut as Option A.

25. (A) Agnosia.
Agnosia is an inability to identify objects despite having normal sensory function. Apraxia is an inability to perform certain motor skills that were previously learned while motor function is intact. Aphasia is an inability to use or understand words. Akinesia is an inability to move despite having a normal motor function.

26. (B) Grade 2.
Grade 0 – No contraction
Grade 1 – A flicker of contraction
Grade 2 – Active movement when gravity is removed
Grade 3 – Movement against gravity but not against resistance
Grade 4 – Movement against both gravity and resistance
Grade 5 – Normal power.

27. (D) Cholinesterase inhibitor.
Donepezil is an acetylcholinesterase inhibitor that prolongs the action of acetylcholine. It is used to improve memory and cognition in patients with Alzheimer's disease. Other examples are tacrine, galantamine and rivastigmine. Examples of NMDA antagonists are amantadine, memantine and dextromethorphan. Examples of selective serotonin receptor blockers are sertraline, escitalopram, fluoxetine, fluvoxamine and citalopram. Examples of acetylcholine receptor blockers are atropine and scopolamine.

28. (C) NMDA receptor antagonist.

Amantadine is an NMDA receptor antagonist used in treating dyskinesia and tremors in patients with Parkinson's disease. It increases the action of both dopamine and acetylcholine. It is not used as monotherapy. Examples of dopamine receptor antagonists are bromocriptine, pramipexole, rotigotine and cabergoline. Examples of acetylcholinesterase inhibitors are physostigmine and neostigmine. Examples of MAO-B inhibitors are selegiline, rasagiline and safinamide.

29. (C) Cullen's sign.

Cullen's sign is seen in acute pancreatitis. Signs seen in acute appendicitis are rebound tenderness, which can be elicited by palpating the McBurney's point; Rovsing's sign, which is tenderness at the right lower quadrant on palpation of the left lower quadrant; the psoas sign, which is tenderness caused by passive extension of the right hip; and the obturator sign, which is tenderness elicited when the thigh is flexed and passively rotated (internal rotation).

30. (B) Clinical evaluation.

Acute appendicitis is often diagnosed by clinical evaluation. In patients with classic features, delaying treatment for imaging tests can worsen the patient outcome and increase the risk of perforation. In patients with unequivocal findings, radiological imaging is done with contrast-enhanced CT scan or ultrasonography.

31. (C) Anorectal fistula.

Anorectal fistulas often present with drainage of purulent or serosanguinous fluid. Hemorrhage is not a usual presentation. Causes of lower GI bleeding include peptic ulcer disease, which presents as melena stools; colorectal cancers, which present as the passage of frank or altered blood; and hemorrhoids.

32. (D) Acanthosis nigricans.
Acanthosis nigricans is a skin manifestation of diabetes mellitus and metabolic syndrome. The skin—particularly skin folds in the neck, groin and axilla—are thickened and hyperpigmented. Stigmata of chronic liver disease include gynecomastia, testicular atrophy, spider nevus, ascites, finger clubbing, lanugo hair, paronychia, sweeping of the parotid gland, jaundice and others.

33. (B) Palpation of the right hypochondrium on deep inspiration.
To elicit the Murphy's sign, the patient is asked to take deep breaths while the right hypochondrium is palpated. The sign is positive when the patient halts during inspiration due to exacerbation of the pain.

34. (C) Increased heart rate.
Theophylline is a phosphodiesterase inhibitor. It is used in treating severe exacerbation of asthma because it stimulates bronchodilation, inhibits the aggregation of leukotrienes and suppresses innate immunity. As an antagonist of the adenosine receptors in the cardiac cells, it increases the ionotropic and chronotropic functions of the heart. It also increases blood pressure. However, in this patient, increased heart rate is not a therapeutic effect.

35. (C) Mechanical ventilation.
This patient requires immediate mechanical support to prevent cardiopulmonary failure. Indications for mechanical ventilation in a patient with severe asthma are PaCo2 that is greater than 60 mmHg, excessive production of respiratory

secretions, decreased consciousness and facial abnormalities that will prevent proper NIPPV.

36. (D) IV amoxicillin.
Antibiotics are not routinely used in the management of asthma unless there is evidence of superseding bacterial infection. Clinical manifestations of bacterial infection are fever and production of purulent sputum.

37. (D) Bronchitis.
Bronchitis is a common cause of wheezing in older patients, not in children. Wheezing is a whistling sound heard mainly during expiration. It is caused by the passage of air through narrow or small to medium airways. Severe wheezing can be heard both during inspiration and expiration. Causes in children are asthma, bronchiolitis, foreign body aspiration, GERD and allergic reactions.

38. (B) Mast cell stabilizer.
Omalizumab is a mast cell stabilizer. It is used to reduce the incidence of asthmatic attacks because it binds to nondegranulated mast cells and prevents activation of IgE-mediated calcium channel blockers. This action prevents the attachment of histamines to the receptors and consequent degranulation. Degranulated mast cells release histamine and other inflammatory mediators.

39. (C) Cigarette smoking.
From the symptoms, this patient has a differential diagnosis of COPD. Cigarette smoking is a primary risk factor for COPD. A history of 40 pack-years is predictive of COPD. Other risk factors are exposure to passive smoking, smoke for indoor cooking, underlying airway disease, occupational hazards (dust) and air pollution.

40. (B) Epinephrine.
Epinephrine is the treatment of choice in anaphylaxis and must be given immediately for relief from all symptoms and clinical signs of anaphylaxis. It can be given subcutaneously or as an intramuscular dose of 0.3 to 0.5 mL. Other treatment includes acute resuscitation with IV fluids, oxygen and vasopressors when indicated. Oral antihistamines are given for pruritus, and nebulized beta-agonists are given for respiratory symptoms.

41. (D) Palpable sigmoid.
Patients with diverticulitis often present with tenderness in the left lower abdominal quadrant. Right-sided pain can be seen in Asian patients. The pain can also be felt in the suprapubic area. However, the sigmoid is often palpable at the left iliac fossa, differentiating it from appendicitis.

42. (C) Lowers excretion of calcium.
Hydrochlorothiazide is a thiazide diuretic given to patients with calcium oxalate calculi. This drug reduces the excretion of calcium in the urine by increasing its reabsorption in the distal convoluted tubule.

43. (B) Constipation.
Aluminum hydroxide is an antacid used in treating GERD. Aluminum hydroxide reacts with HCl and reduces the acidity of the stomach. A side effect of aluminum hydroxide is constipation because aluminum ions prevent contraction of the smooth muscle in the gut, prevent peristalsis and increase stool transit time.

44. (C) Metaplasia of the esophageal mucosa.
Barrett's esophagus is a complication of chronic GERD. Regurgitation of acid from the stomach into the lower esophagus causes metaplasia of the esophageal

mucosa from stratified squamous cells into simple columnar cells. Barrett's esophagus is a premalignant condition of adenocarcinoma of the esophagus and stomach.

45. (B) H. pylori.
H. pylori is a cause of nonerosive gastritis. Common causes of erosive gastritis are NSAID, alcohol and chronic stress. Less common causes are cytomegalovirus infection, Crohn's disease, radiation, vascular injury and direct trauma to the gastric mucosa.

46. (B) Normal reflex.
0 – Absent reflex
1+ – Diminished reflex
2+ – Normal reflex
3+ – A brisk reflex that is more active than normal
4+ – Very brisk and hyperactive reflex.

47. (D) Collapsing pulse.
Typical presentations in a patient with aortic dissection are precordial pain, which is described as tearing or ripping. The pain can also be interscapular. Patients can also present with syncope and features of hypotension. The patient can present with symptoms of end-organ malperfusion. In about 20 percent of patients, there are deficits of arterial pulses in major blood vessels. This can present as a difference in blood pressure between two limbs if more than 30 mmHg. Murmurs of regurgitation can also be heard on auscultation. Collapsing pulse is not an expected presentation.

48. (A) Beta-blockers.

Beta-blockers are first-line antihypertensive drugs in patients with aortic dissection. 5 mg IV metoprolol is given for up to four doses at about 15-minute intervals. Second-line drugs are calcium channel blockers like verapamil or diltiazem. If the systolic blood pressure is persistently above 110 mmHg, an IV infusion of nitroprusside is given. Please note that nitroprusside must not be used as monotherapy. It must be given either with a beta-blocker or a calcium channel blocker to prevent the incidence of reflex activation of the sympathetic system.

49. (A) Tunica intima.

In aortic dissection, there is a surge of blood through a tear in the tunica intima of the blood vessel. There is a separation of the tunica intima and tunica media, leading to a false lumen through which blood flows. Aortic dissection progresses from inflammation of the aortic wall, apoptosis of the cells of the smooth muscle, breakdown of the aortic media to disruption of the elastin fibers and then dissection.

50. (A) External auditory meatus in the same plane as the sternum.

To open the airway, elevate the patient's head so that the external auditory meatus and sternum are in the same plane. In this position, the patient's face is parallel to the ceiling. Position the mandible upward by lifting the lower jaw or pushing the ramus of the mandible upward (jaw lift). The head should not be kept flat unless contraindicated.

51. (B) It should not be taken with alcohol.

When taken with alcohol, metronidazole triggers a disulfiram-like reaction. Symptoms include nausea, vomiting, palpitations, shortness of breath, flushing and hypotension. To reduce the risk of this occurrence, patients are counseled to avoid alcohol throughout metronidazole therapy and for at least two days after completion.

52. (B) Mucus thinner.
Nebulized hypertonic saline is used as a mucus thinner in patients with exacerbated symptoms of cystic fibrosis. The salt molecules in the hypertonic saline are deposited in the respiratory airway and exert an osmotic pressure on the mucosa, absorbing water and thinning out the mucus plugs. This makes the mucus easier to expectorate.

53. (D) Hypoglycemia.
Epinephrine activates sympathetic nervous activity by stimulating adrenergic receptors. Side effects are a result of the stimulation of these receptors. These side effects are hypertension, tachycardia, pulmonary edema (as a result of increased hydrostatic pressure), tremor, arrhythmia and anxiety. Hypoglycemia is not a side effect because epinephrine stimulates glycogenolysis and increases serum glucose.

54. (C) Contractures.
Contractures and the formation of keloids are late complications of burns. They form during healing and fibrosis. Contractures often form at the joints in the feet and hands. They can also form at the perineum.

55. (B) Stress ulcers.
Cimetidine is an H2 receptor blocker. It inhibits the secretion of hydrochloric acid and will be useful in this patient for preventing stress ulcers.

56. (C) Mydriasis.
In organophosphate poisoning, there is stimulation of parasympathetic activity. Clinical features include lacrimation, diarrhea, frequency, miosis, bradycardia, vomiting, salivation and fasciculations.

57. (B) Muscle fasciculations.
Pralidoxime is used to treat neuromuscular symptoms such as muscle fasciculations in patients with organophosphate poisoning. Secretory features (lacrimation, diarrhea, salivation, frequency, vomiting) are treated with atropine. Benzodiazepines are used to treat seizures.

58. (D) Distal leg paresis.
Complications of electrical injury include burns, hemolysis, compartment syndrome, rhabdomyolysis, cardiac arrhythmias, thrombosis, avulsion of muscles or tendons, fractures, dislocations, seizures, involuntary contractions of muscles and others. Distal leg paresis is not a complication.

59. (C) Psychoanalysis.
The components of critical incident stress management include defusing, which is the first stage of management; debriefing, which is the second stage; and follow-up, which is the third stage.

60. (A) Helping patients cope with depressive disorders.
This is not the purpose of critical incident stress management. CISM is not an alternative treatment for patients with psychiatric disorders. It is a form of psychological first aid used to reduce the risk of post-traumatic stress disorder in trauma patients. This therapy helps patients identify the emotions surrounding

the trauma and encourages them to talk about their perceptions without fear of judgment or condemnation.

61. (D) Stage IV colorectal cancer.
Stage IV colorectal cancer is not an example of a critical incident. Critical incidents are stressful events that can cause psychological reactions in the people who witness the events. They are sudden and can overwhelm the witnesses' ability to cope. Critical incidents are often work-related. Examples include the death of a coworker, terrorist attack, natural disaster, workplace assault, workplace injuries, war, states of emergencies, vehicular accidents and others.

62. (D) None of the above.
CISM is often done in groups and handled by specialists trained in crisis intervention. However, simple interventions like giving stressed workers time off to calm down, allowing people to talk about their feelings about the event and making yourself available for conversation can go a long way in helping affected individuals cope. Anyone can perform these simple interventions.

63. (C) Autonomy.
Autonomy means that the patient has the final say in the decision-making of his or her health. This ethical principle gives the patient the right to accept or refuse treatment after thorough education and counseling.

64. (B) Provocative test.
Provocative testing with acetylcholine or ergonovine is used to confirm a diagnosis of variant angina. This test is done during angiography in a cardiac catheterization lab. The test is positive when ST-segment elevation is observed on ECG or when a coronary artery spasm is observed on cardiac catheterization.

65. (D) Reduces heart rate.

Nitroglycerin is a short-acting and potent vasodilator. It dilates arteries, veins and arterioles and thereby reduces left ventricular preload and afterload. Because it reduces the oxygen demand of the cardiac muscle, it reduces cardiac ischemia. It does not reduce heart rate. This function is mediated by beta-blockers.

66. (D) Pulmonary embolism.

This is not an immediate complication in this patient. The three immediate complications are hypovolemic shock, which is secondary to a rupture of the aneurysm. Rupture is most likely to occur below the renal arteries. Morbidity rates are very high. Embolization of a thrombus can include the arteries in the lower limbs, bowel and kidneys. Large aneurysms increase the risk of disseminated intravascular coagulation that is caused by rapid thrombosis and depletion of clotting factors.

67. (C) Abdominal ultrasonography.

Abdominal CT scan or ultrasonography is the investigation of choice for ruptured aneurysms. Bedside ultrasonography provides reliable results for interventions, although its accuracy may be limited by abdominal distension and abdominal gas. For unruptured aneurysms, CT angiography or magnetic resonance angiography is very sensitive and accurate. Abdominal X-rays are not sensitive or accurate but may show aortic calcifications.

68. (B) Myocardial infarction.

For patients who undergo surgery for abdominal aortic aneurysm, acute myocardial infarction is the most common cause of early postoperative death. Kidney injury is the most common cause of late postoperative death.

69. (C) Female sex.

The risk factors of aortic dissection are Black race, including Africans and African Americans; elderly patients; existing hypertension and male sex. The peak incidence of aortic dissection is ages 50 to 65 in the general population and 20 to 40 for patients with connective tissue disorders like Marfan syndrome and Ehlers-Danlos syndrome.

70. (D) Short duration of ingestion of toxic material.

Gastric lavage is not routine management of poisoning due to numerous risks (aspiration, perforation, esophageal injury and epistaxis). The only indication of gastric lavage is when there is a short duration between the ingestion of the material and onset of symptoms (usually less than one hour). This is usually not the case for most patients. Gastric lavage is contraindicated in patients with hydrocarbon poisoning due to the high risk of aspiration pneumonia. Drugs that are absorbed by activated charcoal do not need to be eliminated via gastric lavage. Also, treatment for heavy metal poisoning includes the use of the appropriate chelating agent.

71. (C) Left ventricular hypertrophy.

In a right axis deviation, there is a deviation of the QRS complex to an angle that is more than +90°. Other features of a right axis deviation are the presence of a dominant S wave in Lead I and the presence of a dominant R wave in Lead II, Lead III and aVF. Causes are right ventricular hypertrophy, right bundle branch block, COPD, acute pulmonary embolism, hyperkalemia, myocardial infarction and Wolff-Parkinson-White syndrome.

72. (B) Silent chest.
A silent chest is a sign of severe exacerbation of symptoms. In this case, the patient stops coughing and wheezing due to worsening respiratory function. Immediate assisted ventilation is needed to prevent cardiopulmonary failure.

73. (C) Red meat.
In atrophic gastritis, there is autoimmune destruction of parietal cells, including the proton pump and intensive factor necessary in producing gastric acid and aiding vitamin B12 absorption. Patients with this disease have megaloblastic anemia from cobalamin deficiency. The treatment plan will include supplementation with vitamin B12 and an increase in the intake of foods rich in vitamin B12. Sources of vitamin B12 are meat, especially red meat from beef, pork and offal. Other sources are poultry, dairy and seafood like salmon, mackerel, oysters and clams.

74. (C) Increases HbF.
Hydroxyurea is a myelosuppressive drug used in treating myelosuppressive diseases like leukemia, ovarian cancer and melanoma. In sickle cell anemia, it is used to increase HbF and total hemoglobin level. Since HbF is less prone to sickling in stressful conditions, it reduces the frequency of sickle cell crises by almost 50 percent.

75. (B) Hepatosplenomegaly.
Adults with sickle cell anemia are most likely to have an autosplenectomy due to repetitive infarction of the splenic bed. Hence the spleen is unlikely to be palpable. Splenomegaly is likely to be seen in children with sickle cell disease.

76. (C) Elevated liver enzymes.
Elevated liver enzymes are not responsible for this patient's coagulopathy. In liver disease, coagulopathy is caused by vitamin K deficiency, which affects the function of vitamin K-dependent clotting factors and the clotting cascade. This leads to hypofibrinogenemia. Also, diminished secretion of thrombopoietin causes thrombocytopenia. Elevated liver enzymes are seen in liver disease and point to existing liver pathology.

77. (A) Fibrinogen.
Cryoprecipitate provides concentrated fibrinogen, clotting factor 1. In the coagulation cascade, fibrinogen is converted to fibrin. Fibrin molecules polymerize into a mesh that reinforces the blood clot. Cryoprecipitate is made from fresh frozen plasma that is frozen and thawed repeatedly in the laboratory.

78. (B) Tissue factor.
The tissue factor, also known as Factor III, initiates the extrinsic pathway of the clotting cascade in DIC. The tissue factor activates Factor XI. Factor XI activates the conversion of prothrombin to thrombin. Thrombin activates the conversion of fibrinogen to fibrin.

79. (A) Muscarinic receptor blocker.
Ipratropium bromide is a muscarinic receptor blocker. It is a broncholytic drug used for the symptomatic relief of symptoms in patients with COPD and asthma. It reduces bronchoconstriction and mucus plug formation in the respiratory tree.

80. (C) Impaired consciousness.
The level of consciousness in patients with Alzheimer's is usually intact until delirium sets in. The manifestation of Alzheimer's includes short-term memory

loss; cognitive dysfunction that manifests as impaired judgment; impaired reasoning and inability to perform complex tasks. Dysfunction in language manifests as difficulty in speaking and difficulty recalling words. Visuospatial dysfunction manifests as an inability to recognize familiar faces.

81. (D) Acetaminophen.
Acetaminophen is not used in treating trigeminal neuralgia. Carbamazepine is the drug of choice. If there are contraindications to the use of this drug in the patient, other anticonvulsants like gabapentin, lamotrigine and phenytoin are used. Apart from anticonvulsants, baclofen and amitriptyline are used in place of carbamazepine.

82. (A) Aural irrigation.
This treatment is contraindicated in this patient. The aim of treatment includes keeping the ear canal moist to encourage hemostasis and clot formation and reduce the risk of infections. Irrigation of the ear canal can dislodge clots, prevent hemostasis and encourage infection. Perforations that last for more than eight weeks are surgically closed. Antibiotic therapy is indicated for a dirty or infected ear canal.

83. (B) Abscess.
Ludwig's angina is used to describe cellulitis of the submandibular region of the jaw. However, there is no abscess formation because it is not a true abscess. However, clinical treatment includes incision and drainage. Cellulitis also involves the suprahyoid soft tissues and the submaxillary and sublingual spaces.

84. (A) Sodium.
Patients with Ménière's disease will benefit from a low-salt diet to reduce the buildup of endolymphatic fluid in the inner ear. Other measures include a restriction on alcohol and caffeine intake and the use of diuretics like acetazolamide and hydrochlorothiazide.

85. (D) Nystagmus.
The cardinal symptoms of Ménière's disease are tinnitus, vertigo and sensorineural deafness. Vertigo is often associated with nausea, vomiting, diarrhea, diaphoresis and unsteady gait.

86. (D) Tetracycline.
Tetracycline is not implicated in ototoxicity. A significant side effect of tetracycline is staining and permanent discoloration of the enamel of the teeth. Drugs implicated in ototoxicity are aminoglycosides, antineoplastic drugs, quinine, salicylates and diuretics like furosemide.

87. (B) Paroxysmal.
The pain in trigeminal neuralgia is described as paroxysmal attacks of excruciating and unilateral pain that is triggered by stimulation of facial points.

88. (C) Cutting food into smaller pieces before chewing.
After reducing the dislocated mandible, the mandible is supported with Barton's bandage. The patient is counseled to not open his or her mouth wide for at least six weeks, is advised to cut food into smaller pieces before eating and is advised to use a fist to support the jaw when yawning.

89. (D) Allopurinol.
Myoglobinuria is managed with IV fluids to facilitate excretion, alkalinization of urine with sodium bicarbonate and rapid debridement of necrosed muscle. Allopurinol is used to reduce serum concentrations of uric acid. It is not used in the management of myoglobinuria.

90. (C) Applying a tourniquet.
This intervention is not encouraged in the management of snakebites because it can worsen perfusion and increase the risk of tissue necrosis. Other unacceptable first aid interventions are suctioning the wound, incising the wound and using cauterization, cryotherapy or electric shock.

91. (D) North American.
According to data, children from African American, Native American, Hispanic American and immigrant families are most vulnerable to drowning. This factor is often fueled by low socioeconomic status.

92. (B) New stimulation.
For patients with Alzheimer's disease, new stimulation is inappropriate and should be kept to a minimum. This is necessary to reduce the risk of the patient feeling out of control, restless, anxious or agitated, and it lowers the incidence of behavioral disorders.

93. (A) Lacrimation.
Myasthenic crisis is characterized by severe weakness of the muscles of respiration (manifesting as tachypnea, cyanosis and other signs of respiratory distress/failure) or severe quadriparesis. It is seen in 15 to 20 percent of patients. It is caused by infectious states that stimulate the immune system and drive

autoimmune responses against acetylcholine receptors. Lacrimation is a side effect seen in a cholinergic crisis (caused by high doses of anticholinesterase drugs).

94. (B) Cholelithiasis.
About 95 percent of patients with cholecystitis have cholelithiasis. Impaction of a gallstone in the gallbladder causes chronic obstruction and status of bile. This leads to an inflammatory cascade initiated by inflammatory mediators like phospholipase A and prostaglandins. There may be a supervening bacterial infection. Causes of acalculous cholecystitis include total parenteral nutrition, prolonged fasting, critical illness, vasculitis and immune deficiency. This form of cholecystitis is thought to be caused by bile stasis, infection and ischemia.

95. (C) Brain.
Lactulose in this patient is useful for managing encephalopathy. Lactulose inhibits the production of ammonia in the gut because it is metabolized into lactic acid. Lactic acid converts soluble ammonia into ammonium, thereby inhibiting the absorption of ammonia into the bloodstream.

96. (C) Sedatives.
Sedatives are contraindicated in patients with hepatic encephalopathy because sedatives can worsen outcomes by pushing patients further into a coma. A low-protein diet with protein sourced from plants is more beneficial than a diet that completely excludes protein.

97. (A) Inhibition of glucagon.

Octreotide increases splanchnic vasoconstriction by inhibiting the release of vasodilating hormones like glucagon and vasoactive intestinal peptide. Octreotide is a derivative of somatostatin and is more preferable to vasopressin.

98. (B) TIPS procedure.

Transjugular intrahepatic portosystemic shunt (TIPS) is a life-saving procedure for patients with upper GI bleeding. In this procedure, a bypass is created between the hepatic and portal venous circulation. TIPS is an emergency procedure with a lower morbidity profile than the Sengstaken-Blakemore tube (increased risk of perforation and aspiration). IV octreotide has a better therapeutic effect compared to IV vasopressin.

99. (B) Sterile gloves.

Noroviruses are spread by direct and indirect contact with patients and their surroundings. Viruses are present in the patient's stool and can infect others via feco-oral routes. Contact precautions include handwashing, isolation of the patient, disinfection of the patient's surroundings and use of gowns and gloves. However, these gloves are not necessarily sterile since contact is not made with an exposed mucosa or broken skin.

100. (D) False imprisonment.

In false imprisonment, patients are held against their wishes. Restraints can be chemical, physical or psychological. In this case, psychological restraint has been used. The nurse has lied to the patient to dissuade her from leaving.

101. (B) Effect.

Effect is not a component of malpractice. The components are:

Duty – The nurse must have a professional relationship with the patient that requires the provision of nursing care.
Breach of duty – The nurse does not provide the required standard of care.
Foreseeability – An unfavorable effect from the nurse's inability to provide care.
Causation – An ability to draw a link between the nurse's action and the harm done.
Harm/injury – Injury suffered as a result of the nurse's actions.
Damages – The nurse is accountable for the harm and must compensate for it.

102. (B) Use of structured questionnaires.
This is a characteristic of a quantitative research method. Qualitative research aims to describe data and understand a phenomenon. Sample sizes are often small, and open-ended questions are used in a semiformal or informal format. The researcher is often involved in the research. Therefore, data obtained are subjective and may be biased.

103. (C) Interpreting social interactions.
This is an objective of qualitative research. Quantitative research is done to explain a phenomenon, test a hypothesis, establish a correlation between variables and use this correlation to predict outcomes in the future.

104. (C) Clinical journals.
Evidence-based practice is focused on providing efficient health care that is based on observation and analysis of clinical data.

105. (C) Fresh frozen plasma.
Fresh frozen plasma contains Factors VIII and IX and is useful in providing urgent treatment until the necessary clotting factor is transfused. Red blood cells

are not necessary unless the patient is in hemorrhagic shock. Option B is not useful since hemorrhage is from deficient clotting factors, not platelets. Option D is incorrect because whole blood is not useful in treating this patient.

106. (C) Heparin binder.
Protamine sulfate binds to heparin and forms a stable complex with no anticoagulant function. This complex is readily broken down by the reticuloendothelial system. This antidote readily reverses the action of heparin in five minutes. About 1 to 1.5 mg of protamine is given per 100 IU of circulating heparin.

107. (A) Withhold the next dose of warfarin.
In normal patients, INR that is less than or equal to 1 is normal. In patients on anticoagulant therapy, a range from 2 to 3 is considered therapeutic. A value of 4.5 is considered critical and puts the patient at increased risk of bleeding. The most appropriate response is to withhold the next dose of warfarin, assess the patient's vital signs and assess for bleeding. The attending physician must also be informed. The antidote for warfarin is vitamin K and fresh frozen plasma. Protamine sulfate is used to reverse the effects of heparin.

108. (A) Nasal balloons.
Posterior bleeds are controlled by inserting nasal balloons for tamponade. Anterior bleeds are more common than posterior bleeds. They are also easier to control than posterior balloons. This is because anterior bleeds occur in the Kiesselbach's area, while posterior bleeds occur in the posterior septum and are more serious. Another method for controlling bleeding is the use of a posterior gauze pack. Other measures for severe cases are ligation of the internal maxillary artery or angiographic embolization.

109. (D) Swallowing.

Trigeminal neuralgia is caused by compression of the fifth cranial nerve by an intracranial artery, a vein, multiple sclerosis plaques or a tumor. Clinical features are excruciating and paroxysmal facial pain that is triggered by brushing the teeth, chewing, smiling or sleeping on the affected side of the face. Swallowing is unlikely to cause increased pain.

110. (B) Serum sickness.

Serum sickness is a type III hypersensitivity reaction against antivenoms obtained from animal sources. FAb antivenom comes from sheep antibodies. Clinical features of serum sickness are rashes, fever, pruritus, hypotension, hematuria, splenomegaly, arthralgia, malaise, glomerulonephritis, lymphadenopathy and shock. To reduce the risk of this happening, a loading dose of the antivenom is administered slowly, then the patient is observed for adverse reactions.

111. (C) Clostridium perfringens.

This is a ubiquitous anaerobic bacteria found in feces, air, soil and water. It is mostly spread by contaminated meat in commercial settings. Inside the gut, C. perfringens releases enterotoxins into the small intestine.

112. (C) Oral metronidazole.

Treatment of food poisoning caused by Clostridium perfringens is supportive management of gastroenteritis. Antibiotics are not useful in management.

113. (C) Bile acid sequestrant.
Cholestyramine is a bile acid sequestrant. It binds to intestinal bile acids, thereby preventing their absorption into the bloodstream. The bile acid/cholestyramine complexes are then excreted in the stool.

114. (A) Ribavirin.
Ribavirin is an antiviral drug used in treating infections with hepatitis C, RSV and viruses responsible for some viral hemorrhagic fevers. Acute hepatitis A is a self-limiting infection that requires no specific treatment with antiviral medications. Treatment is mainly supportive to treat nausea, vomiting, fever, abdominal pain and pruritus.

115. (C) Escherichia coli.
Hemolytic uremic syndrome is an acute and rapidly progressive disease characterized by acute kidney injury, hemolytic anemia and thrombocytopenia. It commonly affects children who have been infected by Escherichia coli O157:H7, which releases Shiga toxin. It can also affect adults.

116. (B) Loperamide.
Loperamide is an antidiarrheal drug. It is not used in managing acute watery diarrhea in children less than two years of age. IV crystalloids are used in managing patients with moderate to severe dehydration, while ondansetron is safe for use in children with severe and persistent vomiting. Oral zinc is effective in bulking up the stools and reducing the frequency of stooling.

117. (B) It is more likely to herniate into the scrotum.
This statement is false. Since direct hernias do not transverse through the inguinal canal, they are less likely to be found in the scrotum. Indirect hernias

pass through the inguinal canal and are very likely to be found in the scrotum. Inguinal hernias seen in the scrotum are always indirect. Direct hernias herniate obliquely and appear as a circular sweeping at the external ring.

118. (C) Hemorrhage.
A hemorrhage is not a complication of a strangulated inguinal hernia. This is because the strangulated virus is commonly a bowel loop or peritoneal fat. Complications of strangulated inguinal hernias are intestinal obstruction, dehydration, sepsis/septic shock, hypovolemic shock from severe dehydration, rupture/perforation of the strangulated viscus and fistula formation. A strangulated hernia is a surgical emergency.

119. (B) Rectal bleeding is present.
This statement is false because the rectum is typically spared in Crohn's disease. Therefore, rectal involvement and consequent bleeding are rare, unlike in ulcerative colitis. Other differences include asymmetric involvement of the bowel, unlike in ulcerative colitis, which has asymmetric involvement; and epithelioid granulomas, which are usually seen in Crohn's disease but not in ulcerative colitis.

120. (D) Respiratory droplets.
Giardiasis is a parasitic infection of the bowel. It is not spread by respiratory droplets and oral secretions. It is spread by feco-oral routes via contaminated food and water. Transmission can also occur by contact with feces during sex, ingestion of contaminated water in swimming pools in nurseries when changing diapers of infected children and through poor handwashing hygiene.

121. (A) Distance from the tip of the nose to the tragus of the ear.

The appropriate measurement before inserting a nasopharyngeal airway is the distance from the tip of the nose to the tragus of the ear. The distance for an oropharyngeal airway is measured from the angle of the mouth to the angle of the ramus of the mandible.

122. (C) Inserting the airway with its tip pointing to the floor of the mouth.

This step is incorrect because the airway must be inserted with its tip pointing toward the roof of the mouth (concave up). If a tongue depressor is used, its tip should be pointed toward the floor of the mouth (concave down).

123. (A) Infants.

The Heimlich maneuver should not be done in infants who are less than one year. Infants are resuscitated by back blows. In this maneuver, the infant is held in a prime position with the head down. The head of the infant is supported with the rescuer's nondormant hand while the dominant hand delivers five back blows. After this, the infant is placed on the rescuer's thigh in a supine, head-down position and five chest thrusts are given. A sequence of back blows and chest thrusts are given until the airway is cleared.

124. (A) You should insert an oropharyngeal airway.

This statement is incorrect because oropharyngeal airways are contraindicated in conscious patients with an intact gag reflex. A nasopharyngeal airway should be used in this patient.

125. (B) Atrial flutter.
ECG findings of atrial flutter are the presence of a narrow complex tachycardia, flutter waves that present as sawtooth pattern in leads II, III and aVF, regular atrial activity and absence of isoelectric baseline.

126. (D) Praziquantel.
Praziquantel is not a scabicide. It is the drug of choice for fluke infestation. Scabicides used in the treatment of scabies infestation are permethrin, lindane, ivermectin, sulfur mixed with petroleum jelly and crotamiton lotion.

127. (C) Decontaminating intact skin before wounds.
This is not a principle of decontamination. Wounds must be decontaminated before intact skin. This is because wounds have a higher risk of absorption of radioactive materials than intact skin.

128. (C) Lymphoid cells.
Undifferentiated cells with high mitotic rates are the most vulnerable to radiation. Examples of such cells include cancerous cells and stem cells like lymphoid cells. Differentiated cells in the brain, muscle and spinal cord are the least susceptible to radiation.

129. (B) Veracity.
The ethical principle of veracity requires all health workers to be truthful and honest in their dealings with their patients, even if such honesty can affect the patients' coping mechanisms. The ethical principle of veracity backs up a patient's right to know.

130. (D) Discuss the results of the test with your patient first.
This is the most appropriate response because the patient has a right to autonomy and protection of her health information. Other options listed are inappropriate.

131. (D) Are you sexually active?
This is the most appropriate method of obtaining a sexual history from this patient. Options A and B are judgmental, while Option C is presumptive.

132. (B) Attempting a venipuncture without permission.
Battery is unauthorized and intentional touching or handling of a patient. This act may or may not be harmful. Battery is classified under civil law.

133. (A) Giving a vesicant drug intramuscularly.
Vesicant drugs are not given intramuscularly because they cause tissue necrosis. These drugs are given intravenously in the right dilutions. The route of administration of vesicant drugs is clearly stated. Using an inappropriate method of administration is a form of negligence.

134. (D) It reduces the risk of regurgitation in conscious patients.
This statement is false because regurgitation and aspiration is a complication in patients with intact gag reflexes or patients who have been excessively ventilated. It is not a complication of a laryngeal mask airway. To reduce the risk of regurgitation, drugs should be used to remove the gag response.

135. (A) Sniff position.
In the sniff position, the patient's head is elevated so that the external auditory meatus and sternum are on the same plane. This position is contraindicated in

patients with a suspected cervical spine injury. Therefore, the neck of such patients must not be handled or maneuvered. Acceptable positions are chin lift, jaw thrust and placing the patient in a supine position.

136. (C) Magnesium sulfate.
This patient has drug-induced torsades de pointes. Treatment modalities include electrolyte measurement and correction (hypokalemia), cessation of digoxin and use of lidocaine and magnesium sulfate. About 2 g of MgSo4 is given IV in one to two minutes. If there is no therapeutic response, a second bolus is given over 5 to 10 minutes, then continuous infusion of 3 to 20 mg/minute is started in patients with good renal function.

137. (A) Pulseless ventricular tachycardia.
Pulseless ventricular tachycardia and ventricular fibrillation are the two arrhythmias amenable to direct-current defibrillation.

138. (A) Potassium.
This patient is at risk of digoxin toxicity. Risk for toxicity increases when there is hypokalemia. It is important to monitor his serum potassium to reduce this risk.

139. (B) Cyanosis.
Cyanosis is seen in patients with chronic bronchitis, not emphysema. Patients with emphysema are characteristically called pink puffers. Clinical features of emphysema are cachexia, dome-shaped or hyperinflated chest wall, dyspnea characterized by pursed-lip breathing and use of accessory muscles of respiration and cough.

140. (C) Chronic bronchitis.
Blue bloater is used to describe a patient with chronic bronchitis. This patient presents with central cyanosis, pedal edema, pulmonary hypertension and chronic cough. These patients are usually overweight.

141. (D) Hemorrhoids.
The Schilling test is used to assess cobalamin deficiency, not hemorrhoids. Causes of cobalamin deficiency include decreased intake (malnutrition and vegan diet) and decreased absorption (atrophic gastritis, gastric bypass surgery, inflammatory bowel disease, Celiac disease, peptic ulcer disease and fish tapeworm infestation). Anemia from chronic bleeding (as seen in hemorrhoids) causes iron deficiency anemia.

142. (C) Calcium gluconate.
Calcium gluconate is given to patients with severe hyperkalemia to stabilize the cardiac membrane and reduce the risk of arrhythmia. It does not correct hyperkalemia. Treatment options for correcting hyperkalemia are polystyrene sulfate, salbutamol, dextrose insulin infusion and dialysis in severe hyperkalemia.

143. (A) Conjunctiva.
The conjunctiva is used to assess pallor. It is not suitable for assessing hydration status. To assess this child's hydration status, the buccal mucosa, capillary refill, skin turgidity, blood pressure, heart rate, urine color and output, weight, consciousness and respiratory rate are assessed.

144. (B) Amiloride.
Amiloride is a potassium-sparing diuretic. Hyperkalemia (not hypokalemia) is a side effect of this drug. Another example of a potassium-sparing diuretic is

spironolactone. Potassium-wasting drugs include diuretics like furosemide and thiazides, insulin, salbutamol, albuterol, enemas, laxatives and antipsychotics.

145. (B) Tapping the skin 2 cm in front of the tragus.
The Chvostek sign is seen in hypocalcemia. To elicit this sign, the facial nerve, which is anterior to the zygomatic arch nerve, is stimulated by tapping the skin that is 2 cm anterior to the tragus of the ear. There is an ipsilateral contraction of the face due to stimulation of the facial nerve. This sign confirms muscle tetany. Option A is used to elicit Trousseau's sign (for hypocalcemia). Option C is used to assess the motor function of the facial nerve, while Option D is used to elicit the jaw jerk reflex.

146. (A) Iatrogenic sodium chloride overload.
Iatrogenic sodium chloride overload can cause hypervolemic hypernatremia. Hypovolemic hypernatremia is caused by dehydration and sodium loss. However, the loss of water is greater than the loss of sodium. Most causes include dehydration (i.e., from diuretic therapy and osmotic diuresis caused by glycerol), mannitol, urea and glucose (diabetes mellitus).

147. (C) Hyponatremia.
Diabetes insipidus is a cause of hypernatremia (not hyponatremia). In this disease, there is insufficient secretion of antidiuretic hormone. This leads to the excretion of diluted urine and polyuria. To compensate for the increased serum osmolality, the thirst center is triggered and polydipsia occurs.

148. (D) 3 L.
Adults with diabetic ketoacidosis will require resuscitation with at least 3 L of normal saline in the first five hours of management. When urine flow is adequate

and blood pressure is stable, normal saline can be replaced with 0.45 percent saline. Five percent dextrose water can then be added to 0.45 percent saline when plasma glucose reduces to 200 mg/dL.

149. (C) Salmeterol.
Salmeterol is a long-acting beta-agonist used to manage nocturnal chest symptoms in patients with COPD. Other examples of long-acting beta-agonists are olodaterol, vilanterol, formoterol and arformoterol.

150. (B) Biot's respiration.
In Biot's respiration, there is a regular deep inspiration that is followed by regular/irregular apnea. Cheyne-Stokes respiration is characterized by deep and fast breathing that progresses in nature and then followed by a gradual decrease into apnea. This pattern fluctuates between apnea and hyperpnea. Kussmaul breathing is characterized by deep and labored hyperventilation. It is seen in patients with metabolic acidosis from diabetic ketoacidosis.

151. (C) Increased carbon dioxide excretion.
Pursed-lip breathing increases the exhalation and excretion of carbon dioxide. This method helps the patient control the depth of expiration, thereby reducing the risk of trapped air in the alveoli and improving hypercapnia.

152. (B) Vital capacity – 15 mL/kg.
Worsening respiratory function presents as cyanosis, bradypnea and vital capacity that is below 15 ml/kg. In patients with Guillain-Barré syndrome, respiratory failure due to paralysis of muscles of respiration is a potential complication. Therefore, these patients must be managed in an intensive care

setting with continuous monitoring of their vital signs. Inability to lift the head from the pillow is an early sign of weakness of the diaphragm.

153. (B) Plasma exchange.
Plasma exchange removes circulating plasma components (cryoglobulins and antibodies) responsible for the autoimmune response in Guillain-Barré. This procedure is useful in patients who fail to respond to IV immunoglobulin. Heat therapy is a supportive measure used to relieve pain in elderly patients. Other supportive measures include physiotherapy and anticoagulation therapy with LMWH to reduce the risk of deep vein thrombosis. Baclofen is not used because the paralysis seen in Guillain-Barré syndrome is flaccid.

154. (C) IV corticosteroids.
Corticosteroids may worsen outcomes in a patient with Guillain-Barré. Therefore, their use is contraindicated. IV immunoglobulin is the treatment of choice in this case. Heat therapy is useful in providing analgesia, while low-weight molecular heparin is used for anticoagulation prophylaxis.

155. (A) Emergency CT of the brain.
This is the most appropriate initial response because a CT scan of the brain will reveal the underlying pathology, like tumor, ischemia, bleeding or other causes. The treatment options depend on the cause of the disease. For example, thrombolytics, like IV rt-PA, are contraindicated in patients with hemorrhagic stroke due to the risk of bleeding.

156. (A) Hyperthermia.
Parkinsonian crisis is a rare complication of Parkinson's disease caused by exacerbation of motor symptoms. Hyperthermia is a poor prognostic factor of

recovery. Clinical manifestations of Parkinsonian crisis include severe akinesia, dysphagia, hyperthermia, diaphoresis and elevated muscle enzymes. Risk factors are infections and changes in medication.

157. (C) Angiography.
Angiography may not be useful in controlling bleeding because the stomach has a lot of collateral blood vessels. Treatment options in this patient include acute resuscitation with IV fluids and blood transfusion and endoscopic control of the bleeding. Gastrectomy can be used as a last resort. Proton pump inhibitors are given to correct hyperacidity.

158. (B) Cimetidine.
Cimetidine is an H2 receptor blocker used in treating stomach hyperacidity. However, it is a nonselective antagonist of cytochrome P450 enzymes. It interacts with a lot of drugs, like selective serotonin reuptake inhibitors and tricyclic antidepressants. It inhibits their metabolism and increases their serum levels to toxic states.

159. (C) Pale stools.
Pale stools are not a clinical feature seen in hepatocellular jaundice. Pale stools are seen in obstructive jaundice. In obstructive jaundice, conjugated bilirubin is unable to enter the enterohepatic circulation. Therefore, the stools are pale. However, there is an exception of conjugated bilirubin in the urine and excess conjugated bilirubin manifests as jaundice and pruritus.

160. (C) Inhibits formation of plasmin.
Aminocaproic acid and tranexamic acid are antifibrinolytic drugs that inhibit the formation of plasmin. They do so by binding to plasminogen and inhibiting its conversion to plasmin.

161. (D) Rice.
Rice is a poor source of iron. Cereals and pulses contain phytates that inhibit iron absorption. The mother should be counseled to give her son dark, leafy vegetables; red meat; poultry; pork and dark fruits like mulberries and black currants.

162. (A) Anterior.
Anterior dislocation of the condyle of the mandible is the most common direction of dislocation.

163. (D) Constipation.
Constipation is a common side effect of antacids containing calcium hydroxide, calcium carbonate and aluminum carbonate. The formation of kidney stones is another side effect of calcium-containing antacids.

164. (D) Cod liver oil.
Cod liver oil is an excellent source of vitamin K and is not contraindicated. Patients on anticoagulants are encouraged to consume foods rich in vitamin K to reduce the risk of bleeding. Warfarin is an oral anticoagulant. It interacts with a wide range of orthodox and complementary therapies. Implicated complementary drugs include ginkgo biloba, vitamin E, garlic, ginseng, green tea and St John's wort. Common drugs include aspirin, salicylates, acetaminophen, antacids, NSAIDs and a lot of antibiotics.

165. (C) Damage to the hypothalamus.
The hypothalamus regulates temperature changes to heat. Damage to the hypothalamus (infarct or lesions) affects autoregulation of temperature.

166. (D) Stop Lasix.
The normal range of serum potassium is 3.5 to 5.5 mmol/L. This patient has hypokalemia. The most appropriate response is to stop Lasix therapy because furosemide is a potassium-losing diuretic. After this, the doctor should be informed of the patient's condition and measures taken to increase serum potassium. Some of these measures include oral slow K, increased intake of potassium-rich foods like bone broth and bananas, or IV potassium chloride.

167. (D) Hyperventilation.
The pathophysiology of drowning includes tissue hypoxia, which triggers respiratory and cardiac arrest; metabolic acidosis; cerebral edema and brain death; hypothermia due to submersion in cold water; and aspiration of fluid, which causes pneumonitis and pulmonary edema.

168. (C) High surface area/mass ratio.
This factor contributes to the risk of hypothermia in children, not the elderly. Factors that contribute to the risk of hypothermia in elderly patients are diminished sensation to temperature, diminished subcutaneous fat, impaired communication and mobility, neglect and impaired cognition.

169. (C) Tachypnea.
Tachypnea is unlikely to be seen in a patient who presents to the ER with hypothermia following a near-drowning accident. Hypothermia slows down all physiologic functions of the respiratory, cardiac and nervous systems. It also

slows down metabolism, nerve conduction and mental acuity. Clinical features of hypothermia are lethargy, bradycardia, bradypnea, chills, hallucinations and coma.

170. (A) Erythema migrans.
Lyme's disease is an infection with borrelia mediated by the bite of a tick. Erythema migrans is the typical dermatologic finding in this disease. It is a red macule with a central clearing. It can also present as a reddish macule encircled by a pale ring. It is seen about 3 to 32 days after the tick bite.

171. (B) Doxycycline.
The primary drug of choice for Rocky Mountain spotted fever is doxycycline. Therapy is done for about 5 to 10 days. Early commencement of antibiotics drastically reduces mortality.

172. (D) Probability sampling.
This is a form of data collection for quantitative research. Data collection methods for qualitative research include focus groups, interviews with semiformal or informal questionnaires and direct observation of the data.

173. (C) Ethnographic studies.
In ethnographic studies, the researcher observes the variable in its natural setting. This research aims to observe the environment, culture and unique challenges of the variable. This research method is time- and cost-intensive and requires skill in observing and inferring data.

174. (A) Hair color.
A categorical variable is also called a nominal variable. It is a variable that cannot be intrinsically arranged or ordered. Age, blood pressure and height can be arranged in ascending or descending order. Hair color can be categorized but not ordered.

175. (A) Temperature.
An interval variable describes data that can be arranged on a scale. It is a form of an ordinal variable. These values are arranged equidistant from each other on the scale. Examples of such data include temperature measured in Fahrenheit or Celsius.

Test 2: Questions

1. Which of the following is most useful in distinguishing paralytic ileus from mechanical obstruction?

   A. Abdominal X-ray
   B. Auscultation
   C. Abdominal ultrasound
   D. Serum potassium

2. Which of the following clinical features is highly suggestive of a duodenal ulcer?

   A. Nocturnal pain
   B. Hematemesis
   C. Vomiting
   D. Postprandial pain

3. A 49-year-old male presents to the ER with complaints of severe epigastric pain of 12 hours duration. He said he has GERD and has been on his medication for five years. On examination, he is noticed to have gynecomastia. Which of the following drugs is most likely the cause of gynecomastia?

   A. Omeprazole
   B. Cimetidine
   C. Aluminum hydroxide
   D. Magnesium hydroxide

4. You are giving IV amphotericin B to a patient being managed for systemic histoplasmosis. An hour after commencing the infusion, the patient complains of chills and rigors. Which of the following responses is most appropriate?

A. Switch amphotericin B to fluconazole
B. Administer IV prednisolone and continue with the infusion
C. Stop the infusion
D. Administer IV acetaminophen and premedicate for consequent doses

5. Which of the following substrates is not expected to be present on dipstick urinalysis in a 45-year-old female with diabetic ketoacidosis?

A. Glucose
B. Ketones
C. Protein
D. Bilirubin

6. Which of the following interventions is prioritized in the management of a patient with diabetic ketoacidosis?

A. IV insulin
B. IV normal saline
C. IV potassium
D. IV antibiotics

7. A patient who is being managed for alcoholic ketoacidosis does not present with which of the following?

A. Ketonemia
B. Hyperglycemia
C. Hypokalemia
D. Metabolic acidosis

8. Which of the following is not a clinical feature of pheochromocytoma?

A. Hypertension
B. Postural hypotension
C. Palpitations
D. Diarrhea

9. You are managing a patient with pheochromocytoma. To reduce the risk of paroxysmal hypertension, which of the following interventions is most appropriate?

A. Place the patient in the semi-Fowler's position
B. Avoid abdominal palpation
C. Elevate the foot of the bed
D. Use compression stockings

10. Which of the following drugs is inappropriate for use in a 45-year-old asthmatic male being managed in the ER with malignant hypertension and ischemic cerebrovascular disease?

A. Labetalol
B. Hydralazine
C. Nicardipine
D. Fenoldopam

11. A 67-year-old female who presents to the ER with palpitations and dizziness is being managed with procainamide for supraventricular tachycardia. Which of the following is a common side effect of procainamide?

A. Hypotension
B. Polyuria
C. Tremors
D. Diaphoresis

12. An 89-year-old female who presents to the ER with palpitations is being managed for atrial fibrillation. She is placed on a continuous infusion of amiodarone. Which of the following is a significant side effect of this drug?

A. Color blindness
B. Hepatitis
C. Acute kidney injury
D. Acute diarrhea

13. A 58-year-old male who is very athletic presents to the ER with complaints of nocturnal chest pain. A history of exercise-induced angina is obtained. He is not a known hypertensive. Which of the following drugs is useful in the management of this patient's condition?

A. Nitroglycerin
B. Aspirin
C. Esmolol
D. Hydralazine

14. Which of the following best describes the pathophysiology of carbon monoxide toxicity?

A. Alveolar edema
B. Displacement of oxygen from hemoglobin
C. Depression of the respiratory center
D. Paralysis of muscles of respiration

15. A child who presents to the ER with ingestion of a large number of iron tablets will be managed with which of the following?

A. Succimer
B. Mucomyst
C. Deferoxamine
D. Dimercaprol

16. Which of the following is not a common source of lead poisoning in children?

A. Toys
B. Traditional remedies
C. Contaminated water
D. Fumes from leaded gasoline

17. A person who ingests bitter almond oil is likely to be poisoned with which of the following?

A. Methanol
B. Cyanide
C. Iron
D. Copper

18. Which of the following plants is a source of cardiac glycoside poisoning?

A. Belladonna
B. Oleander
C. Poison ivy
D. Cannabis

19. A 56-year-old male who was admitted into the ER with cachexia, chronic cough and night sweats has just been diagnosed with pulmonary tuberculosis. He is to be commenced on a two-month intensive therapy with all of the following drugs except:

A. Rifampicin
B. Streptomycin
C. Ethambutol
D. Pyrazinamide

20. A 28-year-old female who is being managed with rifampicin, isoniazid, pyrazinamide and ethambutol in a two-month intensive therapy for pulmonary tuberculosis is prescribed supplemental pyridoxine to reduce the risk of which of the following?

A. Pernicious anemia
B. Megaloblastic anemia
C. Paresthesia
D. Optic neuritis

21. A 45-year-old homeless male presents to the ER with a history of fever, shortness of breath of three days duration and a history of a dry, nonproductive cough of three weeks duration. Chest X-ray findings include diffuse perihilar infiltrates on both lungs. Serology reveals antibodies to HIV 1. Which of the following organisms is most implicated in his respiratory symptoms?

A. Histoplasma capsulatum
B. Pneumocystis jirovecii
C. Mycobacterium tuberculosis
D. Staphylococcus aureus

22. A 45-year-old male with pneumonia caused by P. jirovecii will be managed with which of the following antibiotics?

A. Fluconazole
B. Trimethoprim/sulfamethoxazole
C. Pyrimethamine
D. Pyrazinamide

23. Which of the following measures is not useful in reducing the risk of hospital-acquired pneumonia in an emergency setting?

A. Early weaning off the ventilator
B. Ambulation
C. Prophylactic antibiotics
D. Isolation

24. A 21-year-old female is being managed in the ER with sumatriptan for migraines. Which of the following best describes the mechanism of action of this drug?

A. 5-HT receptor agonist
B. Vasodilation
C. Calcium channel blocker
D. Stimulates the release of neuropeptide

25. A 45-year-old male presents to the ER with a history of headaches of five days duration. The patient describes the headaches as excruciating attacks that rapidly peak and subside quickly in an hour. Headaches are on the left side of his head and radiate in an orbitotemporal fashion. They are so severe that the patient paces back and forth until the episode is over. Which of the following diagnoses is most appropriate?

A. Tension headache
B. Cluster headache
C. Migraines
D. Trigeminal neuralgia

26. A 56-year-old female who presents to the ER with diplopia is likely to have a palsy in any of these cranial nerves except:

A. II
B. III
C. IV
D. VI

27. A patient who presents to the ER with headaches, diplopia and bilateral papilledema secondary to raised intracranial pressure is being managed for pseudotumor cerebri. Which of the following best describes the pathophysiology of raised ICP in this patient?

A. Hydrocephalus
B. Cerebral tumor
C. Obstructed venous drainage
D. Meningitis

28. Which of the following best describes the mechanism of action of acetazolamide in the management of idiopathic intracranial hypertension?

A. Osmotic diuretic
B. Carbonic anhydrase inhibitor
C. Na-K-Cl transporter inhibitor
D. Antimineralocorticoid

29. A 65-year-old male who is being managed for STEMI is placed on streptokinase therapy. Which of the following parameters must be monitored during therapy?

A. Hematocrit
B. Partial thromboplastin time
C. Thromboplastin time
D. Platelet count

30. Which of the following is not a major criterion for diagnosing infective endocarditis?

A. Two positive blood cultures of Staphylococcus aureus
B. Two positive blood culture for Coxiella burnetii
C. Oscillating intracardiac mass
D. New onset of valvular regurgitation

31. A 25-year-old male presented to the ER with a history of fever, weight loss and malaise. Significant findings on examination are Osler nodes, Janeway lesions and splinter hemorrhages. History of IV drug abuse was obtained. Which of the following is not required to make a diagnosis of infective endocarditis according to the Duke's criteria?

A. Two major criteria
B. One major and two minor criteria
C. One major and three minor criteria
D. Five minor criteria

32. Which of the following is not a risk factor for developing endocarditis?

A. Prosthetic heart valves
B. Congenital heart disease
C. Sepsis
D. Codeine addiction

33. A 35-year-old male who presents to the ER with fever, pallor and malaise is being managed for infective endocarditis. Which of the following statements is correct about antibiotic treatment in this patient?

A. Antibiotics must be commenced before blood culture samples are collected.
B. Standard antibiotic therapy is given for two to four weeks.
C. Antibiotic therapy must cover gram-negative bacteria, gram-positive bacteria and fungi.
D. Empiric therapy must be according to local patterns of infection.

34. A 35-year-old male who is being managed for infective endocarditis is scheduled to receive IV vancomycin as part of empiric antibiotic therapy. As the nurse injects the drug as an IV bolus, she notices that the injection site is flushed and erythematous. Which of the following responses is most appropriate?

A. Discard the drug and commence a different antibiotic
B. Continue with the drug administration
C. Inform the attending physician
D. Give the drug as an IV infusion

35. A 17-year-old female who was admitted into the ER with an acute asthmatic attack is to be discharged 36 hours later. Part of her discharge requirements is oral prednisolone. Which of the following best describes the use of prednisolone in this patient?

A. Bronchodilator
B. Mucolytic
C. Anti-inflammatory
D. Pneumonia prophylaxis

36. A two-year-old male presents to the ER with a history of cough, fever and body weakness of three days duration. On examination, there is tachycardia, tachypnea and hyperpyrexia. Breath sounds are vesicular and chest expansion is equal on both sides. Percussion sounds are resonant in both hemithoraces. Chest X-ray shows patchy opacities on both lung fields. Which of the following organisms is most implicated in this patient's condition?

A. Mycobacterium
B. Candida
C. Respiratory syncytial virus
D. Haemophilus influenzae

37. Which of the following is not a clinical finding expected to be seen in a 45-year-old male admitted into the ER with community-acquired pneumonia?

A. Contralateral tracheal deviation
B. Bronchial breath sounds
C. Hyporesonant percussion notes
D. Diminished chest expansion

38. Which of the following is not an expected chest X-ray finding in a 56-year-old male who presents to the ER with chronic cough, weight loss, malaise and night sweats of three weeks duration from pulmonary tuberculosis?

A. Flattened diaphragm
B. Hilar adenopathy
C. Cavitations
D. Meniscus sign

39. A 35-year-old male was admitted to the ER with a history of chronic cough, hemoptysis, weight loss, fever and night sweats of three weeks duration. Chest X-ray findings revealed multiple cavities at the perihilar regions, with pleural effusion in the right hemothorax. Tuberculin skin tests revealed an induration that is less than 5 mm 48 hours later. The nurse will interpret the skin test as:

A. Positive
B. Negative
C. False-positive
D. False-negative

40. Which of the following is not a clinical manifestation of dyslipidemia?

A. Arcus cornealis
B. Xanthelasma
C. Pruritus
D. Paresthesia

41. Which of the following religions is least likely to accept organ donation?

A. Jehovah's Witnesses
B. Hinduism
C. Buddhism
D. Catholicism

42. The living will is legally backed by which of the following?

A. State nursing board
B. State law
C. Scope of practice
D. Federal law

43. A Jehovah's Witness who presents to the ER with blunt trauma to the chest refuses acute resuscitation with red blood cells. The patient is expected to provide which of the following?

A. Living will
B. Durable power of attorney
C. Physician orders for life-sustaining treatment
D. Informed consent

44. Nurse M just obtained a sample from a rape victim in the ER. To maintain chain of custody, Nurse M is expected to do which of the following?

A. Send the sample immediately to the lab
B. Hand the patient directly to the forensic officer
C. Hand the specimen immediately to the forensic officer
D. Document and sign the procedure of specimen collection

45. The responsibility for maintaining a chain of custody rests on which of the following?

A. Emergency nurse
B. Emergency physician
C. Police
D. Social worker

46. Which of the following is not a feature of decorticate posturing?

A. Flexion of the arm
B. Extension of the leg
C. Inversion of the feet
D. Extension of the elbows

47. A patient who was brought into the ER with decerebrate posturing has an ongoing pathology in which of the following areas?

A. Thalamus
B. Cerebral hemispheres
C. Red nucleus
D. Brain stem

48. A patient who presents to the ER with acute closure glaucoma is being managed with latanoprost. Which of the following best describes the mechanism of action of this drug?

A. Decreases pupil size
B. Decreases production of aqueous humor
C. Increases outflow
D. Causes mydriasis

49. Before dilating the eyes for ophthalmoscopy, which of the following must be excluded?

A. Retinal detachment
B. Raised intraocular pressure
C. Corneal abrasion
D. Papilledema

50. Which of the following is not a use of a slit lamp examination?

A. Corneal abrasion
B. Measuring the depth of the anterior chamber
C. Assessing the lens of the eye
D. Viewing the fundus of the eye

51. Which of the following ethnicities is most at risk of developing glaucoma?

A. African American
B. Asian American
C. Native American
D. Nordic

52. A patient is being managed with topical prednisolone for allergic conjunctivitis. Long-term use of this drug puts the patient at risk for all of the following except:

A. Corneal ulceration
B. Cataracts
C. Glaucoma
D. Ectropion

53. Which of the following is not a feature of upper motor neuron lesion?

A. Muscle atrophy
B. Hyperactive reflexes
C. Absent muscle fasciculations
D. Positive Babinski's sign

54. Which of the following is given to reduce the risk of contrast nephropathy in a patient scheduled to have a CT angiography?

A. IV normal saline
B. IV allopurinol
C. IV mesna
D. IV acetylcysteine

55. A patient who is being managed for inflammatory bowel disease is being treated with sulfasalazine. The patient will need which of the following micronutrients?

A. Folic acid
B. Nicotinic acid
C. Ascorbic acid
D. Cobalamin

56. You are to discharge a 15-year-old male who had an emergency laparotomy for intussusception. Which of the following is not a preventive method in reducing the risk of recurrence in this patient?

A. Handwashing
B. Food hygiene
C. Rotavirus vaccination
D. Environmental sanitation

57. The stools of patients with intussusception are often described as:

A. Fatty and bulky
B. Tarry
C. Currant jelly
D. Pale

58. A 34-year-old female who is being managed for acute pancreatitis secondary to alcohol intoxication presents to the ER with Grey Turner's sign. Which of the following best describes this sign?

A. Tenderness on palpation of the left hypochondrium
B. Ecchymoses of the umbilicus
C. Tenderness on flexion of the back
D. Ecchymoses of the flanks

59. Which of the following is not a criterion used in confirming a diagnosis of systemic inflammatory response syndrome?

A. Temp <36°C
B. Heart rate >100 bpm
C. Respiratory rate >20 cpm
D. Temp >38.3°C

60. Which of the following statements is false about bowel sounds?

A. They are best heard around the umbilicus.
B. Hyperactive bowel sounds are heard in intestinal obstruction.
C. Bowel sounds should be assessed for at least two minutes.
D. Hypoactive bowel sounds are heard in malabsorption syndromes.

61. A 56-year-old male presented to the ER with headache, difficulty breathing, nausea and seizures following exposure to carbon monoxide. Which of the following best explains the toxic effect of carbon monoxide?

A. Shifting of the oxygen hemoglobin curve to the right
B. Inhibition of mitochondrial respiration
C. Increased alveolar dead space
D. Displacement of carbon dioxide from hemoglobin

62. A 56-year-old male presented to the ER with a history of nonproductive cough and fatigue of three months duration and difficulty breathing of two days duration. He is a foreman who works in a remodeling and renovation company. Which of the following is most likely a risk factor in this patient?

A. Carbon fiber
B. Asbestos
C. Mold
D. Chlorine gas

63. In inserting a chest tube for drainage of pleural effusion, it is important to avoid the neurovascular bundle by doing which of the following?

A. Inserting the needle above the upper edge of the rib
B. Inserting the needle below the rib
C. Identifying the sternal notch
D. Infiltrating the area with lidocaine

64. Which of the following is not a characteristic of an exudate?

A. Protein >3 g/dL
B. Lactate dehydrogenase <200 IU
C. Specific gravity >1.015
D. Cell count >1,000/uL

65. Which of the following is not a clinical manifestation of pleural effusion?

A. Tachypnea
B. Tactile fremitus
C. Diminished chest expansion
D. Pleuritic chest pain

66. Which of the following treatments is most required in managing a patient with Addisonian crisis?

A. Prednisolone
B. Cortisol
C. Hydrocortisone
D. Epinephrine

67. A 56-year-old female with thyroid storm is being managed with propranolol. This drug is required in treating all these symptoms except:

A. Tachycardia
B. Tremor
C. Diarrhea
D. Exophthalmos

68. A 35-year-old female with a thyroid storm is being managed with Lugol's solution. Which of the following is a complication of this treatment?

A. Agranulocytosis
B. Sialadenitis
C. Rebound hypertension
D. Hepatitis

69. In the management of a patient in myxedema coma, the nurse should be careful when doing which of the following?

A. Providing warmth
B. Administering supplemental oxygen
C. Administering enteral foods
D. Administering corticosteroid

70. Which of the following is not a likely complication of hyperpyrexia?

A. DIC
B. End-organ failure
C. Seizures
D. Anemia

71. A 56-year-old female is placed on digoxin therapy for left-sided heart failure. In the case of toxicity, which of the following measures is not useful in the management of this patient?

A. Digoxin fab
B. Magnesium sulfate
C. Lidocaine
D. Calcium gluconate

72. Which of the following principles of management is unsuitable for a 67-year-old female managed for congestive heart failure?

A. Serial weight monitoring
B. Anticoagulant therapy
C. Sodium restriction
D. Salt-poor albumin infusion

73. A 65-year-old hypertensive male presented to the ER with altered consciousness and agitation. Blood pressure on admission was 210/120 mmHg. Which of the following principles of management is inappropriate in this patient?

A. Use of short-acting IV antihypertensives
B. Reduction of MAP to about 30% over two hours
C. Urine input and output monitoring
D. Antipyretics

74. A patient with STEMI secondary to atherosclerosis is being managed with rosuvastatin. Which of the following is an adverse effect in the use of this drug?

A. Flatulence
B. Pruritus
C. Elevated liver enzymes
D. Hyperuricemia

75. A patient who presents to the ER with severe hypertension is being managed with sublingual nitroglycerin and labetalol. Which of the following is the most likely effect of sublingual nitroglycerin in this patient?

A. Postural hypotension
B. Rebound hypertension
C. Pruritus
D. Red man syndrome

76. A patient who has sustained a corneal abrasion will fluoresce which of the following colors after staining?

A. Yellow
B. Orange
C. Green
D. Blue

77. Which of the following interventions must be prioritized in a patient who presents to the ER with a chemical injury to the eye?

A. Irrigation with normal saline
B. Fluorescein staining
C. Visual acuity test
D. Tonometry

78. Eye burns caused by acids tend to be less destructive than their alkali counterparts. Which of the following best explains the reason for this?

A. Acids coagulate eye proteins.
B. Acids have a lower pH than alkalis.
C. Acids are more easily metabolized than alkalis.
D. Acids do not trigger a rapid immune response.

79. A patient who presents to the ER with a corneal abrasion is being managed with homatropine. Which of the following best describes the rationale behind the use of this drug?

A. Lubrication
B. Mydriasis
C. Antibiotics
D. Diuretic

80. To measure the intraocular pressure of the eye, which of the following must first be administered?

A. Bacitracin
B. Fluorescein
C. Proparacaine
D. Tropicamide

81. A patient who presents to the ER with acute acetaminophen poisoning is being managed with N-acetylcysteine. This drug reduces the toxic effects of acetaminophen on which of the following cells?

A. Neurons
B. Hepatocytes
C. Nephrons
D. Cardiomyocytes

82. A four-year-old child who presents to the ER with acute salicylate poisoning is being managed with activated charcoal. Which of the following best describes the mechanism of action of this substance?

A. Induces vomiting
B. Induces diuresis
C. Increases absorption
D. Increases elimination

83. Which of the following interventions is most appropriate in a patient who ingests toilet bowl cleaner?

A. Activated charcoal
B. Gastric lavage
C. Oral sodium bicarbonate
D. IV fluids

84. Which of the following is not a clinical feature of tonsillar herniation?

A. Tachycardia
B. Systolic hypertension
C. Widened pulse pressure
D. Abnormal breathing

85. A 56-year-old male presents to the ER with traumatic brain injury following a fall. As the emergency nurse on call, you are to quickly assess all the brain stem reflexes. Which of the following is not useful?

A. Pupillary reflex
B. Corneal reflex
C. GCS
D. Respiratory pattern

86. A 67-year-old male presents to the ER with traumatic brain death following a home accident. On examination, the pupils are round and mid-sized but do not respond to light. The hemorrhage is most likely located in which of the following areas?

A. Cerebral cortex
B. Midbrain
C. Cerebellum
D. Pons

87. Which of the following describes the doll's eye movement?

A. Conjugate movement of the eyes in the opposite direction when the head is rotated
B. Conjugate movement of the eyes in the same direction of the head when rotated
C. Disconjugate movement of the eyes
D. Flickering of the eyelids

88. Which of the following is not a lateralization sign?

A. Anisocoria

B. Unilateral Babinski's sign

C. Muscle flaccidity

D. Facial asymmetry

89. A 35-year-old female presents to the ER with altered consciousness, vomiting and restlessness secondary to domestic violence. On examination, she is diagnosed with a basilar skull fracture. Which of the following is not a feature of a basilar skull fracture?

A. Raccoon eyes

B. Battle sign

C. Diplopia

D. Anosmia

90. A 35-year-old male presents to the ER with traumatic brain injury following a road traffic accident. On examination, the patient makes incomprehensible sounds in response to depression of his nail beds. However, his eyes remain closed. He also shows a flexion response to pain. What is his GCS score?

A. 4

B. 5

C. 6

D. 7

91. Which of the following is not a source of carbon monoxide poisoning?

A. Automobiles
B. Gas heaters
C. Kerosene heaters
D. Tobacco smoke

92. A patient with carbon monoxide poisoning is being managed with hyperbaric oxygen. Which of the following is a complication of this treatment?

A. Pneumothorax
B. Pulmonary edema
C. Atelectasis
D. Emphysema

93. A middle-aged patient with ischemic stroke is discharged from the ER. This patient should be referred first to which of the following?

A. Neurologist
B. Primary care provider
C. Physiotherapist
D. Speech therapist

94. Which of the following is the most appropriate time to begin a discharge plan?

A. On the first postoperative day
B. On the physician's request
C. After admission
D. As soon as the patient is stable

95. A caregiver who expresses financial constraints in meeting medical bills will be referred to which of the following?

A. Charity organizations
B. Social services
C. Psychologists
D. Hospital administration

96. Nurse P is preparing to discharge a male patient who was admitted with STEMI. Which of the following is not necessary in the discharge summary?

A. Drug prescription
B. Recent vital sign data
C. Advance directives
D. Diet modifications

97. A nurse is preparing to discharge a patient who was admitted into the ER with acute pyelonephritis. Which of the following must first be done?

A. Patient evaluation
B. Patient education
C. Referral to primary care provider
D. Consultation with social services

98. A 15-year-old female is being managed in the ER with acute glomerulonephritis. Which of the following is a likely history in this patient?

A. Recent sexual history
B. Recent history of sore throat
C. History of abdominal trauma
D. Family history of acute glomerulonephritis

99. Which of the following is a typical presentation in a patient with acute glomerulonephritis?

A. Dysuria and flank pain
B. Hematuria and proteinuria
C. Anasarca and oliguria
D. Ascites and hypertension

100. Which of the following is not a biochemical indication for dialysis?

A. Potassium – 6.5 mEq/L
B. Creatinine – 12 mg/dL
C. pH – 7.1
D. Sodium – 130 mEq/L

101. A 56-year-old male with chronic kidney disease presents to the ER with nausea, vomiting and altered sensorium. On examination, he is severely pale and demonstrates a positive asterixis sign. Which of the following interventions is most prioritized in this patient?

A. Hemodialysis
B. Red blood cell transfusion
C. Calcium therapy
D. Erythropoietin

102. A 56-year-old male who had hemodialysis due to acute kidney injury complains of headaches, restlessness, confusion and vomiting. Which of the following best explains the pathophysiology behind these symptoms?

A. Rapid removal of urea
B. Severe hypotension
C. Redistribution of fluid in the nephrons
D. Anxiety disorder

103. A patient who is being managed for severe anemia secondary to chronic kidney disease complains of pruritus. Which of the following is a likely cause?

A. Potassium
B. Urea
C. Bilirubin
D. Uric acid

104. A 54-year-old male has gone into respiratory arrest. You decide to intubate the patient with an endotracheal tube to commence assisted ventilation. Which of the following drugs is most suitable in blunting any potential gag reflex?

A. Succinylcholine
B. Atropine
C. Atracurium
D. Mivacurium

105. Nurse M is about to intubate a 15-year-old male with apnea caused by severe asthma. She decides to use ketamine to sedate her patient. Nurse M must be aware of which of the following side effects of ketamine?

A. Hypotension
B. Hallucinations
C. Malignant hyperthermia
D. Bradycardia

106. Which of the following drugs is not a cause of priapism?

A. Prazosin
B. Sildenafil
C. Amphetamine
D. Spironolactone

107. Which of the following immediate interventions is most appropriate in a 35-year-old male who presents to the ER with priapism secondary to abuse of a recreational drug?

A. Electrophoresis
B. Ice pack therapy
C. Penile shunt
D. Phenylephrine injection

108. Which of the following is an immediate intervention in a patient who presents to the ER with flank pain, fever, nausea and vomiting due to nephrolithiasis?

A. Morphine
B. Potassium citrate
C. Metoclopramide
D. Acetazolamide

109. A 56-year-old male who presents to the ER with severe abdominal pain, nausea and vomiting is being managed with tamsulosin. Which of the following best describes the rationale behind the use of this drug?

A. Alkalinization of the urine
B. Analgesia
C. Dissolution of calculi
D. Excretion of calculi

110. Which of the following features distinguishes testicular torsion from epididymitis?

A. Testicular induration
B. Transillumination
C. Absent cremasteric reflex
D. Urinary frequency

111. Which of the following interventions is appropriate in a patient being managed for corneal ulceration?

A. Antibiotics
B. Eye shield
C. Corticosteroid
D. Irrigation with normal saline

112. Which of the following measures is most appropriate in reducing the risk of spread in a patient with viral conjunctivitis?

A. Eye shield
B. Handwashing
C. Topical antibiotics
D. Cool compresses

113. Which of the following actions is most appropriate in a patient who complains of increasing pain in his limb with a scotch cast?

A. Apply zinc oxide underneath the cast
B. Stretch the muscle
C. Remove cast immediately
D. Inform physician

114. Which of the following is the earliest symptom of compartment syndrome?

A. Pain
B. Paresthesia
C. Paralysis
D. Pulselessness

115. A 55-year-old female who presents to the ER with diaphoresis, fast breathing, cough and hemoptysis has just been diagnosed with left ventricular heart failure. Which of the following is not an expected finding on a chest X-ray?

A. Meniscus sign
B. Kerley B lines
C. Unfolding of the aorta
D. Ground glass appearance

116. A 67-year-old male is being managed for left ventricular failure with preserved ejection fraction. All these drugs are beneficial to this patient except:

A. Losartan
B. Spironolactone
C. Atenolol
D. Furosemide

117. Which of the following is not an expected clinical finding in a 67-year-old female being managed for right-sided heart failure?

A. Distended neck veins
B. Pedal edema
C. Tender hepatomegaly
D. Bilateral crepitations

118. A four-year-old male presents to the ER with a history of sore throat, drooling, fever and irritability of three days duration. On examination, there is hyperpyrexia, tachycardia and tachypnea. The child is also noted to stay in the tripod position. An X-ray of the neck shows a classic thumb sign. Which of the following diagnoses is most likely?

A. Croup
B. Epiglottitis
C. Tonsillitis
D. Pharyngitis

119. Which of the following is not a classic presentation of croup?

A. Barking cough
B. Tripod position
C. Crackles
D. Wheezing

120. A five-year-old male presents to the ER with cough, stridor fever and malaise. On examination of the throat, there is a gray exudate in the tonsillar area. The exudate is fibrinous and difficult to scrape. Scraping causes bleeding. Which of the following organisms is most implicated?

A. Pertussis
B. Haemophilus
C. Corynebacterium
D. Streptococcus

121. You are performing a NIPPV on a 15-year-old male who presents to the ER with severe acute asthma. Which of the following is a sign of too-rapid ventilation?

A. Tachypnea
B. Stomach insufflation
C. Increased oral secretions
D. Increased chest expansions

122. A 45-year-old male who presents to the ER with respiratory failure secondary to severe acute asthma is unlikely to present with which of the following?

A. Altered consciousness
B. Cyanosis
C. Bradypnea
D. Nasal flaring

123. Which of the following is not a treatment modality in managing increased intracranial pressure in a patient being managed for traumatic brain injury secondary to a road traffic accident?

A. Prednisolone
B. Hyperventilation
C. IV hypertonic fluid
D. Furosemide

124. A 55-year-old female with raised intracranial pressure is being managed in the ER. Part of her treatment includes hyperventilation with supplemental oxygen. Which of the following best describes the mechanism of action of hyperventilation on ICP?

A. Vasoconstriction
B. Vasodilation
C. Reduced cerebral perfusion
D. Reduced systemic blood pressure

125. Which of the following is the most appropriate treatment for clostridium difficile–induced diarrhea?

A. Clindamycin
B. Probiotics
C. Vancomycin
D. Metronidazole

126. To reduce the risk of botulism, parents are counseled not to feed their infants which of the following?

A. Unpasteurized milk
B. Raw steak
C. Honey
D. Ice cream

127. Which of the following is most likely to cause foodborne botulism?

A. Home-canned foods
B. Condensed milk
C. Tinned tomatoes
D. Red wine

128. Which of the following is not a complication of measles?

A. Encephalitis
B. Conjunctivitis
C. Pneumonia
D. Shingles

129. You are educating the mother of a four-year-old patient with chicken pox on the varicella vaccine. What type of vaccine is this?

A. Toxoid
B. Antitoxin
C. Immunoglobulin
D. Live attenuated

130. Nurse P is to assess pain in a patient with Alzheimer's. Which of the following approaches is inappropriate?

A. Collecting data from the caregiver
B. Observing facial expressions
C. Eliciting tenderness
D. Using the graphic pain scale

131. Which of the following patients is the most likely candidate for long-term opioid therapy?

A. A patient with osteoarthritis
B. A patient with stage III colorectal cancer
C. A patient with cervical spondylosis
D. A patient with acute lymphoblastic leukemia

132. Which of the following is not an expected complication in a patient recently placed on IV opioids for third-degree burns?

A. Constipation
B. Nausea
C. Itching
D. Respiratory depression

133. Nurse P is monitoring fluid intake in a patient with meningitis to reduce the risk of which of the following?

A. Rebound hypertension
B. Pulmonary edema
C. Cerebral edema
D. Heart failure

134. A patient who is on chemotherapy for acute lymphoblastic leukemia has anorexia. Which of the following interventions is most appropriate in encouraging this patient to eat?

A. Pass a nasogastric tube
B. Serve spicy foods
C. Give IV vitamin B complexes
D. Serve small, frequent meals

135. Which of the following is a standard goal in the management of a patient with raised intracranial pressure?

A. Blood pressure – 150/100–140/90 mmHg
B. ICP – 25–30 mmHg
C. $PaCO_2$ – 26–30 mmHg
D. Cerebral perfusion pressure – 50–70 mmHg

136. Which of the following describes the use of misoprostol in a 45-year-old male being managed for erosive ulcers from chronic use of ibuprofen?

A. Proton pump inhibitor
B. Increases pH of the stomach
C. Increases mucosal resistance
D. Inhibits secretion of somatostatin

137. Which of the following is unlikely to be elevated on dipstick urinalysis in a 25-year-old female who presents to the ER with clinical features of acute pyelonephritis?

A. Nitrites
B. Red blood cells
C. Specific gravity
D. Urobilinogen

138. A 26-year-old female presents to the ER with a history of lower abdominal pain, purulent vaginal discharge and fever. On examination, there is positive cervical motion tenderness and strawberry cervix. Which of the following organisms is most implicated?

A. Gonorrhea
B. Chlamydia
C. Trichomonas vaginalis
D. Candida albicans

139. Which of the following treatment modalities is most suitable for use in managing a 20-year-old male with gonococcal urethritis?

A. Ceftriaxone + azithromycin
B. Ceftriaxone + gentamicin
C. Cefuroxime + gentamicin
D. Doxycycline + gentamicin

140. A 19-year-old female who was managed for acute cervicitis secondary to chlamydial infection is about to be discharged. Which of the following is not useful in reducing the risk of reinfection in this patient?

A. Treating all sexual partners
B. Contraceptives
C. Abstinence
D. Completed antibiotic dose

141. A patient with acute lymphoblastic leukemia is premedicated with allopurinol before the commencement of chemotherapy. Which of the following best explains the rationale behind the use of this drug?

A. Increases excretion of uric acid
B. Reduces production of uric acid
C. Alkalinizes urine
D. Inhibits excretion of calcium

142. A patient who is being managed with cyclophosphamide must be given which of the following as premedication?

A. Pyridoxine
B. Mesna
C. Ondansetron
D. Prednisolone

143. Which of the following is not an indication of reverse barrier nursing?

A. AIDS
B. Aplastic anemia
C. SCID
D. SARS

144. Tumor lysis syndrome is likely to be seen in which of the following conditions?

A. Osteosarcoma
B. Non-Hodgkin's lymphoma
C. Cervical carcinoma
D. Melanoma

145. Which of the following is not used to describe the loss of vision in amaurosis fugax?

A. Unilateral
B. Temporary
C. Painful
D. Severe

146. A 54-year-old female is being managed in the ER with amaurosis fugax. Which of the following causes is unlikely?

A. Transient ischemic attack
B. Atherosclerosis
C. Neovascularization
D. Cataract

147. Which of the following is not a clinical feature of retinal detachment?

A. Decreased vision
B. Eye pain
C. Floaters
D. Photopsia

148. A patient who presents to the ER with retinal detachment will require which of the following investigations to confirm the diagnosis of his or her condition?

A. Tonometry
B. Slit lamp test
C. Ophthalmoscopy
D. Gonioscopy

149. Which of the following interventions is most required in a patient who presents to the ER with hyphema?

A. Irrigation with normal saline
B. Ice pack compress
C. Eye patch on both eyes
D. Cycloplegic

150. Which of the following is not a clinical feature of globe laceration?

A. Leaking of the aqueous humor
B. Positive red reflex
C. Irregular pupils
D. Raised intraocular pressure

151. Which of the following is not a feature of opioid overdose?

A. Miosis
B. Bradycardia
C. Hypotension
D. Diaphoresis

152. A woman who presents to the ER with poisoning with valium may be managed with which of the following?

A. Naltrexone
B. Flumazenil
C. Gabapentin
D. Disulfiram

153. A man who presents to the ER with withdrawal symptoms to nicotine is being managed with bupropion. Which of the following best describes the function of this drug in this patient?

A. Anxiolytic
B. Mood stabilizer
C. Synthetic nicotine
D. Dopamine reuptake inhibitor

154. Which of the following is not a feature of amphetamine intoxication?

A. Psychosis
B. Delirium
C. Hyperthermia
D. Increased appetite

155. Which of the following is the most common cause of Clostridium difficile–induced gastroenteritis?

A. Contaminated water
B. Antibiotics
C. Raw seafood
D. Raw steak

156. Nurse P is about to hand over a specimen to the police officer in a chain of custody. She is expected to do all of the following except:

A. Request identification from the police officer
B. Examine the specimen in front of the police officer
C. Document and sign
D. Have the police officer document and sign

157. Nurse O is to obtain a sample for blood alcohol sampling. Which of the following antiseptics is most suitable for prepping the skin for venipuncture?

A. Povidone-iodine
B. Tincture of iodine
C. Isopropyl alcohol
D. Hydrogen peroxide

158. To assess the severity of pain in an adult male with intact cognition, Nurse P can use any of the following methods except:

A. Verbal scale
B. Visual analog scale
C. Functional pain scale
D. Graphic scale

159. A five-year-old female with febrile seizures presents to the ER. Which of the following interventions has the highest priority?

A. Administering IV acetaminophen
B. Administering IV diazepam
C. Placing the child in the left lateral position
D. Tepid sponging

160. You are counseling the parents of a four-month-old male who presents to the ER with bronchopneumonia. Which of the following statements is false?

A. Handwashing reduces the risk of infections.
B. Breastfeeding should only be continued until the baby is six months old.
C. The baby should be fully immunized.
D. The iron-rich formula should be commenced when the baby is six months old.

161. A 45-year-old female who presents to the ER with a transient ischemic attack will be asked to undergo all of the following radiologic investigations except:

A. Brain CT scan
B. ECG
C. Chest X-ray
D. Brain MRI

162. You are responsible for measuring the blood pressure of a 55-year-old hypertensive male who presents to the ER with an altered sensorium. Which of the following principles is false in obtaining accurate blood pressure reading?

A. The arm used for measuring should be kept at the level of the heart.
B. The cuff should cover about 80 percent of the arm.
C. About three consecutive readings should be obtained.
D. Phase 1 Korotkoff sound is a blowing sound that indicates systolic blood pressure.

163. You are monitoring a 55-year-old female who was admitted with STEMI and commenced on heparin therapy. Which of the following medications is required during heparin therapy?

A. Vitamin K
B. Protamine sulfate
C. Aminocaproic acid
D. Epinephrine

164. A 67-year-old male who presents to the ER with crushing chest pain, diaphoresis and shortness of breath is given oral aspirin as part of supportive care. Which of the following best describes the mechanism of action of aspirin?

A. Dilates peripheral blood vessels
B. Lysis of existing blood clot
C. Inhibits platelet aggregation
D. Inhibits vitamin K-dependent clotting factors

165. A 56-year-old female presents to the ER with difficulty breathing, chest pain and pedal edema. On cardiac examination, a murmur is heard at the second right intercostal space. Which of the following valves is most likely affected?

A. Aortic valve
B. Bicuspid valve
C. Tricuspid valve
D. Pulmonic valve

166. A 35-year-old male who presents to the ER with testicular torsion is having an urgent manual detorsion of the affected testes. In this procedure, the testis will be rotated in which direction?

A. Inward
B. Outward
C. Upward
D. Downward

167. A 35-year-old male presented to the ER with suprapubic pain and sweeping of 12 hours duration following an inability to pass urine. On examination, his bladder was markedly distended. The attending nurse attempted passing size-18 and size-22 catheters, which were both unsuccessful. Which of the following interventions is most immediate?

A. IV analgesia
B. Cystostomy
C. Pass a size-16 catheter
D. Infiltrate the bladder with lidocaine

168. Which of the following measures is most important in preventing a UTI in a 45-year-old male with a urethral catheter for acute urinary retention secondary to fecal impaction?

A. Use of a closed drainage system
B. Change of catheter every two weeks
C. Use of a silicone catheter
D. Prophylactic antibiotics

169. A 56-year-old male with chronic urinary retention presented to the ER with difficulty passing urine of six hours duration. He was immediately catheterized and seen to produce large quantities of dilute urine. This patient must be monitored for which of the following?

A. Hematuria
B. Vasovagal response
C. Postobstructive diuresis
D. Acute kidney injury

170. Which of the following is an indication of a three-way catheter?

A. Bladder cancer
B. Benign prostatic hyperplasia
C. Prostatitis
D. Urethral stricture.

171. A 34-year-old male with septic shock presents with severe hypotension. Which of the following is most appropriate in treating this condition?

A. IV normal saline
B. IV dobutamine
C. Red blood cell transfusion
D. Nitroglycerin

172. Which of the following microorganisms is least implicated in septic shock?

A. Streptococcus
B. Staphylococcus
C. Enterococci
D. Candida

173. Which of the following fluids is not useful in resuscitating a patient with septic shock?

A. Normal saline
B. 5% dextrose saline
C. Albumin
D. Hydroxyethylcellulose

174. You are administering IV vancomycin to a patient with sepsis when you notice that the patient looks red and flushed. Which of the following interventions is most appropriate?

A. Stop vancomycin and give ceftriaxone instead
B. Stop the drug and give IV acetaminophen
C. Give vancomycin as an infusion over 30 minutes.
D. Stop the drug and inform the attending physician

175. Which of the following antibiotics is most suitable for empirical treatment in a 12-minute-old neonate with pathologic jaundice and sepsis?

A. Cefuroxime
B. Ceftriaxone
C. Gentamycin
D. Vancomycin

Test 2: Answers and Explanations

1. (B) Auscultation.
On auscultation, paralytic ileus presents with hypoactive or silent bowel sounds, while mechanical obstruction presents with hyperactive bowel sounds. X-ray findings in both are very similar, especially if the ileus is not from a complication of surgery.

2. (A) Nocturnal pain.
Duodenal ulcers typically present with nocturnal pain that rouses the patient from sleep. And unlike gastric ulcers, duodenal ulcers are relieved by food, although pain can return about three hours after eating. Hematemesis and vomiting are general symptoms that are seen in both ulcers. Other symptoms of a duodenal ulcer are epigastric pain, dyspepsia, nausea and hematochezia.

3. (B) Cimetidine.
Cimetidine is an H2 receptor blocker used in reducing stomach hyperacidity. Gynecomastia is a side effect of its long-term use due to its antiadrenergic effect.

4. (D) Administer IV acetaminophen and premedicate for consequent doses.
Chills and rigors are side effects of amphotericin B. These symptoms typically subside with subsequent doses. Premedication with a steroid or an antipyretic reduces the risk of these side effects.

5. (D) Bilirubin.
Bilirubin is not expected to be present on urinalysis. Protein may be increased in patients with a suspected urinary tract infection (which, in such cases, may be a

trigger for the glycemic event). Nitrates and red blood cells may also be increased.

6. (B) IV normal saline.
Acute volume resuscitation is the priority goal in patients with diabetic ketoacidosis. These patients are severely dehydrated, with an estimated 10 percent deficit in blood volume. Therefore, resuscitation must include volume repletion with at least 3 L of normal IV saline in the first five hours of presentation. Thereafter, other measures, like potassium repletion, insulin and treatment of underlying infections, can be done.

7. (B) Hyperglycemia.
Patients with alcoholic ketoacidosis do not present with hyperglycemia. Those with hyperglycemia may have undiagnosed diabetes mellitus. Biochemical abnormalities present in alcoholic ketoacidosis include ketonemia, metabolic acidosis, hypokalemia, hypophosphatemia and hypomagnesemia.

8. (D) Diarrhea.
Diarrhea is not a clinical feature of pheochromocytoma. Pheochromocytoma is characterized by an excess secretion of adrenergic hormones in the adrenal medulla. These hormones stimulate receptors that mediate the sympathetic nervous. Therefore, clinical features of pheochromocytoma are a result of the sympathetic drive. These features include constipation, palpitations, paroxysmal hypertension, postural hypotension, tachypnea, angina, anxiety, headaches, nausea, vomiting, epigastric pain and paresthesia.

9. (B) Avoid abdominal palpation.

Paroxysmal hypertension can be triggered by palpating the tumor and release of catecholamines. To reduce this risk, abdominal palpations should be avoided or kept to a minimum.

10. (A) Labetalol.

Labetalol is a beta-blocker with mild alpha-1-blocking activity. It causes vasodilation without causing reflex tachycardia. It is used as a bolus or a continuous infusion in patients with malignant hypertension. Its use is contraindicated in patients with asthma due to its antisympathetic activity on the respiratory tree.

11. (A) Hypotension.

Procainamide is a sodium channel blocker and a class 1 antiarrhythmic drug. Side effects of procainamide use are bradycardia, shock and hypotension. Patients may also experience ventricular dysrhythmias, drug-induced lupus-like diseases and other allergic responses.

12. (B) Hepatitis.

Significant side effects of amiodarone are pulmonary fibrosis, thyroid dysfunction and hepatotoxicity. It is important to monitor pulmonary, hepatic and thyroid function during the use of this drug.

13. (A) Nitroglycerin.

This patient has exercise-induced angina, which can be managed with sublingual nitrates. These drugs are potent vasodilators of arteries, veins and arterioles. They reduce preload and afterload without reducing cardiac output and heart rate.

14. (B) Displacement of oxygen from hemoglobin.
Hemoglobin in red blood cells has a higher affinity for carbon monoxide than oxygen. In carbon monoxide poisoning, there is a displacement of oxygen and shift of the oxygen dissociation curve to the left. Other pathophysiologic processes include inhibition of mitochondrial respiration and toxic effects of carbon monoxide on brain tissues.

15. (C) Deferoxamine.
This is a chelating agent used in the management of iron poisoning. IV deferoxamine is given to chelate-free and circulating iron in the blood. The antidote is given as an IV infusion until the patient's blood pressure drops. Patients who are given this drug are managed with IV fluids to improve circulation.

16. (D) Fumes from leaded gasoline.
This is an unlikely source of lead poisoning in children in the United States. Common sources of poisoning include toys, jewelry, contaminated water and soil, lead-based paint chips and dust, lead-glazed pottery and ceramics, traditional home remedies and imported candies.

17. (B) Cyanide.
Bitter almond oil contains hydrocyanic acid, a form of cyanide. Symptoms include tachycardia, hypotension, dizziness, syncope, seizures, acidosis, coma and death. Treatment is with supportive measures and a cyanide kit (including hydroxocobalamin).

18. (B) Oleander.

Common oleander and yellow oleander are sources of cardiac glycoside poisoning. Other sources are woolly foxglove, purple foxglove and lily of the valley. Belladonna is a source of atropine poisoning. Poison ivy induces type III hypersensitivity reaction. Cannabis is a hallucinogenic drug.

19. (B) Streptomycin.

First-line drugs are used for two-month intensive therapy. These first-line drugs are rifampicin, ethambutol, pyrazinamide and isoniazid. Streptomycin is a second-line drug used in the four-to-six-month continuation phase. Other second-line drugs include amikacin, fluoroquinolones, cycloserine, ethionamide, para-aminosalicylic acid and others.

20. (C) Paresthesia.

Peripheral neuropathy is a complication of isoniazid. This is because isoniazid causes pyridoxine deficiency. Peripheral neuropathy manifests as paresthesia, burning, stinging and numbness of the hands and feet. Risk for peripheral neuropathy increases in patients with HIV, diabetes mellitus, alcoholism, cancer and uremia. Pregnant women and elderly patients are also at risk. Pyridoxine supplement is given as 25 to 50 mg daily.

21. (B) Pneumocystis jirovecii.

P. jirovecii is a ubiquitous yeast infection implicated in pneumonia in immunocompromised patients (patients with advanced HIV, patients on a systemic corticosteroid, patients with hematologic cancers and recipients of organ transplants). This infection is suspected in immunodeficient patients with chronic dry cough. It is confirmed with histopathology.

22. (B) Trimethoprim/sulfamethoxazole.
The first-line antibiotic for treating P. jirovecii is trimethoprim/sulfamethoxazole. Second-line drugs are pentamidine, trimethoprim/dapsone, atovaquone and clindamycin/primaquine.

23. (C) Prophylactic antibiotics.
Antibiotics should not be used as prophylaxis to prevent hospital-acquired pneumonia. This is necessary to reduce the rising prevalence of bacterial resistance to antibiotics and MRSA. Useful prevention methods are early weaning from ventilators, early ambulation and chest physiotherapy for bedridden patients and compliance with universal and standard precautions.

24. (A) 5-HT receptor agonist.
Sumatriptan is a 5-HT receptor agonist used in treating migraines. Its mechanisms of action include vasoconstriction of meningeal arteries, inhibition of the vasoactive hormone, neuropeptide and inhibition of neurotransmission of pain within the trigeminal nerve.

25. (B) Cluster headaches.
In cluster headaches, the patient experiences excruciating unilateral pain that spreads in an orbitotemporal fashion. The headaches rapidly peak and subside spontaneously in an hour. Unlike migraines, patients who suffer from cluster headaches are restless, agitated and unable to derive relief from sleep. The patient also experiences autonomic features like rhinorrhea, nasal congestion and facial flushing.

26. (A) II.

Cranial nerve palsy is a common cause of diplopia, which is also known as double vision. Affected nerves include the oculomotor nerve (III), which is responsible for accommodation; the trochlear nerve (IV), which innervates the superior oblique muscle responsible for downward rotation, internal rotation and abduction of the eye; and the abducens nerve (VI), which innervates the lateral rectus muscle responsible for abduction of the eyes.

27. (C) Obstructed venous drainage.

Pseudotumor cerebri is also known as idiopathic intracranial hypertension. In this disease, the reason for the raised intracranial pressure is unknown, although obstructed venous drainage is a likely cause. This disorder is suspected in patients with features of raised ICP without cerebral tumor, malignant hypertension, hydrocephalus or other causes of mass effect.

28. (B) Carbonic anhydrase inhibitor.

Acetazolamide inhibits the action of carbonic anhydrase, an enzyme that stimulates the absorption of sodium, bicarbonate and chloride from the tubules in the kidney. By blocking this enzyme, these electrolytes are excreted in the urine with water. Acetazolamide is used in managing raised intracranial pressure, raised intraocular pressure and pulmonary edema.

29. (C) Thromboplastin time.

Streptokinase is a fibrinolytic agent that cleaves unbound plasminogen into plasmin. This plasmin then breaks down fibrin in blood clots. Thromboplastin time must be monitored and maintained at about two to five times its control value to reduce the risk of hemorrhage.

30. (B) Two positive blood cultures for Coxiella burnetti.

This is not a major criterion for diagnosing infective endocarditis. The criterion is one positive blood culture for Coxiella burnetii. Major criteria for diagnosing infective endocarditis are:

- Two positive blood cultures of organisms typically implicated in infective endocarditis.
- Serologic evidence of Coxiella burnetii presents as markedly elevated IgG antibodies.
- One positive blood culture of Coxiella burnetii.
- Echocardiographic findings, which are cardiac abscess, new onset of valvular regurgitation or dehiscence of prosthetic valves and the presence of an oscillating mass on the heart valves.

31. (B) One major and two minor criteria.

The diagnostic requirements for confirming a diagnosis of infective endocarditis are two major criteria, or one major and three minor criteria, or five minor criteria. A differential diagnosis of infective endocarditis is made with one major and one minor criterion or three minor criteria.

32. (D) Codeine addiction.

Risk factors for endocarditis can be divided into endocardial risk factors and bacteria. Endocardial risk factors include rheumatic valvular disease, congenital heart disease, hypertrophic cardiomyopathy, prosthetic valves and other intracardiac devices. Risk factors for bacteremia are IV drug abuse, sepsis, invasive dental procedures and others.

33. (D) Empiric therapy must be according to local patterns of infection.
Option A is false because antibiotics are withheld until at least two samples of blood are obtained from different body sites. Thereafter, empiric antibiotic therapy can be commenced. Option B is incorrect because standard therapy is for about six to eight weeks. Option C is incorrect because empiric therapy must cover gram-positive and gram-negative organisms. Fungi infections are not usually implicated unless the patient has severe immunosuppression. Thus, only Option D is correct.

34. (D) Give the drug as an IV infusion.
This patient is experiencing red man syndrome, an adverse effect of vancomycin injection. This effect is more likely when the injection is given as a bolus injection. Interventions include flushing the line with IV normal saline and giving the drug as an IV infusion over 30 minutes.

35. (C) Anti-inflammatory.
Prednisolone is a corticosteroid used in the treatment of asthma. As a corticosteroid, prednisolone reduces inflammation of the airway by suppressing the release of inflammatory mediators like leukotriene, histamine and cytokine. Corticosteroids are used as a prophylaxis to reduce the frequency of asthmatic attacks.

36. (C) Respiratory syncytial virus.
From the history, examination and investigation, this patient most likely has bronchopneumonia. Implicated organisms in bronchopneumonia are viruses that are not as virulent as bacteria seen in lobar pneumonia. Because these organisms are not virulent, the inflammatory response is not as intense. Hence typical chest findings on examination and X-ray are not seen.

37. (A) Contralateral tracheal deviation.

Expected chest findings in pneumonia are ipsilateral tracheal deviation due to pulmonary fibrosis and collapse, hyporesonant percussion notes from fibrosis or pleural effusion, diminished chest expansion and bronchial breath sound. Contralateral tracheal deviation, which is the deviation of the trachea away from the site of pathology, is caused by the pressure effect from fluid accumulation (hemothorax, pyothorax) or air accumulation (pneumothorax).

38. (A) Flattened diaphragm.

The typical chest X-ray findings in a patient with pulmonary tuberculosis are hilar adenopathy that presents as calcified nodules at the hilar regions of the lungs. Some cavities present as infiltrates at the apical regions of the lungs; they can also be seen in the middle and lower lung regions. Also, there may be pleural effusion, which presents as a meniscus sign and blunting of the costophrenic angle. A flattened diaphragm is seen in COPD (emphysema) as a result of hyperinflation of the lungs.

39. (D) False-negative.

From the history and chest X-ray findings, this patient has pulmonary tuberculosis. A tuberculin skin test ought to be positive in this patient, with an induration that is more than 5 mm (usually about 10 mm). False-negative results can be seen in immunosuppressed patients, patients with hyperpyrexia, elderly patients and patients with HIV whose CD4 count is less than 200 cells/uL.

40. (C) Pruritus.

Pruritus is not a clinical manifestation of dyslipidemia. It is a clinical feature of conjugated hyperbilirubinemia. Clinical features of dyslipidemia are arcus cornealis, which is lipid deposits in the cornea; xanthelasma, which is deposits of cholesterol in the eyelids; tuberous and tendinous xanthomas; paresthesia; lipemia retinalis and others.

41. (C) Buddhism.
Most Buddhists believe that the spiritual consciousness of a person remains in the body even after death. This belief creates conflicting views on the acceptance of organ donation. Also, some Buddhists accept the Confucian taboos that forbid disfiguring the human body. Other Buddhists who practice Pure Land Buddhism believe that the soul takes its time to leave the body; hence the body should not be disturbed. Although Jehovah's Witnesses are against blood transfusion, they accept organ donation as long as the organ is drained completely of blood. Hindus believe in reincarnation and therefore welcome organ donation. Catholics believe in organ donation.

42. (B) State law.
A living will must conform to the standards set by state law to be valid. This means that state law sets the standard of how it should be written, signed and witnessed. This standard varies from state to state. The state law also confirms the medical condition of patients and their inability to make decisions.

43. (B) Durable power of attorney.
A durable power of attorney is used to show that a patient (the principal) has given another person (a proxy, or agent) the right to make decisions about their health care. Unlike a living will, it can be used even when the principal can still make clinical decisions.

44. (D) Document and sign the procedure of specimen collection.
A chain of custody is used to legally prove that evidence has not been tampered with. A cabin of custody also proves that the evidence is in the possession of an assigned and identified person at all times. Nurse M must record the procedure of collecting the specimen and sign off. She must also confirm that the specimens are properly labeled with a unique identifier. The specimen must remain in her possession until it is handed over to the designated person (who may or may not be the forensic officer).

45. (C) Police.
Collection of the specimen rests on the emergency nurse and physician. However, maintaining the chain of custody rests on the police officer or forensic officer.

46. (D) Extension of the elbows.
The features of decorticate posturing are flexion of the elbows. In this case, the elbows are bent toward the chest, hands are tightened into fists, legs are extended and feet are inverted. Extended elbows are seen in decerebrate posturing, not in decorticate posturing.

47. (D) Brain stem.
Decerebrate posturing is a sign of brain stem damage, especially damage that has occurred below the red nucleus. Decorticate posturing is a sign of damage to the cerebral hemispheres, thalamus, red nucleus or internal capsule.

48. (C) Increases outflow.
Latanoprost is a prostaglandin analog used in the treatment of glaucoma. It increases the permeability of the sclera and improves the uveoscleral outflow of aqueous humor. Miotics like carbachol and pilocarpine are used to decrease

pupillary size. Beta-blockers like timolol and esmolol and carbonic anhydrase inhibitors like acetazolamide and methazolamide reduce the secretion of aqueous humor.

49. (B) Raised intraocular pressure.
Before ophthalmoscopy is performed, the eyes are dilated for a proper view of the fundus of the eye. However, mydriasis can precipitate angle-closure glaucoma if the anterior chamber of the eye is shallow. Therefore, the depth of the anterior chamber should be measured with a slit lamp. Other contraindications to dilation are head injury and globe rupture.

50. (D) Viewing the fundus of the eye.
The fundus and posterior chamber of the eyes are viewed with an ophthalmoscope. The slit lamp assesses the eyelids, cornea, conjunctiva, iris, lens, anterior chamber and anterior vitreous of the eyes. It can also be used to assess the retina and macula with a condensing lens. It is not used to view the fundus.

51. (A) African American.
Glaucoma is six times more common in Africans, African Americans and Hispanics. It is the second-most common cause of irreversible blindness in the United States and the leading cause of blindness in Blacks. It is also more common in people older than 60.

52. (D) Ectropion.
Ectropion is an eversion of the eyelids. A common cause of this disorder is senility. Long-term use of topical corticosteroids places the patient at risk for

ocular herpes simplex infection and consequent corneal ulceration. It also increases the risk of cataracts and glaucoma.

53. (A) Muscle atrophy.
This is a feature of lower motor neuron lesions. Features of upper motor neuron lesions are muscle spasticity, hyperactive reflexes, absent muscle fasciculations and a positive Babinski's sign.

54. (A) IV normal saline.
IV normal saline is given 6 to 12 hours before injection of contrast and then continued 6 to 12 hours after administration. Sodium bicarbonate and acetylcysteine have no proven benefits over normal saline.

55. (A) Folic acid.
Sulfasalazine is a 5-aminosalicylic acid. It is an immunosuppressant that inhibits the synthesis of prostaglandin, leukotrienes and other inflammatory mediators. The sulfa component of the drug inhibits the absorption of folic acid (vitamin B9). Hemolytic anemia is an adverse effect of using this drug. To reduce the risk of this occurrence, patients must take oral folic acid supplements and measure their complete blood counts every six months.

56. (C) Rotavirus vaccination.
Acute watery diarrhea is implicated in the risk of developing intussusceptum. This is because the rates of intussusception peak when cases of viral enteritis increase. However, a previous history of intussusception is a contraindication in taking the rotavirus vaccine because the patient has a higher risk of recurrence.

57. (C) Currant jelly.

Patients with intussusception often present with currant jelly-like stools in the late stage. This term is used to describe stools covered with blood and mucus as a result of rectal bleeding. Fatty and bulky stools are seen in patients with malabsorption syndromes. Tarry stools indicate upper GI bleeding, while pale stools are seen in patients with obstructive jaundice.

58. (D) Ecchymoses of the flanks.

Grey Turner's sign describes ecchymosis of the flanks due to retroperitoneal hemorrhage in the abdominal cavity. Ecchymosis appears as a bluish or purplish diffuse discoloration. Cullen's sign, which is also seen in acute pancreatitis, is ecchymosis around the umbilicus. It is caused by downward gravitation of retroperitoneal hemorrhage.

59. (B) Heart rate >100 bpm.

Criteria used in confirming a diagnosis of systemic inflammatory response syndrome are: Temperature >38.3° C or <36.0° C; respiratory rate >20 cp;, heart rate >90bpm, white blood cell count <4,000/mcL or >12,000/mcL. Diagnosis is made when there are two or more symptoms.

60. (D) Hypoactive bowel sounds are heard in malabsorption syndromes.

This statement is false because hyperactive bowel sounds are heard in malabsorption syndromes and partial mechanical obstruction. Hypoactive bowel sounds are heard in paralytic ileus and peritonitis.

61. (B) Inhibition of mitochondrial respiration.

The mechanism of action of carbon monoxide poisoning are oxygen displacement from hemoglobin due to carbon monoxide's high affinity for hemoglobin, inhibition of respiration in the mitochondria, inhibition of the respiratory drive due to toxic effects on the brain and shifting of the oxygen hemoglobin dissociation curve to the left.

62. (B) Asbestos.
Asbestos is a group of heat-resistant natural silicates used in construction, building, automobile and textile manufacturing. Chronic exposure to asbestos causes asbestosis, a form of pulmonary fibrosis. Risk of exposure increases in home remodelers, miners, shipbuilders, construction workers, those living close to mines and families of workers exposed to asbestos.

63. (A) Inserting the needle above the upper edge of the rib.
Neurovascular bundles of nerve, arteries and veins are arranged just underneath the lower edge of the rib. To avoid piercing this bundle, the needle should be inserted above the rib. To do this, the person performing the procedure must locate the first rib and palpate the intercostal spaces.

64. (B) Lactate dehydrogenase <200 IU.
This is not a characteristic of exudate. The characteristics of exudates are protein >3 g/dL; lactate dehydrogenase >200 IU; specific gravity >1.015 and cell count >1,000/uL.

65. (B) Tactile fremitus.
Clinical manifestations of pleural effusion are tachypnea, dyspnea, absent tactile fremitus, hyporesonant percussion notes and pleural friction rub heard on auscultation. This is a creaking or grating sound heard during inspiration and expiration.

66. (C) Hydrocortisone.

High-dose hydrocortisone is the treatment of choice in Addisonian crisis. 100 mg of hydrocortisone is given IV over one minute. This dose is repeated every six to eight hours in the first 24 hours. Also, the patient must be resuscitated with 1 L of 5% dextrose in 0.9% saline. Delay in commencing treatment with hydrocortisone increases mortality.

67. (D) Exophthalmos.

Symptoms that do not respond to beta-blockers are goiter, weight loss, exophthalmos, increased oxygen consumption and bruit. Propranolol is used in thyroid storms to treat the symptoms of unopposed adrenergic activity. Features that respond to beta-blocker therapy are tachycardia, heat intolerance, sweating, lid lag, proximal myopathy and diarrhea.

68. (B) Sialadenitis.

This is an inflammation of the salivary glands. Other complications of Lugol's treatment are conjunctivitis and eruption of rashes. Agranulocytosis and hepatitis are side effects of propylthiouracil.

69. (A) Providing warmth.

During acute resuscitation, hypothermia should not be rapidly corrected because rapid warming can trigger hypertension and cardiac arrhythmias.

70. (D) Anemia.

Hyperpyrexia is defined as a core temperature that is greater than 41°C. Complications of hyperpyrexia are denaturation of enzymes, end-organ damage, activation of the coagulation cascade and DIC and cardiopulmonary stress. In children, a febrile seizure is a common occurrence.

71. (D) Calcium gluconate.

Digoxin fab is the primary treatment of digoxin toxicity. It is an antibody that consists of fragments of antidigoxin immunoglobulin. Digoxin fab is used to treat severe hyperkalemia and arrhythmias. Other treatment modalities are magnesium sulfate, which is used to treat ventricular arrhythmias; lidocaine, a class 1 antiarrhythmic drug; and phenytoin. Bradyarrhythmias are treated with atropine or catecholamines.

72. (D) Salt-poor albumin infusion.

This treatment is inappropriate in this patient with edema caused by increased hydrostatic pressure. Salt-poor albumin infusion is used in patients with edema caused by decreased oncotic pressure (i.e., hypoproteinemia).

73. (B) Reduction of MAP to about 30% over two hours.

This principle of management is inappropriate because MAP is reduced to about 20 to 25 percent over two hours. In this patient, cerebral autoregulation is lost. This means that blood pressure will have to be high for cerebral perfusion to be maintained. Drastically reducing blood pressure can reduce cerebral perfusion and worsen ongoing brain ischemia. Option A is appropriate because short-acting antihypertensives like labetalol and hydralazine are used to quickly control blood pressure. Option B is appropriate because fluid input and output are monitored to reduce the risk of cerebral edema or acute kidney injury. Antipyretics are used to control the temperature in patients who have lost thermoregulation and patients are given adequate nutrition to improve recovery.

74. (C) Elevated liver enzymes.

Rosuvastatin is an HMG CoA reductase inhibitor that reduces serum concentrations of LDL. Adverse effects of this drug are rare. However, they include myositis, elevated liver enzymes and rhabdomyolysis. Adverse effects are more likely in older patients and patients taking multiple drugs.

75. (B) Rebound hypertension.
Nitrates are direct vasodilators that work on both arterial and venous blood vessels. They are fast-acting vasodilators. They are not used as monotherapy in severe and malignant hypertension due to their high risks of rebound hypertension caused by reflex tachycardia.

76. (C) Green.
The orange fluorescein stain appears green in corneal ulcers on slit lamp examinations. This stain is useful in highlighting the edges and margins of the ulcer.

77. (A) Irrigation with normal saline.
Chemical burns are more extensive than thermal burns. Acids denature and coagulate the proteins in the eye, thereby preventing further absorption of the acids. Alkalis, on the other hand, liquefy the eye proteins and penetrate to affect other tissues, thereby causing more extensive burns. The first intervention is to irrigate the eye with copious amounts of normal saline or a borate buffer solution. Irrigation should ideally be done under ocular anesthesia. Irrigation is necessary to remove all traces of the toxic agent and prevent further ocular injury. Irrigation should continue until the pH of the eye is between 7 and 7.2.

78. (A) Acids coagulate eye protein.
Acids have a less destructive action on the eye than their alkali counterparts because acids denature and coagulate the proteins in the eyes, thereby forming

an impenetrable barrier. However, alkalis are more lipophilic and can penetrate the deeper tissues of the eye.

79. (B) Mydriasis.
Homatropine is a cycloplegic drug used to induce mydriasis (pupillary dilation). As a muscarinic receptor antagonist, it inhibits the action of acetylcholine on the pupillary reflexes responsible for constriction and accommodation.

80. (C) Proparacaine.
Tonometry is done to measure the intraocular pressure of the eye. It must be performed under anesthesia because the cornea of the eye is indented. To minimize pain, local anesthesia must be used.

81. (B) Hepatocytes.
N-acetylcysteine is a precursor of glutathione. When administered, N-acetylcysteine is metabolized to glutathione. Glutathione binds to the toxic metabolite of acetaminophen before it damages the hepatocytes. This bound substrate is then excreted.

82. (D) Increases elimination.
Activated charcoal is used to prevent the absorption of toxic materials into the systemic circulation. Because of its large surface area, activated charcoal absorbs and binds to toxic materials, making them inert and facilitating their excretion via the feces.

83. (D) IV fluids.
Treatment of caustic ingestions is supportive. Gastric lavage and emesis are contraindicated due to the high risk of erosion of the esophageal mucosa. The use

of activated charcoal is contraindicated due to the high risk of worsening gastric erosions. Neutralizing the caustic with an alkaline substance or acidic substance can trigger an exothermic reaction and worsen tissue necrosis. Also, insertion of an NG tube is strongly advised against. The most appropriate intervention involves IV fluids.

84. (A) Tachycardia.
Tonsillar herniation is the herniation of the cerebellar tonsils through the foramen magnum and subsequent compression of the medulla of the cerebellum against the odontoid process. This compression is called coning, which manifests clinically as Cushing's triad. Cushing's triad includes bradycardia, systolic hypertension (widened pulse pressure) and abnormal respiration. Progressive coning leads to cardiopulmonary failure and death. Tachycardia is not a clinical feature of the condition.

85. (C) GCS.
The Glasgow Coma Scale is used to assess the consciousness of a patient. Consciousness is mediated by different parts of the brain, including the brain stem. Hence it is not a test for brain stem function. Tests for brain stem function include assessment of pupillary reflex, ocular reflex, respiratory pattern and ocular movement.

86. (B) Midbrain.
Lesions in the midbrain present as round, midsized pupils that do not respond to light. Pontine lesions cause pinpoint pupils; lesions in the lateral medulla often present as ipsilateral Horner's syndrome.

87. (A) Conjugate movement of the eyes in the opposite direction when the head is rotated.

The doll's eye movement indicates an intact oculocephalic reflex. In this movement, the two eyes move in the opposite direction when the head is rotated. This means that if the head is rotated to the left, the eyes move to the right and vice versa. Please note that this reflex cannot be elicited in an awake patient.

88. (C) Muscle flaccidity.

Muscle flaccidity is not a lateralization sign. Lateralizing signs point to a local (often structural) pathology in the brain. These signs are unequal pupil sizes (anisocoria), unilateral Babinski's sign, facial asymmetry, unilateral focal fits, asymmetric deep reflexes, unilateral hypotonia and movement of the eyes to one side.

89. (D) Anosmia.

Anosmia is a dysfunction of the olfactory nerve and is not a feature of basilar skull fracture. Features of a basilar skull fracture include Battle's sign, which is a fracture of the mastoid process. It presents as bleeding behind the ear and around the mastoid. Other features are raccoon eyes (black eyes), which are periorbital hemorrhage; leakage of cerebrospinal fluid from the ears or nose; hemotympanum; hemoptysis and bleeding from the ears; vomiting; deafness; nystagmus; palsies of the cranial nerve, which present as diplopia; and visual problems.

90. (C) 6.

The patient has an eye response of 1, a verbal response of 2 and a motor response of 3. His total GCS score is 6.

91. (D) Tobacco smoke.

Although tobacco smoke contains carbon monoxide, the amount is not enough to cause poisoning. Sources of carbon monoxide poisoning include furnaces, gas heaters, kerosene heaters, automobiles, charcoal-burning stoves and water heaters.

92. (A) Pneumothorax.

Barotrauma is a potential complication of hyperbaric oxygen therapy. In this patient, barotrauma can present as pneumothorax.

93. (B) Primary care provider.

This patient should first be referred to his primary care provider. The primary care provider is responsible for following up with the patient on consultations with a neurologist, speech therapist and physiotherapist.

94. (B) On the physician's request.

Discharge planning begins as soon as the physician requests it. The discharge planning can be written by a nurse or another member of the health team. It is, however, initiated by the attending physician.

95. (B) Social services.

Social services should be consulted. Social workers are responsible for assessing the social welfare of patients and providing financial and other assistance tailored to patients' needs.

96. (C) Advance directives.

Advance directives are not necessary in this patient because myocardial infarction is not a terminal disease. Advance directives are components of palliative care given to patients with a terminal illness.

97. (B) Patient education.

The patient must first be educated on the levels of prevention of the condition; the dose, indications and side effects of medications; diet modifications and information on home health services, among other things. Patient evaluation is required before discharge planning is commenced. Referrals and consultations are done after patient education.

98. (B) Recent history of sore throat.

Postinfectious glomerulonephritis caused by group A beta-hemolytic streptococcus is a common cause of glomerulonephritis. A recent history of sore throat or impetigo (about 6 to 21 days) before the occurrence of renal symptoms is typically seen.

99. (B) Hematuria and proteinuria.

Clinical features of acute glomerulonephritis are hematuria, proteinuria and hypertension. Clinical features come in a spectrum. Patients with extreme cases present with oliguria and acute kidney injury. Dysuria and flank pain are common findings in urinary tract infections. Anasarca and oliguria are findings in nephrotic syndrome, while ascites and hypertension are seen in acute kidney injury.

100. (D) Sodium – 130 mEq/L.
Mild hyponatremia is not an indication of dialysis. The biochemical indications for dialysis are severe hyperkalemia that is equal to or greater than 6.5 mEq/L and is refractory to other treatment; uremia with clinical features such as gastritis, uremic encephalopathy, uremic gastritis and pericarditis; serum creatinine that is equal to or greater than 12 mg/dL and acidosis.

101. (B) Red blood cell transfusion.
This patient has severe anemia secondary to chronic kidney disease and needs an urgent transfusion. The definitive treatment is renal replacement therapy with dialysis and renal transplant. However, his hematocrit must be optimized before hemodialysis is done. Erythropoietin therapy can be commenced after blood transfusion.

102. (A) Rapid removal of urea.
This patient is experiencing disequilibrium syndrome caused by the rapid removal of urea from the blood. Urea has a small osmotic effect on the plasma. Hence it is rapidly removed. However, the rate of clearance is faster than its diffusion in the blood-brain barrier. This creates a gradient between the plasma and brain cells and leads to cerebral edema.

103. (B) Urea.
Uremia is a common cause of pruritus in patients with chronic kidney disease (CKD). This form of pruritus is worse at night and is severe enough to disrupt sleep. Areas that are often involved are the abdomen, back, arms and head. Increased serum calcium and phosphorus are other causes of pruritus in patients with CKD.

104. (A) Succinylcholine.

Succinylcholine is a reversible neuromuscular blocker with a very rapid onset of action (30 seconds to 1 minute). This pharmacokinetic property makes it suitable for use in emergency cases to blunt a potential gag reflex. However, the use of succinylcholine is contraindicated in patients with eye injuries, renal failure, crush injuries, spinal cord injuries and burns. Atracurium and mivacurium are nondepolarizing neuromuscular blockers with a long onset of action and long duration.

105. (B) Hallucinations.

Ketamine causes dissociative anesthesia. Side effects are hallucinations, delirium, frightening dreams and nightmares. Because ketamine stimulates the cardiac centers, hypertension and tachycardia are also side effects. Ketamine has bronchodilation effects that are therapeutic in this patient.

106. (D) Spironolactone.

Spironolactone is not a cause of priapism. It is a loop diuretic used in managing patients with hypertension, heart failure and hypertensive heart disease. A common side effect of this drug is gynecomastia due to its antiadrenergic effect. Drugs that are implicated in priapism are drugs used for erectile dysfunction; alprostadil and phosphodiesterase 5 inhibitors; recreational drugs like cocaine and amphetamine; alpha-blockers like prazosin and tamsulosin; antipsychotics; antihypertensives like nifedipine, warfarin, lithium and corticosteroids; and hypoglycemic agents like tolbutamide.

107. (D) Phenylephrine injection.

Treatment for ischemic priapism must be commenced immediately to reduce the risk of penile gangrene. Immediate treatment involves aspiration of blood to the base of the corpora cavernosa with a nonheparinized syringe and saline irrigation with an injection of phenylephrine into the cavernous. If these interventions are unsuccessful (i.e., priapism lasts more than 48 hours), a surgical shunt between the corpus cavernosum and glans penis is quickly created. Ice pack therapy is used for patients with nonischemic priapism. Plasma electrophoresis is used in patients with priapism secondary to sickle cell disease.

108. (A) Morphine.
Analgesia such as morphine is an immediate intervention in this patient, who is in severe distress. After adequate analgesia, other measures, like antipyretics, antiemetics and fluid administration, can be commenced. Definite treatment is the removal of the calculi either via surgery, radiology or drugs.

109. (D) Excretion of calculi.
Tamsulosin is an alpha-receptor blocker and muscle relaxant useful in enhancing the passage of large calculi. Studies have shown that tamsulosin is more effective than calcium channel blockers in enhancing the excretion of urinary calculi.

110. (C) Absent cremasteric reflex.
The clinical features of testicular torsion and epididymitis often overlap, as they may both present with scrotal pain, fever, urinary frequency, scrotal edema and induration. However, in testicular torsion, the cremasteric reflex on the affected testes is usually absent.

111. (A) Antibiotics.
Ulcerations are treated with broad-spectrum antibiotics for empiric therapy (usually fluoroquinolones). Corticosteroids are rarely used due to the risk of triggering a latent ocular herpes simplex infection. Eye shields are

contraindicated because of the risk of proliferating the infective microorganism via providing warmth. Irrigation with normal saline is not useful.

112. (B) Handwashing.
Handwashing is very useful in reducing the risk of spread of viral conjunctivitis. Patients are counseled to wash their hands after touching their eyes and face. All health workers and caregivers in direct contact with the patient must wash their hands after visitation. Viral conjunctivitis is self-limiting; hence antibiotics and antivirals are not useful. The eyes of affected patients must not be patched to reduce the risk of prolonged infection and viral replication. Cool compresses are not used to reduce the risk of spread. They are used to provide symptomatic relief.

113. (B) Stretch the muscle.
Exaggerated pain is an early sign of compartment syndrome. Before any intervention is done, the muscles in the affected area are passively stretched. In patients with compartment syndrome, the elicited pain is exaggerated. Pulse may still be normal in this patient. Pulselessness is a late sign of compartment syndrome. The attending physician is then informed and the cast is removed. The pressure in the fascia is measured with a pressure monitor. If the symptoms worsen, urgent fasciotomy is done and the muscles are inspected for viability.

114. (A) Pain.
Worsening pain is the earliest sign of compartment syndrome. The patient often complains of pain that is greater than the degree of injury. This pain can also be elicited by passively stretching the muscles in the affected compartment. Pallor and pulselessness are late signs.

115. (D) Ground glass appearance.
Ground glass appearance is typically seen in interstitial fibrosis of the lungs. Chest X-ray features of heart failure are pleural effusion (meniscus sign); boot-shaped heart (enlarged cardiac size); Kerley B lines, which are seen in the lower lung field; unfolding of the aorta; fluid in the major fissure; and alveolar edema.

116. (C) Atenolol.
Atenolol is a beta-blocker that reduces cardiac output by reducing the rate of the pumping action of the heart. In patients with heart failure with preserved ejection fraction, this effect of beta-blockers is harmful. This is because patients with this disorder already have severe diastolic function. Their cardiac output is therefore dependent on the heart rate. Reducing their heart rate can worsen their symptoms.

117. (D) Bilateral crepitations.
Bilateral crepitations are a clinical finding in left-sided heart failure. In this condition, there is a backflow of blood from the left ventricle into the pulmonary veins. This causes pulmonary edema and congestion that manifests as breathlessness, chest tightness, hemoptysis and bilateral crepitations at the basal lung fields.

118. (B) Epiglottitis.
Although the clinical features of croup and epiglottitis may overlap, the thumb sign seen on the X-ray of the neck confirms epiglottitis. Please note that acute epiglottitis requires immediate securing of the airway by qualified personnel in an operating room. This is because the risk of respiratory obstruction is very high.

119. (D) Wheezing.

Croup is an infection of the upper and lower airway by the parainfluenza virus. Clinical presentations include fever, sore throat, difficulty swallowing and drooling. There is a characteristic barking cough that is worse at night. There is also hoarseness and inspiratory stridor. On auscultation, there are crackles and diminished breath sounds. To get relief, the child may sit upright and lean forward, thrust his jaw forward and keep his mouth open (tripod position). Wheezing is heard when there is obstruction of small airways (bronchioles).

120. (C) Corynebacterium.

Corynebacterium diphtheriae is implicated in infections of the nasopharynx. Clinical features include sore throat, fever, malaise, tachycardia, headaches, chills and dysphagia. On throat examination, there is a characteristic exudate in the tonsillar area. This exudate is initially white and glossy but becomes grayish and fibrinous. It is so adherent to the underlying mucosa that scraping causes bleeding.

121. (B) Stomach insufflation.

Evidence of hyperventilation through an endotracheal tube includes stomach insufflation, tension pneumothorax and aspiration.

122. (D) Nasal flaring.

Nasal flaring is a sign of respiratory distress. In respiratory distress, the patient tries to compensate for failing respiratory function by increasing respiratory effort. Other signs include the use of accessory muscles of respiration, grunting, tachypnea, restlessness and anxiousness. In respiratory failure, the respiratory effort and drive are reduced.

123. (A) Prednisolone.

Prednisolone is an IV corticosteroid used in suppressing the immune response. However, it is effective for raised ICP caused by brain abscesses and tumors. Corticosteroids are not useful in cytotoxic edema caused by cell death (which is seen in traumatic brain injury). This is because of the potential of increasing serum glucose and worsening cerebral hypoxia. Hyperventilation causes hypocapnia, which stimulates vasoconstriction. IV hypertonic fluids like mannitol cause movement of fluid from the tissue space to the intravascular space, while diuretics like furosemide are used with mannitol to reduce the risk of pulmonary edema, a side effect of mannitol use.

124. (A) Vasoconstriction.

Hyperventilation with supplemental oxygen washes out carbon dioxide and induces hypocapnia. As a result of this, the cerebral arteries constrict to reduce cerebral blood perfusion, cerebral blood volume and consequently reduced intracranial pressure.

125. (C) Vancomycin.

Oral vancomycin is given as a gut antiseptic. Since it is not absorbed into the systemic circulation, it remains in the gut and exerts its antimicrobial properties on the gut mucosa. Probiotics have not been proven to be useful as treatment, although they are usually used. Oral metronidazole is no longer indicated in the treatment of clostridium difficile–induced diarrhea.

126. (C) Honey.

Infants under 12 months are not fed honey due to the risk of infections with clostridium botulinum. However, most cases of infant botulism are idiopathic.

127. (A) Home-canned foods.

Because home-canned foods are not heated to the appropriate temperature, they are likely to contain spores of clostridium botulinum. Foods like vegetables, fish, poultry, fruits, pork and dairy products are most implicated. In recent times, noncanned foods have been implicated in outbreaks in restaurants.

128. (D) Shingles.

Reactivation (shingles) is not a complication of measles infection. It is a complication of chicken pox infection. Complications of measles are encephalitis, conjunctivitis, pneumonia, purpura, sepsis and hepatitis.

129. (D) Live attenuated.

The chicken pox vaccine is a live attenuated vaccine made up of a wild strain of varicella with amounts of neomycin and gelatin.

130. (C) Eliciting tenderness.

This approach may be objective, but it does not promote patient comfort and safety. Suitable methods of assessing pain in patients with impaired cognition are observing facial expressions, body positions and mood; collecting information from the caregiver and using appropriate pain scales, such as the graphic pain scale.

131. (B) A patient with stage III colorectal cancer.

Long-term opioid therapy is indicated in palliative care, end-of-life care or terminal illness. This is because the benefits outweigh the risk of addiction and tolerance.

132. (D) Respiratory depression.

This is not an expected complication because the appropriate dose of opioid is given based on the patient's current physiology. Respiratory depression is a consequence of overdose and abuse, which are both rare in a controlled setting like a hospital.

133. (C) Cerebral edema.

Although fluid overload can increase the risk of pulmonary edema and heart failure, in this patient with an existing cerebral pathology, the risk of cerebral edema is greater.

134. (D) Serve small, frequent meals.

This intervention is most appropriate. Small meals can reduce the risk of nausea and vomiting, and serving food frequently can encourage the patient to eat. Option A is incorrect because passing a nasogastric tube should be a last resort and in the face of malnutrition. Spicy foods can worsen the patient's appetite. IV vitamin B complexes may not stimulate the patient's appetite. Moreover, vitamin B complexes like folic acid can stimulate the growth of cancer cells.

135. (D) Cerebral perfusion pressure – 50–70 mmHg.

In the management of raised ICP, both cerebral and intracranial perfusion pressure must be monitored. The goal of monitoring is to keep ICP at or below 20 mmHg and cerebral perfusion pressure at 50–70 mmHg. Option A is incorrect because the blood pressure of patients with malignant hypertension should not be crashed. Patients with hypotension are rapidly managed to improve cerebral perfusion. Option C is incorrect because hypocapnia is not a goal of treatment unless the managing physician decides to commence hyperventilation as a treatment option.

136. (C) Increases mucosal resistance.
Misoprostol is a synthetic prostaglandin analog that is used to reduce the risk of bleeding in patients with erosive ulcers. Prostaglandin is used in making the protective lining that cushions the stomach mucosa from the effects of hydrochloric acid. Prostaglandin also reduces the secretion of gastrin from the G cells in the antrum of the stomach. Gastrin stimulates the release of gastric acid from the parietal cells.

137. (D) Urobilinogen.
Urobilinogen is a byproduct of bilirubin formed by the action of bacterial flora in the gut. It is not expected to be increased in acute pyelonephritis unless there is existing liver disease or increased hemolysis. Nitrites are increased in acute pyelonephritis due to bacterial action on nitrates in the urine. Bacteria that release nitrate reductase are E. coli and Klebsiella. Red blood cells can be increased if there is hemolysis. Increased specific gravity means there are increased solutes in the urine due to either increased excretion of these solutes or dehydration. In acute pyelonephritis, there is excessive excretion of protein, red blood cells and white blood cells that can increase the urine's specific gravity.

138. (C) Trichomonas vaginalis.
Strawberry cervix is used to describe an erythematous cervix with a papilliform and punctate appearance. The most implicated organism is Trichomonas vaginitis, flagellate protozoa.

139. (A) Ceftriaxone + azithromycin.
In uncomplicated gonococcal infections, a stat dose of ceftriaxone 250 mg IM with 1 g of oral azithromycin is the preferable treatment. An alternative regimen

is a stat dose of 400 mg of oral cefixime with 1 g of oral azithromycin. In patients with allergies to azithromycin, doxycycline is used instead. Patients with allergies to cephalosporins like ceftriaxone are treated with either gentamicin or Gemifloxacin. Monotherapy is not used due to the increasing prevalence of antibiotic resistance.

140. (B) Contraceptives.
Contraceptives can prevent unwanted and unplanned pregnancies. However, they do not protect from sexually transmitted diseases. To reduce the risk of recurrence, all sexual partners in this patient must be screened and treated. They should also abstain from all sexual activities until they have completed their treatment regimen (which is about seven days).

141. (B) Reduces production of uric acid.
Allopurinol is a xanthine oxidase inhibitor that prevents the conversion of metabolites of nucleic acid to uric acid. It is given to patients with massive tumor load, at least two days before commencement of chemotherapy.

142. (B) Mesna.
Hemorrhagic cystitis is a complication of cyclophosphamide. To reduce the risk of this occurring, all patients must be premedicated with mesna. Mesna is a water-soluble agent that concentrates in the urine and binds with acrolein, a urotoxic metabolite, to form a stable and inactive compound that is readily excreted in the urine.

143. (D) SARS.
Reverse barrier nursing is indicated for patients with severe neutropenia and immunosuppression. This form of isolation is done to protect the patient from

getting infected by people and the environment. Principles used in reverse barrier nursing are the provision of a positive pressure isolation room, handwashing and use of adequate PPE when visiting the patient.

144. (B) Non-Hodgkin's lymphoma.
Tumor lysis syndrome is a metabolic syndrome characterized by hyperkalemia, hyperuricemia, hyperphosphatemia and hypocalcemia. It is caused by the rapid destruction of malignant blood cells and the release of their inflammatory intracellular components into the bloodstream. It occurs mainly in non-Hodgkin's lymphoma and acute leukemias.

145. (C) Painful
Loss of vision in amaurosis fugax is painless. Other features of loss of vision are sudden, temporary and severe unilateral or bilateral loss.

146. (D) Cataract.
Causes of amaurosis fugax include embolization from atherosclerotic plaque, endocarditis, atrial myxoma and fat. Other causes include sudden occlusion of the retinal arteries from transient ischemic attack and bleeding from neovascularization. Cataracts are an unlikely cause of the condition.

147. (B) Eye pain.
Retinal detachment is a painless eye condition. Symptoms include blurred vision, photopsia and floaters. Peripheral and central vision may be lost in severe cases. As the detachment worsens, the patient complains of grayness or veiling of the affected visual field.

148. (C) Ophthalmoscopy.

Retinal detachment is diagnosed via indirect ophthalmoscopy facilitated with dilatation of the pupils. This investigation not only diagnoses the detachment but differentiates the different types of detachment. Tonometry is used to determine intraocular pressure and diagnose glaucoma; a slit lamp test is used to diagnose ulcers and abrasions of the cornea; gonioscopy is used to assess the iridocorneal angle and diagnose angle-closure glaucoma.

149. (C) Eye patch on both eyes.

Immediate intervention includes placing a patient in the high Fowler's or semi-Fowler's position and using an eye shield to protect and rest the eyes. Also, intraocular pressure is monitored and controlled, and an ophthalmologist is consulted.

150. (B) Positive red reflex.

In globe laceration, the red reflex is absent. Other features of globe laceration are visible lacerations of the sclera or cornea, shallowness of the anterior chamber, raised intraocular pressure, nausea and vomiting.

151. (D) Diaphoresis.

Diaphoresis is a sign of opioid withdrawal. Features of opioid overdose are hypotension, bradycardia, respiratory depression, miosis, urinary retention, coma and death.

152. (B) Flumazenil.

Flumazenil is a benzodiazepine receptor blocker. It is given in acute intoxication to reverse sedation and respiratory depression.

153. (D) Dopamine reuptake inhibitor.
Bupropion is a norepinephrine and dopamine reuptake inhibitor. It increases circulating levels of norepinephrine and dopamine, improves mood and helps patients cope with symptoms of nicotine withdrawal.

154. (D) Increased appetite.
Features of amphetamine intoxication are delirium, toxic psychosis, tachycardia, nausea, vomiting, hyperthermia, seizures, stroke, arrhythmias and hypertension. In severe cases, rhabdomyolysis and acute kidney injury can occur. Increase appetite is not a feature of the condition.

155. (B) Antibiotics.
Clostridium difficile is an anaerobic bacteria found in the intestine. Infections occur when there is an overgrowth. This overgrowth is usually triggered by an alteration in the normal flora of the gut. The most implicated antibiotic is a cephalosporin (especially third generation), clindamycin, fluoroquinolones and penicillins.

156. (B) Examine the specimen in front of the police officer.
This is not appropriate because specimens are stored in tamperproof containers and packaged as soon as they are collected. The nurse must be sure she hands over the specimen to the designated person. To do this, she can ask for identification. She must document and sign off as she hands over and must have the recipient do the same.

157. (D) Hydrogen peroxide.
Hydrogen peroxide is appropriate for prepping the skin for venipuncture. To reduce the risk of obtaining a false-positive result, alcohol-containing antiseptics

are avoided. These antiseptics include isopropyl alcohol, povidone-iodine and tincture of iodine.

158. (D) Graphic scale.
The graphic scale, which often can include images of faces that range from grimacing to smiling or fruits of varying sizes, is typically only used for children or adults with impaired cognition or limited literacy.

159. (C) Placing the child in the left lateral position.
This intervention has the highest priority because it reduces the risk of aspiration. After the child is positioned appropriately, IV benzodiazepines and acetaminophen are administered. Tepid sponging is contraindicated.

160. (B) Breastfeeding should only be continued till he is six months old.
This statement is false. Exclusive breastfeeding should be done till the infant is six months old. Thereafter iron-rich formula and baby food is initiated. Breastfeeding should be continued till the child is two years.

161. (D) Brain MRI.
A brain CT scan is preferable because it is faster than an MRI. Also, CT scans are the first choice for CVAs. A brain MRI can then be done if the physician wants a better view of the nerves, blood vessels and other soft tissues. In this woman with a TIA, brain lesions are unlikely to be seen on CT scans. An ECG and a chest X-ray are necessary to diagnose an underlying cardiovascular pathology like hypertensive heart disease.

162. (D) Phase 1 Korotkoff sound is a blowing sound that indicates systolic blood pressure.

This statement is false because phase I Korotkoff sound is a thud. Phase II Korotkoff sound is a blowing or swishing noise. There are five different Korotkoff sounds heard during the deflation of the cuff. The first sound indicates systolic blood pressure, while the phase V sound indicates diastolic blood pressure.

163. (B) Protamine sulfate.
Protamine sulfate is a nonreversible antagonist of heparin. It is used for heparin overdose. It is also used to counter the effects of heparin, especially during surgery. Protamine is given IV as 1.0 to 1.5 mg for every 100 IU of circulating heparin. It is important to monitor PTT during the commencement of protamine sulfate.

164. (C) Inhibits platelet aggregation.
Aspirin is a potent NSAID used to reduce the risk of mortality in patients experiencing a myocardial infarction. Low-dose aspirin inhibits the production of thromboxane A2 in platelets. This effect reduces platelet aggregation and the formation of a platelet plug. About 325 mg of oral aspirin is given for immediate antiplatelet action. Patients are advised to chew or swallow the drug.

165. (A) Aortic valve.
The aortic valve is auscultated at the second right intercostal space. The pulmonic valve is auscultated on the second left intercostal space. The mitral valve is auscultated on the fifth intercostal space in the midclavicular line, while the tricuspid valve is auscultated on the third/fourth intercostal space at the sternal border.

166. (B) Outward.

The testes rotate inward during torsion. As a result of this, during manual detorsion, the testes are rotated outward. Success rates are variable, and more than one rotation may be required. If detorsion is unsuccessful, immediate surgery is required.

167. (B) Cystostomy.

An urgent suprapubic cystostomy must be immediately done by qualified personnel (most likely a surgeon) to avoid the risk of bladder rupture and to give relief to the patient. This patient most likely has a urethral stricture as the cause of his urinary retention.

168. (A) Use of a closed drainage system.

A closed drainage system (i.e., the urethral catheter is connected to a urine bag) is the most important measure in preventing a UTI. Prophylactic antibiotics, use of a silicone catheter and frequent changing of the catheter are not useful in this patient because his catheterization is short-term management until the fecal impaction is treated.

169. (C) Postobstructive diuresis.

Postobstructive diuresis is polyuria (urine excretion of at least 200 cc for at least two hours) after treatment of urinary retention. It also includes urine excretion of more than 3,000 cc in 24 hours. Causes include poor concentration effect of the kidneys, decreased reabsorption of sodium ions, urea retention and accumulation of atrial natriuretic peptide.

170. (A) Bladder cancer.
Bladder cancer is often characterized by painless hematuria and subsequent urinary retention from blood clots. A three-way catheter is needed for urine excretion and bladder irrigation to dislodge blood clots. A three-way catheter has three lumens: one for inflating the balloon, one for urine drainage and one for irrigation.

171. (B) IV dobutamine.
In shock, severe hypotension is caused by vasodilation of peripheral blood vessels. This vasodilation is triggered by an immune response to overwhelming sepsis. To counteract the toxins, inflammatory mediators released by the bacteria, white blood cells are released into the tissue spaces. For this to happen, there is dilation and increased permeability of the blood vessels. As sepsis worsens, cardiac output drops. Dobutamine increases the contraction of the heart and is useful in increasing cardiac output.

172. (D) Candida.
Septic shock is caused by hospital-acquired gram-negative or gram-positive bacteria. Fungi like Candida are rarely implicated. Routes of entry of these bacteria are via wounds, surgical incisions and invasive procedures like catheterization, thoracostomy, thoracocentesis and others. The risk for infection is high in neonates, elderly patients, bedridden patients and immunosuppressed patients.

173. (D) Hydroxyethylcellulose.
Isotonic crystalloids like normal saline, Ringer's lactate and 5% dextrose saline are the ideal fluids for resuscitation. In some cases, albumin is added to the initial

bolus used for acute resuscitation. Starchy fluids like hydroxyethyl cellulose should never be used for resuscitation because they worsen the outcome.

174. (C) Give vancomycin as an infusion over 30 minutes.
This patient is experiencing red man syndrome. To reduce the risk of this happening, vancomycin should not be given as a bolus injection but as an infusion over 30 minutes. In case of occurrence, the drug is to be stopped and the line flushed with normal saline. Then the remaining drug should be given as an infusion.

175. (A) Cefuroxime.
Cefuroxime is a second-generation cephalosporin suitable for empirical treatment in a neonate with jaundice. Ceftriaxone is unsuitable for neonates with jaundice. Gentamycin is unsuitable for neonates who have not made sufficient urine. This is because urine output must first be quantified to rule out kidney injury. Gentamycin is a nephrotoxic drug.

Test 3: Questions

1. Which of the following is the most common form of shoulder dislocation?

   A. Anterior

   B. Posterior

   C. Superior

   D. Inferior

2. Which of the following is not a complication of an anterior dislocation of the shoulder joint?

   A. Injury to the brachial plexus

   B. Injury to the axillary nerve

   C. Tear to the rotator cuff muscles

   D. Injury to the serratus anterior muscle

3. Which of the following structures will not be affected by an elbow dislocation?

   A. Brachial artery

   B. Ulnar nerve

   C. Median nerve

   D. Radial nerve

4. Which of the following age groups is most prone to subluxation of the radial head?

   A. Elderly

   B. Toddlers

   C. Neonates

   D. Teenagers

5. Which of the following structures is unlikely to be affected in a fracture of the proximal head of the humerus?

A. Radial nerve

B. Axillary artery

C. Axillary nerve

D. Brachial artery

6. A 45-year-old male who presents to the ER with cough, chest pain and difficulty breathing had an emergency chest tube thoracostomy for pulmonary tuberculosis. Which of the following is an indication for removal of the tube?

A. Drainage of 80 mL/day

B. When the fluid changes from purulent to serosanguinous

C. When chest X-ray is free from cavitations

D. As soon as anti-Koch's are commenced

7. Which of the following principles of management is inappropriate for a female patient who has just had a tracheostomy?

A. Place in the semi-Fowler's position

B. Frequent suctioning of oral secretions

C. Provision of a bell and a writing pad

D. Vital sign monitoring

8. Which of the following interventions is not useful in preventing the risk of aspiration in a patient with a tracheostomy?

A. Providing humidified oxygen

B. Provision of small semiliquid feeds

C. Placing the patient in a semi-Fowler's position

D. Infrequent suctioning after feeds

9. Which of the following treatment modalities is not useful in reducing the risk of infections in a patient with a tracheostomy?

A. Monitoring of temperature
B. Monitoring of white blood cell count
C. Stoma care
D. Prophylactic antibiotics

10. The emergency nurse is worried about the risk of shock in a 15-year-old male being managed in the ER with a tension pneumothorax. Which of the following best describes the pathophysiology of this complication?

A. Acute blood loss
B. Increased intrathoracic pressure
C. Decreased afterload
D. Impaired cardiac contractility

11. Which of the following is not a complication of mumps?

A. Orchitis
B. Conjunctivitis
C. Pancreatitis
D. Meningitis

12. You are counseling the mother of a two-week-old infant with bronchopneumonia on the benefits of breast milk in preventing infections. Which of the following is not an antibacterial benefit?

A. IgA transmission
B. Bifidus factor
C. Omega 3 fatty acid
D. Lactoferrin

13. A five-year-old male who is being managed for mumps may be given all of the following foods except:

A. Semisolids
B. Citruses
C. Green vegetables
D. Mashed foods

14. Which of the following patients is least at risk of developing tetanus?

A. A patient with third-degree burns
B. An IV drug abuser with infectious endocarditis
C. A patient with a gunshot injury
D. A patient with caustic poisoning

15. Which of the following is not a complication of meningococcal meningitis?

A. SIADH
B. DIC
C. Gangrene
D. Left ventricular heart failure

16. Which of the following bacteria is least likely implicated in a two-week-old female with acute bacterial meningitis?

A. E. coli
B. Listeria monocytogenes
C. Haemophilus influenzae
D. Streptococcus agalactiae

17. Which of the following best describes Waterhouse-Friderichsen syndrome?

A. Excess secretion of ADH
B. Insufficient plasma cortisol
C. Excess secretion of aldosterone
D. Insufficient plasma insulin

18. Which of the following patients in the children's ER is least at risk of developing febrile seizures?

A. A three-month-old male with meningitis.
B. A four-year-old female with acute tonsillitis
C. A six-month-old female with acute pharyngitis
D. A two-year-old female with chicken pox

19. A 67-year-old male who presents to the ER with crushing chest pain has an emergency ECG that reveals ST elevation in leads II, III and aVF. Which of the following arteries is most likely to be occluded?

A. Right coronary artery
B. Left coronary artery
C. Right subclavian artery
D. Left subclavian artery

20. A 55-year-old male is having an emergency ECG for crushing chest pain, nausea and headaches. Which of the following statements is false about the P wave?

A. It is usually less than 0.11 seconds.
B. It indicates atrial depolarization.
C. It indicates electrical impulses from the AV node.
D. It is upright in a normal sinus rhythm.

21. Which of the following is not a component of Beck's triad seen in a 25-year-old male who presents to the ER with blunt trauma to the chest?

A. Distended neck veins
B. Hypotension
C. Muffled heart sounds
D. Pulsus paradoxus

22. A 55-year-old male who is being managed for myocardial infarction has been stable in the past 48 hours. The patient is being worked up for discharge when the nurse notices on the monitor that the patient is in ventricular tachycardia. On examination, the patient is alert and conscious. There is no cyanosis. Which of the following interventions is most appropriate for this patient?

A. IV epinephrine
B. IV procainamide
C. Defibrillation
D. IV atropine

23. Nurse M notices that her patient, who is being managed for STEMI, has gone into atrial fibrillation. She quickly proceeds to perform a carotid massage. Which of the following best describes the mechanism of action of this procedure?

A. Vasovagal nerve stimulation
B. Baroreflex stimulation
C. Valsalva maneuver
D. Increases intrathoracic pressure

24. You are monitoring a patient who was brought into the ER with altered sensorium secondary to opioid overdose. You notice on the cardiac monitor that the patient is in ventricular fibrillation. Which of the following interventions is most appropriate?

A. Defibrillation
B. Cardiac pacemaker
C. Endotracheal intubation
D. IV dobutamine

25. A 56-year-old male is being managed for supraventricular tachycardia. The nurse teaches the patient how to perform the Valsalva maneuver when he anticipates an impending attack. Which of the following best describes the correct way the patient should perform the Valsalva maneuver?

A. Massage his sternal notch
B. Hold his breath for 30 seconds
C. Inhale air, pinch his nose, close his mouth, and attempt to expel the air through his mouth
D. Pinch his nose, close his ears and attempt to cough

26. Which of the following conditions is unlikely to cause a transudative pleural effusion?

A. Left ventricular heart failure
B. Nephrotic syndrome
C. Liver cirrhosis
D. Pulmonary embolism

27. Which of the following is a contraindication to cricothyrotomy?

A. Severe facial edema
B. Failed orotracheal intubation
C. Toddlers
D. Obesity

28. Emergency cricothyrotomy is being performed on a 45-year-old female who presents to the ER with respiratory failure secondary to upper airway infection. Which of the following is not an acute complication of this procedure?

A. Hemorrhage
B. Apnea
C. Subglottic stenosis
D. Vocal cord injury

29. Which of the following is a contraindication to noninvasive positive pressure ventilation?

A. Obstructive sleep apnea
B. Acute asthma
C. Pulmonary edema
D. Epiglottitis

30. Which of the following is not a clinical feature of Horner's syndrome?

A. Ptosis
B. Mydriasis
C. Anhidrosis
D. Enophthalmos

31. Which of the following is a contraindication to testing the oculovestibular reflex?

A. Cervical spine injury
B. Hemotympanum
C. Vomiting
D. Raised ICP

32. Which of the following describes a positive Kernig sign?

A. Flexion of the knee joint when the neck is passively rotated
B. Flexion of the knees when the neck is passively flexed
C. Inability to extend the knee when the hip and knees are both flexed at 90°
D. Inability to stand with the legs apart and the eyes closed

33. Which of the following is most required before commencing a lumbar puncture in a patient with meningitis?

A. Tonometry
B. Fundoscopy
C. Lumbar X-ray
D. Hematocrit

34. A 25-year-old female who is being managed for ectopic pregnancy is most likely to have the embryo implanted in which of the following areas?

A. Uterine cornua
B. Ovary
C. Fallopian tube
D. Cervix

35. Which of the following is not a risk factor of ectopic pregnancy?

A. Previous ectopic pregnancy
B. Pelvic inflammatory disease
C. Progestin-only pill
D. Multiple sex partners

36. Which of the following is the definitive treatment in a female patient who presents to the ER with a ruptured ectopic pregnancy?

A. Methotrexate
B. Salpingotomy
C. Salpingectomy
D. Bilateral tubal ligation

37. Which of the following is not an absolute indication of a caesarean section?

A. Major degree placenta previa
B. Previous history of myomectomy
C. Two previous caesarean sections
D. Twin gestation

38. You are about to discharge a patient who presented to the ER with a history of febrile seizures secondary to acute pharyngitis. Which of the following does not increase the child's risk of developing a seizure disorder in the future?

A. Complex febrile seizures
B. Delay of developmental milestones
C. History of seizures in siblings
D. Older children

39. Which of the following drugs is unsuitable for use in a four-year-old male being managed for a persistent complex febrile seizure?

A. Lorazepam
B. Valproate
C. Phenobarbital
D. Fosphenytoin

40. Which of the following antipyretics is unsuitable for use in a five-year-old male who is being managed for varicella-zoster infection?

A. Aspirin
B. Ibuprofen
C. Acetaminophen
D. Celecoxib

41. Which of the following antiseizure drugs is unsuitable for use in a 35-year-old female with a BMI of 28 kg/m2?

A. Lamotrigine
B. Valproic acid
C. Ethosuximide
D. Carbamazepine

42. Which of the following antiseizure drugs is suitable in a 24-year-old G2 P 0+1 who was managed in the ER with generalized tonic-clonic seizures and is set for discharge?

A. Ethosuximide
B. Carbamazepine
C. Lamotrigine
D. Valproate

43. Which of the following positions is most appropriate in a patient who has just had a lumbar puncture for suspected meningitis?

A. Fowler's position
B. Semi-Fowler's position
C. Supine position
D. Prone position

44. A 45-year-old male who is being managed for meningitis has a CSF analysis report showing lymphocytosis, elevated protein in the CSF and reduced CSF glucose. Which of the following organisms is most likely implicated?

A. Streptococcus pneumonia
B. Histoplasma capsulatum
C. Neisseria meningitidis
D. Listeria monocytogenes

45. Which of the following clinical findings differentiates tension pneumothorax from cardiac tamponade in a 25-year-old male who presents to the ER with tachypnea and distended neck veins secondary to blunt trauma to the chest?

A. Muffled heart sounds
B. Hypotension
C. Hyperresonant hemithorax
D. Pulsus paradoxus

46. A 58-year-old female presented to the ER with diaphoresis, shortness of breath and crushing chest pain that radiates to the left shoulder. Blood pressure at presentation was 160/100 mmHg. A differential diagnosis of myocardial infarction was made, and the patient commenced tabs aspirin and sublingual nitroglycerin. Which of the following is most required to quickly detect the location of the infarct?

A. Angiography
B. Electrocardiogram
C. Echocardiogram
D. Cardiac enzymes

47. A 56-year-old female who presents to the ER with shortness of breath, cough and hemoptysis has a blood pressure of 160/100 mmHg. Which of the following is most responsible for the high diastolic blood pressure in this patient?

A. Cardiac output
B. Stroke volume
C. Vascular resistance
D. Baroreceptors

48. A 65-year-old female presents to the ER with diaphoresis, crushing chest pain and shortness of breath. On examination, BP is 169/90 mmHg and PR is 90 bpm. Emergency chest X-ray reveals ST elevation. The attending physician requests a cardiac enzyme assay. The emergency nurse expects which of the following cardiac enzymes to be first elevated?

A. Lactate dehydrogenase
B. Troponin I
C. Creatinine kinase
D. Myoglobin

49. Which of the following is an immediate complication of compartment syndrome?

A. Contractures
B. Rhabdomyolysis
C. Hyperkalemia
D. Tissue necrosis

50. Which of the following is not a cause of compartment syndrome?

A. Fracture
B. Snakebite
C. Crush injuries
D. Rhabdomyolysis

51. You expect the doctor to order a serum assay of which of the following enzymes in a patient with rhabdomyolysis?

A. Myoglobin
B. Lactate dehydrogenase
C. Creatine kinase
D. Pyruvate kinase

52. Which of the following is an immediate complication in a patient who is being managed for rhabdomyolysis?

A. Acute kidney injury
B. Hypokalemia
C. Elevated liver enzymes
D. Hyperpyrexia

53. Which of the following drugs is used in managing a patient with malignant hyperthermia?

A. Flumazenil
B. Dantrolene
C. Baclofen
D. Lorazepam

54. Which of the following questions is most suitable in clarifying a patient's ethnicity?

A. Are you an immigrant?
B. What year did you come to America?
C. What is your ethnic group?
D. What country do you come from?

55. Which of the following ethnic groups is most likely to involve the extended family and relatives before making health-related decisions?

A. Asian
B. West African
C. Nordic
D. British

56. Which of the following treatment modalities is inappropriate in a 17-year-old patient with pelvic inflammatory disease?

A. Contact tracing
B. Empirical antibiotics
C. Psychological evaluation
D. Cervical cancer screening

57. Which of the following is not a risk factor for candidal vaginitis?

A. Diabetes mellitus
B. Obesity
C. Contraceptive
D. Menopause

58. Which of the following bedside investigations is required in differentiating COPD from pulmonary edema in a 45-year-old female who presents to the ER with cough, dyspnea, diaphoresis and cyanosis?

A. Pulse oximetry
B. Serum BNP/NT-proBNP
C. Chest X-ray
D. Angiography

59. Which of the following clinical features is most important in differentiating a case of pulmonary edema from a case of exacerbated COPD?

A. Fever
B. Hemoptysis
C. Crepitations
D. High blood pressure

60. A 56-year-old male who is being managed for acute left ventricular heart failure is being placed in the high Fowler's position for relief of dyspnea. Which of the following best explains the function of this position?

A. Decreased intrathoracic pressure
B. Decreased work of breathing
C. Decreased preload
D. Increased cerebral perfusion

61. A patient who presents to the ER with acute pulmonary edema secondary to congestive heart failure is being managed with supplemental oxygen, furosemide and digoxin. Which of the following is important for monitoring to reduce the risk of shock?

A. Fluid status
B. Serum potassium
C. Hematocrit
D. BUN

62. Which of the following is a primary mechanism of pulmonary edema in a 16-year-old female being managed for acute glomerulonephritis?

A. Increased hydrostatic pressure
B. Increased oncotic pressure
C. Increased capillary permeability
D. Obstructed lymphatic drainage

63. Which of the following is a cause of cor pulmonale?

A. Ventricular septal defect
B. Chronic bronchitis
C. Congestive heart failure
D. Eisenmenger syndrome

64. Which of the following is most appropriate in excluding an ectopic pregnancy from a ruptured ovarian cyst?

A. Hematocrit
B. B-HCG
C. Abdominopelvic ultrasound
D. Speculum examination

65. A 25-year-old female who is being managed for rape is to return after six weeks for all of these follow-up tests except:

A. Hepatitis
B. HIV
C. Chlamydia
D. Pap smear

66. A 25-year-old female who is being managed for rape is set to commence postexposure prophylaxis. During the history, it was discovered that the patient has been immunized against the hepatitis B virus. To confer protection against hepatitis from blood and semen exposure from the assailant, which of the following interventions is most appropriate?

A. Ribavirin
B. Hepatitis B immune globulin
C. Repeat vaccination
D. Follow-up test at six weeks

67. Which of the following contraceptive methods is most appropriate for a patient who presents to the ER with a history of rape three days before presentation?

A. Levonorgestrel
B. Copper IUD
C. Estrogen-only pill
D. BTL

68. After hemodynamic control, which of the following interventions must be prioritized in a 25-year-old patient who presents to the ER with vaginal bleeding at 26 weeks gestation?

A. Pelvic examination
B. Pelvic ultrasound
C. Partial thromboplastin time
D. Complete blood count

69. Which of the following is not a complication of abruptio placentae?

A. DIC
B. Rh sensitization
C. Eclampsia
D. Birth asphyxia

70. Which of the following is not a risk factor for placental abruption?

A. Hypertension
B. Previous caesarean section
C. Polyhydramnios
D. Abdominal trauma

71. Which of the following is not a disease-modifying antirheumatic drug?

A. Methotrexate
B. Diclofenac
C. Leflunomide
D. Hydroxychloroquine

72. In which of the following conditions is osteomyelitis secondary to salmonella infection most likely?

A. Hemodialysis
B. Diabetes mellitus
C. Pressure ulcers
D. Sickle cell anemia

73. Which of the following is the initial management of a patient who presents to the ER with neck pain following a fall?

A. Analgesia
B. Cervical collar
C. Physiotherapy
D. Cervical spine X-ray

74. Which of the following is the most common area of fractures in children?

A. Wrist
B. Clavicle
C. Elbow
D. Tibia

75. A patient who presents to the ER with sciatica has just been placed on gabapentin. Which of the following best describes the function of this drug in this patient?

A. Muscle relaxant
B. Anxiolytic
C. Anticonvulsant
D. Analgesia

76. Which of the following is not a function of heat therapy in pain relief?

A. Decreases blood flow
B. Reduces tissue edema
C. Decreases muscle spasm
D. Increases muscle extensibility

77. Which of the following interventions is unnecessary in a patient with a sprain of the ankle?

A. Elevation
B. Compression
C. Rest
D. Heat therapy

78. During the assessment of circulation in a trauma patient, which of the following is correct?

A. Capillary refill is the best assessment for circulation.
B. Cyanosis is best appreciated in the nail bed.
C. Cold, clammy extremities are signs of shock.
D. Hyperpyrexia increases pulse rate, respiratory rate and blood pressure.

79. A patient who just had an emergency exploratory laparotomy for peritonitis is placed on oral Oxycodone. Which of the following side effects is most unlikely to occur in this patient?

A. Nausea
B. Constipation
C. Dizziness
D. Anorexia

80. A 20-year-old female who presents to the ER says that a vampire has been stalking her. She is seen to be clicking her fingers and grimacing constantly. Which of the following diagnoses is most appropriate?

A. Catatonic schizophrenia
B. Major depression
C. Mania
D. Bipolar disorder

81. A 35-year-old woman with a known history of cannabis abuse presents to the ER and states that Michael Jackson is forcing her to marry him. Which of the following diagnoses is most appropriate?

A. Voyeurism
B. Delusion of grandeur
C. Delusion of persecution
D. Erotomania

82. Which of the following is not a risk factor for suicide?

A. Male sex
B. Age less than 40 years
C. Unemployment
D. Alcohol abuse

83. Which of the following is a feature of acrocyanosis in a 35-year-old female who presents to the ER with bluish discoloration of her fingers, a burning sensation and paresthesia?

A. Trophic changes
B. Persistent cyanosis
C. Tenderness of the fingers
D. Absent pulses

84. Which of the following is not a risk factor of peripheral arterial disease?

A. Cigarette smoking
B. Atherosclerosis
C. Female sex
D. Diabetes

85. Which of the following is not a skin manifestation of peripheral arterial disease?

A. Necrosis
B. Dependent rubor
C. Skin atrophy
D. Lichenification

86. Which of the following interventions is suitable to delegate to a nursing assistant in a patient with chronic bronchitis?

A. Monitoring of vital signs every four hours
B. Positioning the patient in the high Fowler's position
C. Teaching the patient how to use a metered-dose inhaler
D. Administering oral antibiotics

87. Which of the following interventions is not suitable for a licensed nurse in the management of a patient with upper GI bleeding secondary to perforated peptic ulcer disease?

A. Assessment of pulse rate and blood pressure
B. Administration of IV omeprazole
C. Assessment of the patient's buccal mucosa and nail beds for pallor
D. Encouraging the patient to eat

88. The nursing assistant informs you that the patient on IV fluids complains of swelling and tenderness of the cannulated arm. Which of the following interventions is most appropriate?

A. Ask the nursing assistant to check the patient's pulse rate
B. Ask the nursing assistant to administer IV acetaminophen
C. Inspect and remove the infiltrated line
D. Wait for the infusion to be over

89. Which of the following patients is most suitable to assign to a newly employed emergency nurse?

A. A 56-year-old male with STEMI
B. A 75-year-old female with pulmonary edema
C. A 45-year-old male with chronic bronchitis
D. A 24-year-old female with acute PID

90. A patient with peripheral arterial disease is being managed with clopidogrel, an antiplatelet drug. Which of the following best describes the mechanism of action of this drug?

A. Glycoprotein IIb/IIIa inhibitor
B. Cyclooxygenase inhibitor
C. ADP inhibitor
D. Leukotriene receptor blocker

91. Which of the following is not a risk factor of venous insufficiency of the lower limbs?

A. Obesity
B. Dyslipidemia
C. Pregnancy
D. Elderly age

92. A patient who presents with a chronic venous ulcer will benefit from which of the following interventions?

A. Antiplatelet drugs
B. Venous ligation
C. Compression stockings
D. Skin grafting

93. A patient who was admitted into the ER with agitation, psychosis and violent behavior was given IM diazepam and haloperidol. You notice later that the patient is unable to move. Which of the following interventions is most appropriate?

A. Flumazenil
B. Baclofen
C. Benztropine
D. Naltrexone

94. A 45-year-old female presents to the ER with agitation, distress and racing thoughts. She is a known bipolar patient who has not been compliant with her drugs. The attending physician decides to commence her on lithium. Which of the following is not necessary for monitoring in lithium therapy?

A. Thyroid function
B. Creatinine
C. Liver function
D. Urea

95. Which of the following is not a contraindication of ECT?

A. Pneumonia
B. Recent STEMI
C. Goiter
D. Arrhythmia

96. Which of the following conditions is suitable for ECT?

A. General anxiety disorder
B. Major depressive disorder
C. Psychosis
D. Dissociative disorder

97. Which of the following conditions is unsuitable for cognitive behavioral therapy?

A. Generalized anxiety disorder
B. Nicotine addiction
C. Anorexia nervosa
D. Schizophrenia

98. Dryness of the mucosa of the mouth and blurred vision are side effects of antipsychotics due to blockage of which of the following receptors?

A. Histamine
B. Dopamine
C. Acetylcholine
D. Norepinephrine

99. A 35-year-old male who presents to the ER is being managed with a tricyclic antidepressant for depression. Which of the following is not an example of this class of drug?

A. Amitriptyline
B. Clomipramine
C. Doxepin
D. Fluoxetine

100. The mother of a five-year-old female with chicken pox wants to know if her daughter can be reinfected with chicken pox. You tell her that this is unlikely due to which of the following?

A. Active natural immunity
B. Passive natural immunity
C. Active artificial immunity
D. Passive artificial immunity

101. A patient with tetanus infection is being managed with tetanus immune globulin. Which of the following best describes the purpose of this drug?

A. Active immunity
B. Neutralization of circulating toxins
C. Prevention of further release of toxins
D. Sedation

102. Which of the following is not an intervention in a patient with tetanus?

A. Frequent turning
B. Hyperalimentation
C. Treatment in a bright room
D. Mechanical ventilation

103. Which of the following is a risk factor of herpes zoster infection?

A. HIV
B. Pregnancy
C. Diabetes mellitus
D. Sickle cell anemia

104. Which of the following strains of the human papillomavirus is implicated in cervical cancer?

A. HPV 6
B. HPV 8
C. HPV 18
D. HPV 11

105. A child who presents to the ER with infectious mononucleosis is at risk of developing which of the following cancers?

A. Acute lymphoblastic leukemia
B. Acute lymphocytic leukemia
C. Non-Hodgkin's lymphoma
D. Burkitt's lymphoma

106. A 56-year-old female who presents to the ER with chronic anemia and vaginal bleeding secondary to uterine bleeding is being managed with IV tranexamic acid. Which of the following best describes the mechanism of action of this drug?

A. GnRH agonist
B. Androgen receptor agonist
C. Estrogen receptor modulator
D. Antifibrinolytic

107. Which of the following interventions is contraindicated in a 78-year-old female who presents to the ER with severe vaginal bleeding secondary to cervical cancer?

A. Blood transfusion
B. Vasopressors
C. Speculum examination
D. Vaginal packing

108. A 38-year-old female who presents to the ER with vaginal bleeding is being worked up for a myomectomy. Part of her pretreatment includes leuprolide. Which of the following best describes the rationale behind the use of the drug?

A. Shrinks fibroids
B. Antifibrinolytic
C. Estrogen receptor blocker
D. Androgen receptor agonist

109. Which of the following is not a cause for menorrhagia?

A. Family history
B. Hyperthyroidism
C. Infection
D. Anorexia nervosa

110. To reduce the incidence of MRSA in hospital settings, which of the following is not useful?

A. Handwashing
B. Isolation procedures
C. Empirical therapy
D. Sensitivity studies

111. In the Mantoux test, protein-derived tuberculin is administered to trigger which of the following hypersensitivity reactions?

A. Type I
B. Type II
C. Type III
D. Type IV

112. A patient who presents to the ER with symptoms of withdrawal from valium will be managed with which of the following?

A. Gabapentin
B. Benzodiazepines
C. Naltrexone
D. Bupropion

113. Which of the following samples is most appropriate for collection in a two-year-old female with suspected tuberculosis?

A. Sputum
B. Stool
C. Gastric acid
D. Saliva

114. Which of the following is not a symptom of withdrawal from opioids?

A. Lacrimation
B. Rhinorrhea
C. Diarrhea
D. Increased appetite

115. A patient who presents to the ER with symptoms of withdrawal from opioid abuse is being managed with methadone. What is the mechanism of action of this drug?

A. Opioid receptor antagonist
B. Opioid receptor agonist
C. Dopamine receptor agonist
D. Dopamine reuptake inhibitor

116. Which of the following is a definitive treatment of endometriosis?

A. Surgical resection
B. Total abdominal hysterectomy
C. Leuprolide
D. Danazol

117. Which of the following is not a goal of treatment in the management of a rape victim?

A. HIV PEEP
B. Emergency contraceptives
C. Psychological evaluation
D. Religious counseling

118. Which of the following is not a clinical feature of a manic episode of bipolar disorder?

A. Grandiosity
B. Hypersomnia
C. Distractibility
D. Talkativeness

119. Which of the following best describes stereotyping?

A. Nurse M serves a kosher diet to a Jewish patient.
B. Nurse M places a Muslim patient on the east side of the ER.
C. Nurse M assumes that a geriatric patient cannot use a glucometer.
D. Nurse M encourages an end-of-life patient to talk to a priest.

120. Which of the following does not contribute to high mortality rates in homeless patients?

A. Premorbid conditions
B. Malnutrition
C. Inefficient access to health care
D. Insufficient health funds

121. A 23-year-old woman presents to the ER in distress. She complains that her right arm is rotten and smelly, although this is not the case. Which of the following drugs is most appropriate for use in this patient?

A. Citalopram
B. Risperidone
C. Lithium
D. Amitriptyline

122. A 35-year-old female who presents to the ER with psychosis and agitation is being managed with olanzapine. Which of the following best describes the mechanism of action of this drug?

A. Dopamine receptor agonist
B. Serotonin receptor agonist
C. Norepinephrine receptor antagonist
D. Dopamine receptor antagonist

123. Which of the following is not a side effect of antipsychotics?

A. Dry mouth
B. Tardive dyskinesia
C. Blurred vision
D. Diarrhea

124. A patient with polycythemia vera is at increased risk of all of the following except:

A. Deep venous thrombosis
B. Iron deficiency
C. Stroke
D. Peripheral arterial disease

125. Which of the following is not useful in reducing the risk of deep vein thrombosis in an obese patient who presents to the ER with STEMI?

A. Early ambulation
B. Subcutaneous heparin
C. Compression stocking
D. Physiotherapy

126. Unfractionated heparins are more suitable for use than lower-weight molecular heparin in which of the following conditions?

A. Liver failure
B. Renal failure
C. Myocardial infarction
D. Stroke

127. Which of the following surgeries has the least risk of DVT?

A. Hip arthroplasty
B. Knee arthroplasty
C. Elective neurosurgery
D. Appendectomy

128. A patient who presents to the ER with peripheral arterial disease is being managed with cholestyramine for atherosclerosis. Which of the following best describes the mechanism of action of this drug?

A. Increases serum HDL
B. Inhibits absorption of cholesterol in the intestine
C. Inhibits absorption of bile acids
D. Inhibits production of cholesterol

129. Which of the following is not a purpose of therapeutic communication techniques?

A. To ease a patient's anxiety
B. To give moral advice
C. To educate the patient
D. To form a nurse-patient relationship

130. Which of the following is not a therapeutic communication technique?

A. Use of open-ended questions
B. Use of silence
C. Active listening
D. Probing

131. A patient who presents to the ER has just been diagnosed with pancreatic cancer. This patient, however, refuses to accept this diagnosis and tells his visiting friends that he has stomach flu. Which of the following defense mechanisms is being demonstrated?

A. Suppression
B. Denial
C. Regression
D. Sublimation

132. A patient who has just received a diagnosis of advanced lung cancer has become aggressive and impatient toward his wife. Which of the following defense mechanisms is being demonstrated?

A. Denial
B. Regression
C. Displacement
D. Reaction formation

133. According to West African culture, which of the following gestures is deemed offensive?

A. Direct eye contact
B. Sitting with the legs crossed
C. Offering your left hand for a handshake
D. Snapping your fingers

134. Which of the following nationalities is likely to avoid direct eye contact during a conversation?

A. Japanese
B. Nigerian
C. Indian
D. British

135. A 19-year-old female who presents to the ER with fever, malaise and polyarthritis is being managed for acute rheumatic fever. Which of the following is not a component of the major criteria according to the modified Jones criteria?

A. Pancarditis
B. Sydenham chorea
C. Hyperpyrexia
D. Subcutaneous nodules

136. Which of the following is an unlikely cause of rheumatic fever in a 17-year-old female who presents to the ER with fever, polyarthritis and difficulty breathing?

A. Overcrowding
B. Malnutrition
C. Incomplete vaccination
D. Poor personal hygiene

137. Which of the following is not a principle of management in a 17-year-old female who is being managed for acute rheumatic fever?

A. Eradication of existing pathogen with penicillin G
B. Inhibition of platelet aggregation with aspirin
C. Immunosuppression with prednisolone
D. Antibiotic prophylaxis till age 40

138. A 25-year-old female presented to the ER with a history of burning sensation, paresthesia and pallor of her fingers. On examination, there was pallor and cyanosis of the ring, middle and little fingers on both hands. A diagnosis of Raynaud's syndrome was made. Which of the following drugs is unsuitable in the management of this patient?

A. Prazosin
B. Nitroglycerin
C. Atenolol
D. Nifedipine

139. A 25-year-old male is being managed in the ER for hemothorax secondary to a road traffic accident. On admission, the patient was in shock, and two units of packed cells were transfused. However, the patient remains in a hemodynamically unstable state. Which of the following treatment modalities is required in this patient?

A. Thoracocentesis
B. Tube thoracostomy
C. Thoracotomy
D. Pericardiocentesis

140. Which of the following is not a pathophysiologic process in a patient who is being managed in the ER for respiratory acidosis secondary to emphysema?

A. Loss of elastic recoil
B. Airway remodeling
C. Loss of alveolar septa
D. Compression of the lung parenchyma

141. A 56-year-old female who is being managed for pulmonary edema secondary to left ventricular heart failure was given IV morphine. Which of the following is not an important effect of morphine for this patient?

A. Reduces anxiety
B. Vasodilation
C. Reduces work of breathing
D. Increases heart rate

142. A 45-year-old female presents to the ER with anxiousness, cyanosis, difficulty breathing, cough and diaphoresis. On examination, BP is 100/60 mmHg and PR is 120 bpm. On auscultation, bilateral crepitations are heard. A differential diagnosis of pulmonary edema is made. Which of the following is an expected finding on a chest X-ray to confirm this diagnosis?

A. Kerley B lines
B. Meniscus sign
C. Unfolding of the aorta
D. Ground glass appearance

143. A 45-year-old female with a known seizure disorder was admitted into the ER with focal seizures. During the discharge, her attending physician counsels her to visit her primary care physician to change her prescription due to enlargement of her gums. Which of the following antiseizure drugs is unlikely to cause this?

A. Phenytoin
B. Valproic acid
C. Lamotrigine
D. Ethosuximide

144. Which of the following is not a clinical feature of shunt obstruction in a 13-year-old female being managed for hydrocephalus secondary to meningitis?

A. Personality problems
B. Projectile vomiting
C. Head enlargement
D. Headaches

145. A 16-year-old female presents to the ER with a history of fever, vomiting, headaches and loss of consciousness of three days duration. She had a ventricular shunt procedure six weeks ago for hydrocephalus secondary to acute bacterial meningitis. Which of the following organisms is most likely to cause an infection in her shunt?

A. Staphylococcus aureus
B. Staphylococcus epidermidis
C. Streptococcus agalactiae
D. Candida albicans

146. A four-year-old presents to the ER with a history of vomiting, headaches and irritability. The child had a VP shunt inserted six months ago for hydrocephalus. On examination, the child is afebrile, with elevated blood pressure and heart rate. The shunt track is also swollen. Which of the following dysfunctions is most likely?

A. Infection
B. Obstruction
C. Overdrainage
D. Subdural hematoma

147. Which of the following is not a complication of overdrainage of ventriculoperitoneal shunts?

A. Chiari malformation
B. Slit-like ventricles
C. Subdural hematoma
D. Ascites

148. Which of the following is not a side effect of lithium use?

A. Polyuria
B. Polydipsia
C. Weight loss
D. Tremors

149. A 54-year-old female presents to the ER with a history of nausea and a metallic taste in her mouth. She was recently placed on a drug for bipolar disorder. Which drug is most likely the cause of her symptoms?

A. Sodium valproate
B. Lithium
C. Olanzapine
D. Lamotrigine

150. Which of the following is not a sign of lithium toxicity?

A. Tinnitus
B. Seizures
C. Hyporeflexia
D. Arrhythmias

151. A 35-year-old patient who presents to the ER with depression is placed on tricyclic antidepressants. Which of the following best describes the mechanism of action of this drug?

A. Dopamine reuptake inhibitor
B. Dopamine receptor antagonist
C. Serotonin receptor agonist
D. Serotonin reuptake inhibitor

152. Which of the following is not a side effect of ECT?

A. Memory loss
B. Confusion
C. Vomiting
D. Hallucinations

153. A patient who presents to the ER is being managed with probenecid for gout. Which of the following best describes the mechanism of action of this drug?

A. Analgesia
B. Immunomodulator
C. Inhibits production of uric acid
D. Increases excretion of uric acid

154. A patient who is being managed for acute gouty attacks should avoid all these foods except:

A. Offal
B. Beer
C. Seafood
D. Skim milk

155. A five-year-old male who is being managed for infectious mononucleosis is most at risk of which of the following complications?

A. Splenic rupture
B. Heart failure
C. Glomerulonephritis
D. Meningitis

156. A patient who was managed in the ER for a severe scabies infestation will be counseled to do all these except:

A. Sun-dry and store all clothes in airtight bags
B. Contact tracing
C. Avoid sharing bedsheets and towels
D. Avoid sharing utensils

157. To reduce the incidence of vancomycin resistance, vancomycin should not be used in which of the following conditions?

A. MRSA-mediated endocarditis
B. Clostridium difficile–induced diarrhea
C. Multidrug-resistant streptococcus pneumoniae
D. Pulmonary tuberculosis

158. Which of the following features of Staphylococcus aureus contributes to its rising prevalence of resistance to beta-lactam antibiotics?

A. Penicillinase
B. Coagulase
C. Exotoxin
D. Peptidoglycan

159. Which of the following ethnic groups is most at risk of type 2 diabetes mellitus?

A. Hispanics
B. Native Americans
C. African Americans
D. Nordics

160. An African American has an increased risk of all of the following conditions except:

A. Hypertension
B. Fibroids
C. Diabetes mellitus type 2
D. Cystic fibrosis

161. Which of the following approaches is most effective in reducing the incidence of patient boarding in emergency rooms?

A. Employing more emergency nurses
B. Providing more primary care providers
C. Providing more beds in emergency rooms
D. Creating more emergency rooms

162. Which of the following is not an effect of patient boarding?

A. Increased turnover of radiological reports
B. Assault to staff
C. Medication errors
D. Sepsis

163. Nurse M is about to commence her night shift. For an effective handover, Nurse M is expected to do all of the following except:

A. Repeat received information
B. Review current vital sign data
C. Question the caregivers on nursing interventions done so far
D. Inquire about the most acutely ill patients

164. Nurse P is about to transfer a patient with opioid overdose from the ER to a rehabilitation facility. Which of the following is not required for documentation in the transfer report?

A. Drug allergies
B. Clinical presentation
C. Food preferences
D. Socioeconomic status

165. Which of the following is a contraindication to vaginal birth after caesarean section?

A. One previous history of vertical uterine incision
B. The fetus having a cephalic presentation at term
C. The fetus weighing 3.5 kg
D. The fetus having a heart rate of 135 bpm in the first stage of labor

166. Which of the following is not a useful method of inducing labor in a 35-year-old female with moderate preeclampsia at 34 weeks gestation?

A. Misoprostol
B. Mifepristone
C. Ergometrine
D. Foley's catheter

167. A patient who presents to the ER with preeclampsia at 33 weeks gestation has just been placed on IV oxytocin for inducing labor. On examination, the nurse discovers that the uterine contractions are six every 10 minutes and last for about a minute. Which of the following interventions is most appropriate?

A. Stop oxytocin infusion
B. Perform a cervical examination
C. Administer a tocolytic
D. Reduce the rate of oxytocin infusion

168. Which of the following is not a component of the active management of the third stage of labor?

A. Controlled cord traction
B. IV oxytocin
C. Uterine massage
D. Episiotomy

169. A 45-year-old G6 P5+1 who presents to the ER with prelabor rupture of membrane at 35 weeks gestation has been induced into labor with IV oxytocin. Which of the following elevates the patient's risk of postpartum hemorrhage?

A. Infections
B. Atony
C. Retention of placenta
D. Bleeding disorder

170. Which of the following is not a metabolic cause of delirium?

A. Vitamin B12 deficiency
B. Hypoglycemia
C. Hyperglycemia
D. Hypernatremia

171. A 15-year-old presents to the ER with a history of weakness and syncope. On examination, the patient is markedly wasted, with lanugo hair. A differential diagnosis of anorexia nervosa is made. According to ICD-10, what is the criterion for diagnosing this patient according to her body weight?

A. Below 10%
B. Below 15%
C. Below 5%
D. Below 25%

172. A 15-year-old female who is being managed in the ER for anorexia nervosa is most likely to have which of the following abnormal blood biochemistries?

A. Hypermagnesemia
B. Hyponatremia
C. Hypokalemia
D. Hypercholesterolemia

173. A patient who presents to the ER is noticed to initiate and involuntarily repeat the actions of the nurse attending to him. What is the name of this abnormality?

A. Apraxia
B. Echopraxia
C. Dysdiadochokinesia
D. Tardive dyskinesia

174. Which of the following is not a priority in a female patient who presents to the ER with seizures and altered consciousness secondary to anorexia nervosa?

A. Provision of warmth
B. Enteral feeding
C. Monitoring of serum biochemistry
D. ECG monitoring

175. A patient with dementia is unlikely to present with which of the following?

A. Personality change
B. Disorientation in time
C. Hallucinations
D. Delusions

Test 3: Answers and Explanations

1. (A) Anterior.
More than 95 percent of shoulder dislocations are anterior. Inferior and posterior shoulder dislocations are rare. Superior shoulder dislocation is not a medical condition.

2. (D) Injury to the serratus anterior muscle.
This statement is false because the anterior dislocation of the shoulder does not damage the serratus anterior. The serratus anterior muscle originates from the upper surface of the eighth and ninth ribs and inserts into the medial margins of the scapula. Anterior dislocation of the shoulder can cause injuries to the brachial plexus and rotator cuff muscles. It can also cause a fracture of the greater tuberosity.

3. (D) Radial nerve.
The radial nerve is unlikely to be damaged in a dislocated elbow. Because it is posterior, injury to the radial nerve is most often caused by a fracture of the humerus. The brachial artery, ulnar nerve and median nerve are anterior to the elbow joint and are therefore at risk for injury.

4. (B) Toddlers.
In toddlers, the width of the radial head is the same as the radial neck. This makes it easy for the radial head to slip through the ligaments in the elbow. Subluxation often occurs when the forearm is pulled upward, such as when the toddler is caught by the wrists to break a fall.

5. (D) Brachial artery.
The brachial artery is likely to be affected by a fracture of the distal head of the humerus, not the proximal head.

6. (A) Drainage of 80 mL/day.
For pleural effusion and hemothorax, the chest tube is removed when drainage is less than 100–200 mL/day.

7. (B) Frequent suctioning of oral secretions.
This management modality is not only inappropriate but also harmful. Suctioning should be done only when secretions are copious. Placing the patient in the semi-Fowler's position allows adequate lung expansion and therefore improves respiration. A bell and a writing pad make communication easy, alerts the managing team to the patient's needs and removes straining of the vocal cords. Regular monitoring of vital signs assesses the patient's respiratory function and alerts the nurse to conditions like distress, fever, pain and others.

8. (A) Providing humidified oxygen.
This intervention is not useful in reducing the risk of aspiration. It is, however, useful in reducing the risk of respiratory distress caused by copious, thick or crusted secretion. Because tracheostomy bypasses the nose, inspired air is neither warm nor humidified. Humidification of oxygen maintains ciliary function and reduces the risk of crusted secretions.

9. (D) Prophylactic antibiotics.
Prophylactic antibiotics are not useful in preventing infection in a patient with tracheostomy. Antibiotics should be used only when there is a suspected or

confirmed infection. Prophylactic antibiotics increase the incidence of bacterial resistance to antibiotic therapy.

10. (B) Increased intrathoracic pressure.
In tension pneumothorax, there is a one-way movement of air into the pleural space. Because of this, there is an accumulation of air in the lungs, leading to mass mediastinal shift, compression of the contralateral lung and increased intrathoracic pressure. This pressure reduces venous return and increases the risk of shock.

11. (B) Conjunctivitis.
Conjunctivitis is not a complication of mumps infection. Complications include orchitis, oophoritis, pancreatitis, meningitis and encephalitis. Rare complications are hepatitis, polyarthritis, mastitis and nephritis.

12. (C) Omega 3 fatty acids.
Omega 3 fatty acids do not have an antibacterial effect. Breast milk is rich in omega 3 and omega 6 fatty acids that are useful in building the infant's developing brain and improving cognition.

13. (B) Citruses.
Acidic foods like citruses and vinegar can worsen pain in patients with swollen parotid glands. Patients should be fed semisolid or mashed foods that will minimize effort spent in chewing and swallowing.

14. (D) A patient with caustic poisoning.
Caustic poisoning does not increase the risk of tetanus. The risk increases when the skin is broken (e.g., burns, gunshot injuries, lacerations, wounds and IV drug

abuse). Risk also increases in nonapparent wounds (e.g., postpartum tetanus and neonatal tetanus such as involving the umbilical cord).

15. (D) Left ventricular heart failure.
Left ventricular heart failure is not a complication of meningococcal meningitis. Meningococcal meningitis is a form of acute bacterial meningitis with high morbidity and mortality rates. This disease is caused by an infection with Neisseria meningitidis, gram-negative diplococci. Complications include DIC, SIADH, tissue necrosis and gangrene, seizures, septic shock, multiple organ dysfunction and cranial nerve deficits.

16. (C) Haemophilus influenzae.
Haemophilus influenzae is not likely to be implicated in a two-week-old's acute bacterial meningitis. Implicated organisms in meningitis in neonates and infants are group B streptococcus (including Streptococcus agalactiae), Listeria monocytogenes and E. coli. These organisms are often obtained via the birth canal. Implicated bacteria in older infants and young adults are Streptococcus pneumoniae, Haemophilus influenzae, Neisseria meningitidis and Staphylococcus aureus. Implicated bacteria in older adults are Streptococcus pneumoniae, S. aureus and N. meningitidis.

17. (B) Insufficient plasma cortisol.
Waterhouse-Friderichsen syndrome is adrenal insufficiency caused by overwhelming meningococcemia. The pathophysiology includes hemorrhage in the adrenal glands, leading to insufficient secretion of adrenal hormones like plasma cortisol and aldosterone.

18. (A) A three-month-old male with meningitis.

This patient is least at risk because febrile seizures occur in patients who are six months to five years old with a temperature that is greater than 38°C. For a diagnosis of febrile seizures to be made, affected patients must not have an underlying pathology of the CNS and also must have no prior history of afebrile seizures.

19. (A) Right coronary artery.

The right coronary artery is most likely to be occluded as it supplies the right ventricle and inferior and posterior walls of the left ventricle. In ECG, leads II, III and aVF represent the inferior surface of the heart, while leads V1–V4 represent the anterior surface. Leads I, V5, V6 and aVL represent the lateral side of the heart.

20. (C) Indicates electric impulses from the AV node.

This statement is false because the P wave indicates impulses from the SA node. The P wave indicates atrial depolarization and lasts less than 0.11 seconds. It is seen just before the QRS complex and is upright in a normal sinus rhythm.

21. (D) Pulsus paradoxus.

Pulsus paradoxus, which is described as a decrease in systolic blood pressure (by more than 10 mmHg) during inspiration, is also seen in cardiac tamponade. It is, however, not a component of Beck's triad. Beck's triad is seen in cardiac tamponade. Clinical features are hypotension; increased venous pressure, which presents as neck distention; and muffled heart sounds.

22. (B) IV procainamide.
Treatment of this patient involves the use of an antiarrhythmic drug, like procainamide, lidocaine or digoxin. Epinephrine will increase this patient's heart rate and is therefore contraindicated. Defibrillation is indicated for pulseless ventricular tachycardia. IV atropine is not useful in controlling an abnormal cardiac rhythm.

23. (B) Baroreflex stimulation.
Carotid massage stimulates the baroreceptors in the carotid sinus. Stimulation of the baroreceptors causes reflex bradycardia.

24. (A) Defibrillation.
Defibrillation must be urgently performed to restore normal heart rhythm. Fibrillation momentarily sensitizes the heart to repeat depolarization. This occurrence makes it easy for the intrinsic pacemaker (the SA node) to initiate cardiac rhythm.

25. (C) Inhale air, pinch his nose, close his mouth, and attempt to expel air through his mouth.
The Valsalva maneuver is used in restoring normal heart rhythm from tachycardia. To do this maneuver, the patient inhales air, pinches his nose, closes his mouth and attempts to expel the air through the mouth. The forceful expulsion stimulates the heart into a normal sinus rhythm. The Valsalva maneuver can also be used to unclog the ears.

26. (D) Pulmonary embolism.
Pulmonary embolism is unlikely to cause a transudative pleural effusion. They are caused by an increase in hydrostatic pressure, a decrease in oncotic pressure,

or both. Heart failure is the most common cause of transudative pleural effusion. Other causes are nephrotic syndrome and liver cirrhosis.

27. (C) Toddlers.
Cricothyrotomy is contraindicated in children under eight years of age. Relative contraindications are transection of the distal trachea, which can be partial or complete; and inability to identify landmarks because of injury to the cricoid, thyroid cartilage and larynx. Cricothyrotomy is indicated when there are multiple failed attempts to perform orotracheal or nasotracheal intubation with an inability to use alternative methods and when there are contraindications to nasotracheal and orotracheal intubation (facial trauma, edema, hemorrhage and other mass effects).

28. (C) Subglottic stenosis.
This is a chronic (not acute) complication that is seen weeks after the cricothyrotomy is performed. Acute complications of this procedure include hemorrhage; erroneous intubation of surrounding tissues in the neck and consequent apnea; and injury to the trachea, thyroid, vocal cords and larynx. Late complications are airway obstruction caused by the formation of stoma granulation tissue, subglottic stenosis, wound infection and voice changes.

29. (D) Epiglottitis.
Noninvasive positive pressure ventilation is contraindicated in patients with upper airway obstruction. Patients with epiglottitis ought to be rapidly intubated by qualified personnel and in an operating room. Other contraindications to NIPPV are cardiopulmonary arrest, severe upper GI bleeding, unstable hemodynamic states, vomiting, copious oral secretions, loss of consciousness and

any condition that can impair gastric emptying (pregnancy, paralytic ileus, or bowel obstruction).

30. (B) Mydriasis.
This is not a clinical feature of Horner's syndrome, which is caused by the disruption of the cervical sympathetic output. This leads to unrestrained parasympathetic activity on the affected side. The classic signs of Horner's syndrome are ptosis (drooping of the eyelid), miosis (constriction of the pupils), increased sweating, sinking of the eyeball (enophthalmos) and hyperemia.

31. (B) Hemotympanum.
The oculovestibular reflex is tested to assess the function of the brain stem. This test is not performed on a patient with a ruptured tympanic membrane because water is poured into the ear during the test. Irrigation with water can dislodge blood clots from the ear and slow down the healing process of the eardrum.

32. (C) Inability to extend the knee when the hip and knees are both flexed at 90°.
Kernig's sign is used to examine meningeal irritation. To do this test, the patient is placed in the supine position with hip and knees flexed at 90°. The patient resists the extension of the flexed knee by flexing the other knee.

33. (B) Fundoscopy.
A fundoscopy is required to rule out papilledema, a feature of raised intracranial pressure. To prevent brain herniation and coning, lumbar puncture must not be done on patients with raised intracranial pressure.

34. (C) Fallopian tube.

The fallopian tube is most likely to be the site of implantation. About 80 percent of embryos implant in the ampulla of the fallopian tube, 22 percent in the interstitial, 5 percent in the fimbrial end and 2 percent in the interstitial part of the fallopian tube. Two percent of ectopic pregnancies are nontubal (i.e., outside the fallopian tubes). These sites include the cervix, ovary, or intra-abdominal.

35. (C) Progestin-only pill.

Progestin-only contraceptives increase the risk of mastalgia, weight gain and depression. Risk factors responsible for the development of ectopic pregnancies are a previous history of ectopic pregnancy, history of tubal or abdominal surgeries, use of IUD, infertility, history of induced abortion, cigarette use and multiple sexual partners.

36. (C) Salpingectomy.

Salpingectomy, which involves excision of the ruptured fallopian tissue, is the definitive treatment for this patient. Salpingotomy is done to preserve the tube by extracting the products of conception. Methotrexate is used for unruptured ectopic pregnancies and is a more conservative approach. Indications for salpingectomy are ruptured ectopic pregnancy, persistent bleeding after salpingostomy and ectopic pregnancy occurring as a result of previous BTL.

37. (D) Twin gestation.

Twin gestation is a relative (not absolute) indication of caesarean section. Vaginal delivery can be attempted if the leading twin has a normal presentation at term. Absolute indications for caesarean section are major degree placenta previa, two previous caesarean sections, previous history of myomectomy, major cephalopelvic disruption and obstructed labor, severe fetal distress in the first stage of labor, retroviral positive mother, bad obstetric history and others.

38. (D) Older children.

The risk of seizure disorders increases in patients who are less than one year old and in patients with other risk factors, like history of complex febrile seizures, delay of developmental milestones and history of febrile seizures in first-degree relatives.

39. (A) Lorazepam.

Lorazepam is inappropriate for this patient. It is a short-acting antiseizure drug used to treat acute seizures. It is given IV as 0.05 to 0.1 mg/kg every 5 to 10 minutes to a maximum of three doses. Drugs used to treat persistent seizures are valproate, phenobarbital and fosphenytoin.

40. (A) Aspirin.

Salicylates like aspirin are contraindicated for use in children, especially children with varicella-zoster infection due to the risk of developing Reye's syndrome, a rare cause of hepatic encephalopathy.

41. (B) Valproic acid.

Weight gain is a side effect of valproic acid (although not typically listed as a common side effect). Studies have shown that valproic acid increases the secretion of insulin. Insulin is an anabolic hormone that increases appetite, food intake, energy conservation and weight gain. This side effect is mostly seen in women.

42. (C) Lamotrigine.
Older antiseizure drugs, like phenytoin, carbamazepine, valproate and phenobarbital, are unsafe in pregnancy due to the high risk of congenital defects and neurologic conditions in the developing fetus. New-generation antiseizure drugs, like levetiracetam and lamotrigine, are widely prescribed for pregnant patients because of their safety profile.

43. (C) Supine position.
After a lumbar puncture, the patient must stay in a supine position for at least an hour. This position is necessary to reduce the distribution effects occurring in the cerebrospinal circulation. Standing or sitting can cause a quick redistribution of CSF and cause spinal headaches.

44. (B) Histoplasma capsulatum.
Histoplasma capsulatum is most likely implicated. The CSF analysis of acute bacterial meningitis includes marked leukocytosis, proteinuria and markedly reduced glucose. Also, CSF is usually turbid on inspection. CSF findings in viral meningitis include elevated leukocytes and protein. CSF glucose is, however, normal. In fungal meningitis, there is lymphocytosis and proteinuria with decreased CSF glucose.

45. (C) Hyperresonant hemithorax.
Although the clinical features of cardiac tamponade and tension pneumothorax may overlap, features that distinguish tension pneumothorax from cardiac tamponade are hyperresonance and absent breath sounds on the affected hemithorax. Pulsus paradoxus is not usually seen in tension pneumothorax.

46. (B) Electrocardiogram.

An electrocardiogram is the quickest and least invasive method for assessing the location of the infarct. Although angiography detects the location of the infarct, it is invasive and not as fast as an ECG. An echocardiogram is used to assess the integrity of the cardiac wall after a myocardial infarction, while cardiac biomarkers confirm a diagnosis of myocardial infarction but do not show the location.

47. (C) Vascular resistance.

This is the amount of pressure in the peripheral blood vessels against which the heart must pump out blood. Vascular resistance determines diastolic blood pressure, while cardiac output influences systolic blood pressure.

48. (B) Troponin I.

Troponin I is very sensitive for myocardial infarction and rises about one hour after an episode of MI. Creatinine kinase rises about three to eight hours after the onset of myocardial infarction. Lactate dehydrogenase rises in about 24 to 48 hours.

49. (D) Tissue necrosis.

This is an immediate complication of compartment syndrome. As tissue edema persists, the blood supply to the muscles is hindered. Necrosis of the tissues triggers infection, rhabdomyolysis, hyperkalemia, hypotension, shock and death. Contractures and limb amputations are late complications of patients who survive.

50. (D) Rhabdomyolysis.

Rhabdomyolysis is a complication of compartment syndrome, not a cause. The most common causes of compartment syndrome are fractures, reperfusion injuries, crush injuries and contusions of the muscles. Less common causes are cocaine overdose, burns, snakebites and the use of tight bandages and casts.

51. (C) Creatine kinase.

Creatine kinase is elevated in patients with rhabdomyolysis due to its massive release from necrose muscles. A serum level that is greater than five times the upper limit of normal is diagnostic. Myoglobin is also measured in the urine.

52. (A) Acute kidney injury.

Acute kidney injury is the most common immediate complication of rhabdomyolysis. This is because the destruction of myocytes triggers the release of intracellular components, enzymes, inflammatory mediators and potassium into the intravascular space. Dehydration, sepsis, acidosis and hyperkalemia worsen the outcomes of patients.

53. (B) Dantrolene.

Dantrolene is a muscle relaxant used in treating the excitability of muscles in patients with malignant hyperthermia. It blocks the release of calcium ions from the sarcoplasmic reticulum. Flumazenil is an antidote to benzodiazepine poisoning. Baclofen is a muscle relaxant used for the relief of muscle spasticity. Lorazepam is a benzodiazepine receptor agonist.

54. (C) What is your ethnic group?

This is the most suitable question for clarifying a patient's ethnicity. Option A is derogatory. Options B and D are presumptive.

55. (A) Asian.
Because Asians have a culture that values ties with extended families and communities, they are most likely to involve extended families and relatives before making a health-related decision.

56. (C) Psychological evaluation.
Psychological evaluation is not a goal of treatment in this patient. This patient will, however, benefit from thorough sex education and counseling that highlights the danger of sexually transmitted infections, unwanted/unplanned pregnancies and cervical cancer. All sexual partners must be traced and treated before the commencement of sexual activities.

57. (D) Menopause.
Candidal vaginitis is rare in postmenopausal women. Atrophic vaginitis is more likely in this group. Risk factors for candidal vaginitis include diabetes mellitus, obesity, use of intrauterine contraceptives, pregnancy, use of corticosteroids, immunosuppression and use of tight and nonbreathable underwear.

58. (B) Serum BNP/NT-proBNP.
In this patient, a chest X-ray is diagnostic for both respiratory disorders and useful in differentiating both. It is, however, not a bedside investigation. Serum BNP/NT-proBNP is usually normal in exacerbated COPD but elevated in pulmonary edema.

59. (C) Crepitations.
Crepitations are usually heard in pulmonary edema. These sounds differentiate pulmonary edema from COPD. Crepitations are cracking sounds best heard at the

base of the lungs. They are caused by the presence of excess fluids in the airways. It is important to note that a patient with pulmonary edema may have variable blood pressure. Therefore Option D is false.

60. (B) Decreased work of breathing.
In the high Fowler's position, the excess fluid in the lungs settles at the base of the lungs due to gravity. This makes it possible for respiration to occur in the middle and apical zones of the lungs.

61. (A) Fluid status.
This patient is on furosemide, a loop diuretic required in reducing the amount of fluid in the interstitial space. It is important to monitor the fluid status of this patient (fluid input and output and signs of dehydration) to reduce the risk of hypovolemic shock.

62. (C) Increased capillary permeability.
Pulmonary edema in acute glomerulonephritis is caused by either decreased oncotic pressure from proteinuria or increased capillary permeability due to deposition of immune complexes on the capillaries and consequent carditis. Noncardiogenic causes of pulmonary edema are not caused by increased hydrostatic pressure.

63. (B) Chronic bronchitis.
Cor pulmonale is pulmonary hypertension caused by a primary pathology in the lungs. Pathophysiologic mechanisms include loss of pulmonary capillary beds, chronic vasoconstriction, increased alveolar pressure and hypertrophy of pulmonary arterioles. Other causes of cor pulmonale include massive pulmonary embolism, ARDS, obesity, systemic sclerosis and neuromuscular diseases.

64. (B) B-HCG.
B-HCG will be elevated in ectopic pregnancy and normal in a ruptured ovarian cyst. Since the clinical presentation of the two conditions overlaps, it is important to rule out/confirm pregnancy by analyzing serum B-HCG levels.

65. (B) HIV.
Follow-up for HIV is done 90 days after the incident. Follow-up tests done at six weeks include hepatitis, chlamydia, syphilis, hepatitis, gonorrhea and HPV (including Pap smear). At six months, follow-up is done for syphilis, HIV and hepatitis.

66. (D) Follow-up test at six weeks.
The most appropriate action is a follow-up test after six weeks. For patients who have had complete immunizations before the incident, a repeat vaccination is not required. Also, treatment with hepatitis B immune globulin or ribavirin is not required.

67. (B) Copper IUD.
A Copper IUD is an emergency contraceptive if it is used within five days of intercourse. The failure rate with this method is about 0.1 percent. Levonorgestrel is another emergency contraceptive if it is used not more than 72 hours after intercourse. It has a failure rate of 2–3 percent. All other methods are unsuitable for emergency contraception.

68. (B) Pelvic ultrasound.
An ultrasound scan must be done to rule out placenta previa. This must be done before pelvic examination because of the increased risk of bleeding in the

placenta previa. Please note that ultrasound scan findings do not exclude abruptio placentae. Diagnosis of abruptio placentae requires clinical evaluation, which is then supported with laboratory and ultrasound scan findings.

69. (C) Eclampsia.
Eclampsia is not a complication of abruptio placentae. It is an obstetric emergency characterized by hypertension, proteinuria, seizures and hematologic abnormalities. Complications of abruptio placentae include hemodynamic instability, DIC, Rh sensitization, fetal distress, birth asphyxia and fetal demise.

70. (B) Previous caesarean section.
This is not a risk factor for placental abruption. This is a risk for placenta previa. Risk factors for placental abruption are hypertension, polyhydramnios, abdominal trauma, old maternal age, chorioamnionitis, vasculitis, previous history of abruption, drug and tobacco abuse.

71. (B) Diclofenac.
NSAIDs are not disease-modifying rheumatic drugs (DMARDs) because they do not slow down the progression of disease. They are given to patients with rheumatoid arthritis for symptomatic relief from joint pain. Examples of DMARDs are leflunomide, methotrexate, sulfasalazine and hydroxychloroquine.

72. (D) Sickle cell anemia.
In patients with sickle cell anemia, immunodeficiency, liver disease and salmonella infection of the bone are most likely. Elderly patients, patients who are bedridden and patients receiving hemodialysis are likely to have osteomyelitis caused by Staphylococcus aureus.

73. (B) Cervical collar.

The neck must first be stabilized to prevent further injury to the cervical spine. For all patients with neck pain following trauma, injury to the cervical spine must be suspected and ruled out only after a radiologic investigation.

74. (A) Wrist.

The wrist is the most common area of fractures in children and makes up more than half of fractures in children.

75. (C) Anticonvulsant.

Gabapentin is an anticonvulsant used in treating focal seizures. It is the drug of choice in the treatment of neuropathic pain (e.g., sciatica).

76. (A) Decreases blood flow.

This statement is false because heat therapy increases blood flow and thereby decreases edema, exudates, pain, joint stiffness and muscle spasms. It also increases the extensibility of muscles.

77. (D) Heat therapy.

This intervention is unnecessary in this patient. Interventions include rest, elevation, compression, protection of the joint and application of ice. Immobilization is used for severe cases.

78. (C) Cold, clammy extremities are signs of shock.

In shock, vasodilation of peripheral blood vessels causes the dissipation of heat. The upper and lower limbs are cool and clammy to the touch. Option A is incorrect because circulation is assessed with pulse rate, blood pressure and capillary refill. Option B is incorrect because cyanosis is assessed in the buccal mucosa, lips and nail beds. Option D is incorrect because hyperpyrexia increases heart rate and respiratory rate but not blood pressure.

79. (D) Anorexia.
Oxycodone is an opioid used in pain management. Common side effects are constipation, nausea, vomiting, dizziness, hypersomnolence, pruritus and xerostomia. Very rare side effects are diarrhea, anorexia, urine retention, difficulty breathing and hiccups.

80. (A) Catatonic schizophrenia.
This disorder is characterized by repetitive, inappropriate and bizarre motor movement; delusions; disorganized speech; and hallucinations. Patients with major depression present with suicidal ideation, fatigue, psychomotor agitation, insomnia or hypersomnia, inability to concentrate and weight gain or weight loss. Patients with mania present with grandiosity, flight of ideas, the pressure of speech, distractibility, increased busyness and engagement in high-risk behaviors

81. (D) Erotomania.
In erotomania, patients believe that someone of a higher status (a celebrity most times) is in love with them. Voyeurism is a paraphilic disorder in which sexual arousal and satisfaction are obtained by watching people disrobing, bathing, or engaging in sexual activities. In delusions of grandeur, patients believe they are important or of a higher status than they actually are. In delusions of persecution, patients believe that people are out to get them.

82. (B) Age less than 40 years.
This is not a risk factor for suicide. The risk for suicide increases in people who are older than 40 years. Other risk factors are male sex, a major stressful event

like divorce or unemployment, psychiatric disorders, alcohol and substance abuse, history of suicide in the family and previous history of suicidal attempts.

83. (B) Persistent cyanosis.
In acrocyanosis, there is a persistent bluish discoloration of the fingers even after the fingers are warmed. Unlike Raynaud's syndrome, there are no trophic changes, ulcers and tenderness. Pulses are also present.

84. (C) Female sex.
About 12 percent of the US population has peripheral arterial disease. Peripheral arterial disease is higher in men than in women. Other risk factors are cigarette smoking, elderly age, atherosclerosis, dyslipidemia, family history, obesity, diabetes, hypertension and high serum levels of homocysteine.

85. (D) Lichenification.
This is a skin manifestation of peripheral venous (not arterial) disease. Chronic venous insufficiency causes stasis dermatitis, which is characterized by hyperpigmentation; lichenification; induration; and shallow ulcers that are often located around the medial malleolus. These ulcers are usually moist and do not penetrate the deep fascia. The ulcers in peripheral arterial disease present as black necrotic tissue, which may be wet due to bacterial infection. Also, these ulcers tend to extend into the deep fascia and expose the tendon and bone.

86. (B) Positioning the patient in the high Fowler's position.
This is the most appropriate task for a nursing assistant because it is within the scope of practice. Options A and C can be done by a licensed nurse, while Option D is done by a registered nurse.

87. (B) Administration of IV omeprazole.
Administration of IV drugs is beyond the scope of a licensed nurse. A licensed nurse can examine patients, make assessments, collect vital sign data and administer oral drugs under direct supervision.

88. (C) Inspect and remove the infiltrated line.
This is the most appropriate response. Checking the pulse rate does not offer relief to the patient's discomfort. Administration of IV drugs is not the duty of the nursing assistant; moreover, it will only worsen the patient's condition. Option D will worsen the patient's condition.

89. (D) A 24-year-old female with acute PID.
This patient has the least risk of mortality and therefore can be assigned to the newly employed emergency nurse.

90. (C) ADP inhibitor.
Clopidogrel is metabolized into an active metabolite that inhibits an ADP receptor responsible for activating platelet aggregation. A loading dose of 300 to 600 mg of clopidogrel is given as an oral tablet of 75 mg daily. Examples of glycoprotein IIb/IIIa inhibitors are abciximab (ReoPro), tirofiban (Aggrastat)and eptifibatide (Integrilin). Aspirin is a cyclooxygenase inhibitor. All these drugs, except leukotriene receptor antagonists, are examples of antiplatelet drugs.

91. (B) Dyslipidemia.
Dyslipidemia is a risk factor for peripheral arterial disease, not venous insufficiency. Risk factors of venous insufficiency are deep venous thrombosis (the most common risk factor), obesity, trauma, elderly age, pregnancy and standing or sitting for long periods.

92. (C) Compression stockings.

The underlying pathophysiology of venous ulcers is the pooling of blood in the peripheral venous due to impaired efficiency of the valves in the veins. Compression stockings improve peripheral circulation by increasing pressure, thereby improving ulcers and edema. The use of drugs like antiplatelets, anticoagulants and antidiuretic drugs does not produce significant effects in the treatment of venous ulcers. Surgical interventions like venous ligation and valve reconstruction also are not effective. Skin grafting produces no effect if the underlying pathophysiology is not corrected.

93. (C) Benztropine.

First-generation antipsychotics like haloperidol have antagonistic effects on D2 dopamine receptors, causing extrapyramidal motor effects like dystonia, akathisia, tremor, bradykinesia and tardive dyskinesia. Benztropine is an antimuscarinic agent used in treating these extrapyramidal effects. It inhibits cholinergic neurons in the basal ganglia and inhibits the reuptake of dopamine. Therefore, it increases dopaminergic activity.

94. (C) Liver function.

Liver function monitoring is not required during lithium therapy. Lithium is a mood stabilizer used in treating patients with bipolar disorder. Hypothyroidism is a side effect of chronic use of this drug. Therefore, thyroid function must be monitored when lithium is commenced and then monitored annually for patients with a family history of thyroid disorder, or in alternate years for patients with no family history. Renal necrosis of the distal tubule is another adverse effect of long-term use. Renal function and BUN must be monitored on commencement of the drug and two to three times in the first six months of use. Monitoring can then be done twice a year.

95. (C) Goiter.
A goiter is not a contraindication of ECT. Contraindications are increased intracranial pressure from edema, tumors and other causes of pressure effect and respiratory and cardiac disorders. Other contraindications are severe liver disease, unstable dentition, retinal detachment and pheochromocytoma.

96. (B) Major depressive disorder.
Electroconvulsive therapy is used to treat patients with major depressive disorder and bipolar disorder that is refractory to pharmacotherapy.

97. (D) Schizophrenia.
CBT is useful in patients with depression, anxiety disorders, substance abuse disorders and eating disorders. It is not useful in patients with schizophrenia whose cognition and perception of stimuli are altered. In cognitive-behavioral therapy, clients are encouraged to explore and identify the underlying thoughts that have negative impacts on their actions and behaviors. When these thoughts are identified, the clients are encouraged to change them for better ones.

98. (C) Acetylcholine.
Antagonistic effects on acetylcholine receptors cause constipation, blurred vision, dry mouth and extrapyramidal effects. Antagonistic effects on dopamine cause reduced libido and gynecomastia. Antagonistic effects on histamine cause sedation, drowsiness and dry mouth. Antiadrenergic effects cause postural hypotension. Hematologic side effects include agranulocytosis and thrombocytopenia, endocrine changes include weight gain, type 2 diabetes

mellitus and metabolic syndrome. Cardiovascular changes include arrhythmia and stroke.

99. (D) Fluoxetine.
Fluoxetine is a selective serotonin reuptake inhibitor. Tricyclic antidepressants are serotonin and norepinephrine reuptake inhibitors, which increase the synaptic concentrations of these two neurotransmitters. Examples are amitriptyline, clomipramine, imipramine, doxepin, lofepramine, iprindole and desipramine.

100. (A) Active natural immunity.
This patient is unlikely to be reinfected with chicken pox due to active natural immunity. In this case, memory cells are exposed to the chicken pox antigen and produce antibodies that can be used to fight off infections in the future.

101. (B) Neutralization of circulating toxins.
Tetanus immune globulin is given to neutralize the unbound circulating toxin. Active immunity is conferred via tetanus antitoxid. Further release of toxins is done by rapid debridement of the wound and commencement of antibiotics. Benzodiazepines are used as sedatives.

102. (C) Treatment in a bright room.
Patients with tetanus should be treated in a quiet and dark room to prevent unnecessary stimulation of the nervous system. Frequent turning is needed to prevent bedsores. IV hyperalimentation is used to prevent aspiration from parenteral feeding. Mechanical ventilation is needed for severe cases with respiratory failure.

103. (A) HIV.

The risk of herpes zoster infection increases in older patients with HIV infection. Risk also increases in patients with severe immunosuppression (e.g., patients with leukemia or SCID).

104. (C) HPV 18.

Carcinogenic strains of HPV implicated in cervical cancer are HPV 16 and HPV 18. These strains are not only implicated in cervical cancers but also cancers affecting the oral cavity, penis, anus, vulva and vagina.

105. (D) Burkitt's lymphoma.

Infectious mononucleosis is caused by infection with Epstein-Barr virus. This virus has been associated with increased risk of developing Burkitt's lymphoma, B cell tumors, gastric cancer, nasopharyngeal carcinoma and some forms of Hodgkin's lymphoma.

106. (D) Antifibrinolytic.

Tranexamic acid is a synthetic derivative of lysine. It is an antifibrinolytic that binds to lysine receptors and inhibits the conversion of plasminogen to plasmin and consequently prevents the breakdown of fibrin molecules. This effect reduces vaginal bleeding in patients with symptomatic uterine fibroids.

107. (C) Speculum examination.

Speculum examination is contraindicated in this patient due to the risk of increased bleeding. In cervical cancer, contact bleeding occurs due to the friability of tissues and mucosa. These tissues can bleed on contact. Treatment modalities in this patient include acute resuscitation with IV fluids, blood products and vasopressors. Also, the vagina should be packed to stimulate clotting.

108. (A) Shrinks fibroids.
Leuprolide is a GnRH agonist that reduces the size of uterine fibroids and uterine bleeding. It does this by reducing the secretion of estrogen. These drugs are given preoperatively to reduce the risk of hemorrhage during surgery. Also, they reduce the size of the uterus and the fibroids. They are not used for long-term management.

109. (D) Anorexia nervosa.
Anorexia nervosa is not a cause for menorrhagia. It is an eating disorder characterized by fear of weight gain, restriction of food and calorie intake and malnutrition. Amenorrhea and oligomenorrhea are complications of malnutrition. Other causes of menorrhagia are the use of nonhormonal IUDs, fibroids, adenomyosis, endometriosis, thyroid disorders, hormonal imbalance, cancers, anticoagulants and inherited bleeding disorders.

110. (C) Empirical therapy.
Empirical use of antibiotics does not reduce the incidence of MRSA in hospital settings. Empirical therapy helps in providing prompt intervention and treatment in patients. However, it may increase the risk of antibiotic resistance.

111. (D) Type IV.
Type IV hypersensitivity reaction is also called delayed cell-mediated hypersensitivity reaction. In this case, T cells, macrophages and monocytes are released to contain the offending antigen. This reaction takes days to develop.

112. (B) Benzodiazepines.

Patients with acute withdrawal symptoms from sedatives will be managed with IV benzodiazepines.

113. (C) Gastric acid.

Sputum may not be easily obtained in young children who do not know how to expectorate. Because of this, gastric aspirate is obtained by gastric lavage. These samples are typically obtained in the morning, just before eating.

114. (D) Increased appetite.

This is not a symptom of withdrawal from opioids. Symptoms are anxiety, yawning, diaphoresis, lacrimation, mydriasis rhinorrhea, tachycardia, hypertension, chills, anorexia, diarrhea and fever. These symptoms are caused by stimulation of the central nervous system. Increased appetite is an effect of cannabis.

115. (B) Opioid receptor agonist.

Methadone is an opioid receptor agonist. It is used in treating patients with opioid withdrawal symptoms. It is also used for opioid detoxification. This is because it has a long half-life and fewer euphoric and sedative effects.

116. (B) Total abdominal hysterectomy.

Total abdominal hysterectomy is the definitive treatment for endometriosis. The other options listed are all symptomatic treatments. In endometriosis, there is ectopic implantation of functional endometrial tissue. Implantation occurs within the pelvic cavity. This pathophysiology occurs during menstruation. Definitive treatment involves the removal of the uterus.

117. (D) Religious counseling.

This is not a goal of treatment of rape victims. However, religious counseling can be offered if the patient requests it. The goals of treatment of rape victims include medical evaluation and rapid management of injuries, pregnancies and sexually transmitted infections; psychologic evaluation and support; collection of evidence and crisis intervention (with the expressed consent of the victim).

118. (B) Hypersomnia.

This is not a clinical feature of a manic episode of bipolar disorder. In the manic phase of bipolar disorder, affected patients experience insomnia. For a diagnosis of mania to be made, the patient must exhibit at least three of these symptoms for more than one week: grandiosity, insomnia, talkativeness, excessive involvement in activities that may be high risk (gambling, drinking, sexual activities), distractibility and racing of ideas.

119. (C) Nurse M assumes that a geriatric patient cannot use a glucometer.

In stereotyping, assumptions are made based on the individual's race, age, ethnic group, sexual orientation or religious beliefs. Options A and B are examples of cultural awareness. Option D is an example of imposition.

120. (D) Insufficient health funds.

In the United States every citizen has a right to health care. This means that no one is denied access due to a lack of funding.

121. (B) Risperidone.

This patient has visual and olfactory hallucinations, which are clinical features of psychosis. An antipsychotic drug such as Risperidone is needed for treating her condition. Citalopram is a selective serotonin reuptake inhibitor used in the treatment of depression and anxiety disorders. Lithium is a mood stabilizer used in the treatment of bipolar disorders. Amitriptyline is a tricyclic antidepressant used in treating depression and anxiety disorders.

122. (D) Dopamine receptor antagonist.
Olanzapine is an atypical antipsychotic. It is a dopamine receptor antagonist, serotonin receptor antagonist and serotonin receptor inverse agonist. It is used to treat psychotic symptoms in schizophrenia.

123. (D) Diarrhea.
Constipation, not diarrhea, is a side effect of antipsychotics. The side effects of antipsychotics arise from their antagonistic effects on dopamine, serotonin and acetylcholine receptors. Antagonistic effects on acetylcholine receptors cause constipation, blurred vision, dry mouth and extrapyramidal effects. Antagonistic effects on dopamine cause reduced libido and gynecomastia. Antagonistic effects on histamine cause sedation, drowsiness and dry mouth. Antiadrenergics cause postural hypotension. Hematologic side effects include agranulocytosis and thrombocytopenia; endocrine changes include weight gain, type 2 diabetes mellitus and metabolic syndrome. Cardiovascular changes include arrhythmia and stroke.

124. (D) Peripheral arterial disease.
Polycythemia vera is characterized by excessive production of red blood cells, white blood cells and platelets. Complications include bleeding; thrombosis; gout; iron-deficiency anemia and hyperviscosity syndromes characterized by deep vein thrombosis, transient ischemic attacks, ocular migraine erythromelalgia, retinal artery occlusion, splenomegaly and splenic infarction and myocardial infarction.

125. (D) Physiotherapy.
Physiotherapy is not a useful intervention in this patient, who is not bedridden. To reduce the risk of DVT, the patient must be ambulated as soon as possible. To do so, the nurse should encourage the patient to take small walks with walking aids. Prophylactic anticoagulants like oral aspirin, oral clopidogrel, oral warfarin, or subcut heparin must be given. Compression stockings can also be applied as soon as the patient wakes up in the morning to inverse venous pressure and improve venous return.

126. (B) Renal failure.
Unfractionated heparin is more suitable for use than LMWH in patients with renal failure. This is because unfractionated heparin is excreted by the kidneys.

127. (D) Appendectomy.
Surgeries of the hip, pelvis and lower limbs have the highest risks of deep vein thrombosis, followed by surgeries of the CNS and spinal cord and major surgeries requiring general anesthesia.

128. (C) Inhibits absorption of bile acids.
Cholestyramine is a bile acid sequestrant that binds to bile acids and inhibits their absorption. This increases the uptake of LDL used in making bile acids. As more bile acids are synthesized from LDL, it is excreted. This mechanism reduces serum LDL in the long run. The use of this drug is, however, limited due to its gastrointestinal symptoms like bloating, flatulence, diarrhea and nausea. This drug reduces the absorption of thyroxine, digoxin and warfarin.

129. (B) To give moral advice.

This is not a purpose of therapeutic communication in a health setting. A health worker is not responsible for giving patients moral advice. They are, however, responsible for giving patients health education, health care and health advocacy. Forming a healthy patient-nurse relationship can help fulfill this goal.

130. (D) Probing.

Probing hinders therapeutic communication. Probing patients for answers to questions that are not necessary for their health care and its management is not only uncomfortable but offensive. Patients may react to this technique by being defensive, suspicious and uncooperative with future health-care plans.

131. (B) Denial.

Denial is a defense mechanism in which the person refuses to admit reality.

132. (C) Displacement.

In displacement, the patient redirects anger or feelings of frustration to a substitute that is not responsible for the condition/response.

133. (C) Offering your left hand for a handshake.

This gesture is deemed offensive in West African culture. The right hand is often associated with good luck, while the left hand is associated with bad luck.

134. (A) Japanese.

The Japanese avoid direct eye contact during conversations as a show of respect. They are likely to speak with their heads bowed.

135. (C) Hyperpyrexia.

According to the modified Jones criteria, major criteria are pancarditis, Sydenham chorea, erythema marginatum, polyarthritis and subcutaneous nodules. Minor criteria are polyarthralgia, hyperpyrexia, prolonged PR interval, elevated ESR and elevated C reactive protein.

136. (C) Incomplete vaccination.

Incomplete vaccination is an unlikely cause because rheumatic fever is caused by group A beta-hemolytic streptococci. Protection from this bacteria is not conferred by immunization. Risk factors for infection include overcrowding; malnutrition; low socioeconomic status; poor perineal hygiene, which includes poor respiratory hygiene; and insufficient handwashing.

137. (B) Inhibition of platelet aggregation with aspirin.

Aspirin is not appropriate for this patient. Aspirin is used for quick and symptomatic relief of fever, polyarthritis and polyarthralgia. About 5 to 20 mg/kg of oral aspirin is given to patients for two to four weeks.

138. (C) Atenolol.

Atenolol is unsuitable in the management of this patient. Vasodilators are used for symptomatic relief. These drugs include calcium channel blockers like nifedipine, felodipine, amlodipine, or isradipine; adrenergic blockers like prazosin; and nitrates like nitroglycerin applied topically on the fingers. Vasoconstrictors like beta-blockers, ergot derivatives and clonidine are contraindicated.

139. (C) Thoracotomy.
Urgent thoracotomy is required in patients with massive bleeding (greater than 1500 mL initially) or blood loss that is more than 200 ml/HR for two to four hours. It is also required in patients who need repeated transfusions of blood. For hemodynamically stable patients, fluid resuscitation and insertion of a chest tube are needed.

140. (D) Compression of the lung parenchyma.
The pathophysiologic processes seen in COPD are airway remodeling and narrowing caused by bronchospasm, mucus production and mucus plug, mucosal edema and fibrosis. Also, there is loss of elastic recoil and alveoli septa with enlargement of the alveolar spaces, which may coalesce into bullae. There is increased airway resistance, which causes hyperinflated lungs and increases energy spent on breathing.

141. (D) Increases heart rate.
Morphine is an opioid used in the acute management of pulmonary edema caused by left ventricular heart failure. It acts as an anxiolytic, providing relief from the restlessness and anxiousness seen in patients with pulmonary edema. It is a vasodilator, which reduces preload and afterload. It also improves respiratory function by reducing the work of breathing. It is not given to increase heart rate.

142. (A) Kerley B lines.
Kerley B lines are also known as septal lines. They are seen when the interlobular septa in the pulmonary tissue become prominent. Kerley B lines are a sign of interstitial edema in the lungs. Other features of pulmonary interstitial edema are thickening of the interlobar fissures, perihilar haze and peribronchial cuffing.

143. (B) Valproic acid.

Valproic acid is unlikely to have caused these symptoms. Antiseizure drugs are implicated in drug-induced gingival hyperplasia, a fibrotic type of gingival hyperplasia characterized by increased secretion and action of tumor growth factors and other cellular components. Implicated drugs include antiseizure drugs like phenytoin, lamotrigine, phenobarbital, vigabatrin, topiramate, ethosuximide and primidone; calcium channel blockers like amlodipine, nifedipine and verapamil; and immunosuppressants like cyclosporine.

144. (C) Head enlargement.

Head enlargement is not a presentation of hydrocephalus in teenagers and adults. This is because the sutures of the skull are rigid and do not allow expansion even in the face of increased intracranial pressure. In infants and toddlers, these sutures are pliable, allowing the head to increase in size.

145. (B) Staphylococcus epidermidis.

About 5 percent to 10 percent of shunts tend to become infected within a month of insertion. This occurrence is most likely in children and young adults. The most implicated organism is the commensal Staphylococcus epidermidis (about 60 percent of cases), followed by Staphylococcus aureus (about 30 percent of cases.)

146. (B) Obstruction.

Obstruction is a common malfunction of a shunt. Blockage can come from blood cells, tissue debris, or microorganisms. Blockage of the distal end of the shunt is a common occurrence in adults. In this case, a ventricular tap is not useful. Symptoms of obstruction in children are headaches, vomiting, nausea, restlessness and irritability. Fever is usually absent unless there is a superseding infection. The shunt track is often swollen.

147. (D) Ascites.
Ascites is not a complication of overdrainage of ventriculoperitoneal shunts. Complications are slit-like ventricles, which occur when the brain and its surrounding meninges pull away from the skull. This is seen in adults who have had a shunt since they were children. Another complication is Chiari I malformation, which is characterized by crowding of the posterior fossa and tonsillar herniation. Subdural hematoma also occurs when there is trauma to the subdural meninges and its surrounding tissue.

148. (C) Weight loss.
Weight gain (not loss) is a side effect of lithium use. Other side effects are polyuria, polydipsia, fine tremors, edema and fasciculation. These effects are transient and usually resolve when the dose is slightly reduced.

149. (B) Lithium.
Lithium is a mood stabilizer used for managing patients with bipolar disorder. Nausea and metallic taste are side effects of its use. Other side effects are weight gain, polyuria, polydipsia, tremors, fasciculations, neutropenia and hypothyroidism.

150. (C) Hyporeflexia.
Hyporeflexia is not a sign of lithium toxicity. Clinical features of acute lithium toxicity are brisk tendon reflexes, tremors, nausea, vomiting, seizures and arrhythmias. The risk for toxicity increases in elderly patients, patients with poor renal function and patients with hyponatremia.

151. (D) Serotonin reuptake inhibitor.
Tricyclic antidepressants are serotonin and norepinephrine reuptake inhibitors. They block the transportation of serotonin and norepinephrine and thereby increase the concentrations of these neurotransmitters in the synapses. They do not inhibit the reuptake of dopamine. Some of these TCAs also antagonize serotonin, adrenergic and NMDA receptors.

152. (D) Hallucinations.
Hallucinations are not a side effect of electroconvulsive therapy (ECT). ECT is used to treat patients with depression that is unresponsive to drugs. Common side effects are retrograde and anterograde amnesia, headaches, confusion, nausea and vomiting, arrhythmia and muscle soreness.

153. (D) Increases excretion of uric acid.
Probenecid is a uricosuric drug that increases the excretion of uric acid. Another example of a uricosuric drug is lesinurad. NSAIDs are given for analgesia, while colchicine is given as an immunomodulator. Allopurinol and febuxostat inhibit the production of uric acid.

154. (D) Skim milk.
The goal of a diet plan in patients with gout is to reduce foods that are high in purines (precursors of uric acid). Some of these foods are red meat, offal, seafood, alcohol made from grain and foods high in fructose (fruit juices, candy, ice cream and confectionery products). Suitable foods include skim milk and low-fat yogurt, complex carbohydrates, nuts and citruses.

155. (A) Splenic rupture.
Splenomegaly is a complication of infectious mononucleosis due to mass aggregation and release of lymphocytes. Splenic rupture can cause massive hypotension and increase morbidity. To reduce the risk of rupture after discharge, patients are advised to avoid contact sports and lifting heavy objects for one month.

156. (D) Avoid sharing utensils.
The patient will not be counseled to avoid sharing utensils because scabies is not spread via the feco-oral route. It is spread by prolonged direct contact (hugging, sex, sleeping on the same bed) and indirectly via fomites (clothes, bedsheets, towels, underwear). All close contacts of the patient must be traced and treated, and all of the patient's clothes and personal materials must be washed, sun- or air-dried, ironed and stored in air-tight bags for at least three days. This must also be done to the personal items of clothing of close contacts.

157. (D) Pulmonary tuberculosis.
Vancomycin is used neither as a first-line nor a second-line treatment of pulmonary tuberculosis. It is used to treat MRSA-mediated endocarditis, clostridium difficile–induced diarrhea, multidrug-resistant streptococcus pneumoniae, beta-lactam-resistant enterococci, viridans streptococci and corynebacteria.

158. (A) Penicillinase.
MRSA has penicillinase that inactivates beta-lactam antibiotics. Some of these beta-lactam antibiotics include penicillin, cephalosporins, carbapenems and monobactams. These beta-lactam antibiotics inhibit the synthesis of the bacteria's cell walls, thereby making them susceptible to lysis. Coagulase is

responsible for coagulating blood and is a feature of Staphylococcus aureus. Exotoxins are responsible for scalded skin syndrome, food poisoning and toxic shock syndrome.

159. (A) Hispanics.
Hispanics/Latinos have the highest risk of type 2 diabetes mellitus. According to the CDC, Hispanic adults have a 50 percent risk of developing diabetes mellitus in their lifetime. These risks are supported by cultural perceptions of food, genetics and lifestyle.

160. (D) Cystic fibrosis.
African Americans don't have an increased risk of cystic fibrosis. CF is a genetic condition affecting the exocrine glands and gastrointestinal and respiratory systems. It is commonly seen in Caucasians. In the United States, the incidence in Caucasians is 1:3, 300 live births.

161. (B) Providing more primary care providers.
A primary cause of patient boarding in the emergency room is the presentation of nonemergency cases in the ER as a result of primary care physicians and providers being overwhelmed. If more primary care providers are employed, patients are more likely to present to them before their condition deteriorates or before they become anxious.

162. (A) Increased turnover of radiological reports.
This statement is false because patient boarding decreases the turnover time for emergency radiologic reports like X-rays, CT scans and ultrasound scans.

163. (C) Question the caregivers on nursing interventions done so far.
This is not appropriate in this context. For an effective hand-off, the nurse should inquire and attend to the acutely ill patients first; repeat or read back received oral information for clarity and recall; review all data about care, presentation and treatment of the patients; and question and receive information from the giver of the handoff information.

164. (D) Socioeconomic status.
Socioeconomic status does not require documentation in the transfer report because it does not affect the mode or form of treatment that will be given in the rehabilitation center.

165. (A) One previous history of vertical uterine incision.
In VBAC, a trial of labor is not done on women with a previous history of vertical uterine incision. Other contraindications to VBAC are a previous history of uterine rupture and persisting conditions to vaginal delivery.

166. (C) Ergometrine.
Ergometrine is an oxytocic used in stimulating contractions. However, the contractions stimulated by ergometrine are frequent and sustained, and this characteristic makes it unsuitable for inducing labor. Ergometrine is used only after delivery of the fetus and for controlling postpartum hemorrhage. It is not used in patients with hypertension and other cardiovascular disorders.

167. (A) Stop oxytocin infusion.
This patient has hyperstimulation of her uterus. In this condition, there is a high risk of fetal distress and demise and uterine rupture. Hyperstimulation occurs when there are more than five contractions in 10 minutes. Management

principles include discontinuing oxytocin infusion, measuring fetal heart rate, encouraging the patient to turn to the left side and giving supplemental oxygen and IV fluids to increase oxygen circulation to the fetus.

168. (D) Episiotomy.
This is not a component of the active management of the third stage of labor, which involves the use of measures that minimize bleeding after the fetus is delivered. Components of the active management of the third stage of labor include controlled cord traction in delivering the placenta, rubbing off contractions by massaging the fundus of the uterus and administering IV oxytocin as soon as the fetal shoulder is delivered.

169. (B) Atony.
Uterine atony elevates the risk of postpartum hemorrhage in this patient, who is a grand multipara (with five or more viable pregnancies). Chorioamnionitis also puts her at risk of uterine atony. To reduce this risk, the principles of the active management of labor must be strictly adhered to.

170. (A) Vitamin B12 deficiency.
A deficiency of vitamin B12 causes megaloblastic anemia. Wernicke encephalopathy is a metabolic cause of delirium. The underlying pathophysiology is a deficiency of vitamin B1, thiamine, in the presence of alcohol intoxication. Metabolic causes of delirium include hyperglycemia, hypoglycemia, hypernatremia, acid-base disturbances, hyponatremia, hypocalcemia, hypercalcemia, hypomagnesemia, uremic encephalopathy, hepatic encephalopathy, dehydration and hypoxia.

171. (B) Below 15%.
According to the International Classification of Diseases, the criterion for diagnosing this patient is having a body weight below 15 percent of the expected body weight.

172. (C) Hypokalemia.
Hypokalemia is a common biochemical finding in patients with anorexia nervosa. This is a common cause of presentation in the ER. Other abnormal biochemical results are hypoglycemia, hypoalbuminemia and hypomagnesemia.

173. (B) Echopraxia.
Echopraxia, also known as echokinesis, is the involuntary imitation and repetition of the actions of another person. It is often seen in Tourette's syndrome, schizophrenia and autism spectrum disorders. Apraxia is a difficulty in performing previously acquired skills. Dysdiadochokinesia is the inability to perform rapidly alternating movements, while tardive dyskinesia is an extrapyramidal symptom characterized by involuntary movement of the tongue, face, lips, trunk and extremities.

174. (B) Enteral feeding.
This is not a priority in this patient because she requires acute resuscitation with IV fluids and glucose. Also, serum biochemistry and cardiac function must be monitored. You should note that this patient is at risk of having refeeding syndrome.

175. (C) Hallucinations.
Patients with dementia are unlikely to present with hallucinations. Typical presentations are disorientation in time, person and place; memory loss;

language impairment; delusional beliefs; and personality change. Hallucinations are seen in psychosis.

Test 4: Questions

1. Which of the following is the most significant history to be obtained from a 25-year-old male who presents to the ER with a history of intermittent claudication in the arch of his left foot and left leg?

A. Family history of diabetes
B. Smoking history
C. Drug history
D. Medical history

2. A 56-year-old obese female who presents to the ER with tenderness of the right calf, fever and leg pain is currently being managed for deep vein thrombosis. Which of the following best explains the use of heparin over warfarin in the acute management of this patient?

A. Wider therapeutic window
B. Availability of its antidote
C. The short onset of action
D. Less risk of hemorrhage

3. A 45-year-old female who presents to the ER with a history of chest pain, dizziness and severe hypotension is being managed for aortic disruption secondary to blunt trauma to the chest. Which of the following is not an expected finding on a chest X-ray?

A. Widened mediastinum
B. Unfolding of the aorta
C. Obliterated aortic knob
D. Pleural cap

4. Which of the following interventions is paramount in a 35-year-old male who presents to the ER with Beck's triad following penetrating trauma to the chest?

A. Pericardiocentesis
B. Thoracotomy
C. Thoracocentesis
D. Tracheostomy

5. A 56-year-old female is being managed in the ER for heart failure due to severe mitral stenosis. The attending physician requests monitoring of the pulmonary artery pressure, including pulmonary capillary wedge pressure. Which of the following areas of management is affected by the value of the pulmonary capillary wedge pressure?

A. Fluid input
B. Dose of antihypertensive
C. Blood transfusion
D. Anticoagulant therapy

6. A 65-year-old male presents to the ER with chest pain, cough and hemoptysis. Blood pressure on admission is 170/100 mmHg. As part of the patient's management, the attending physician orders insertion of a Swan-Ganz catheter. Which of the following best describes the purpose of this catheter?

A. Detection of occluded coronary arteries
B. Diagnosis of valvular insufficiency
C. Measurement of pulmonary wedge pressure
D. Measurement of left ventricular systolic pressure

7. You are preparing to discharge a patient who had an emergency CABG for STEMI. Which of the following discharge instructions is false?

A. Avoid heavy lifting
B. Cardiac rehabilitation program
C. Expect pedal edema
D. Expect low-grade fever one to two weeks after surgery

8. A 56-year-old male who presents to the ER with intermittent claudication and ulcers at the ankle had a femoropopliteal bypass for peripheral vascular disease. Which of the following parameters is most important for monitoring after the procedure?

A. Capillary refill
B. Tenderness
C. Pulse rate
D. Paresthesia

9. Nurse M is to measure the pulmonary capillary wedge pressure in a 55-year-old male who presents to the ER with left ventricular heart failure. After measuring the pressure, Nurse M is expected to do which of the following?

A. Ask the patient to lie in the semi-Fowler's position
B. Deflate the balloon quickly
C. Flush the catheter with normal saline
D. Administer oral analgesia

10. Which of the following treatment modalities is inappropriate in a 35-year-old male who presents to the ER with cardiogenic shock secondary to left ventricular failure?

A. IV vasopressors
B. Liberal IV fluids
C. Emergency PCI
D. Balloon pump

11. Which of the following best describes the mechanism of action of dobutamine given to a 67-year-old male being managed for cardiogenic shock secondary to myocardial infarction?

A. Alpha and beta-agonist
B. Beta-agonist
C. Adrenergic receptor blocker
D. Calcium channel agonist

12. A 25-year-old male presented to the ER with blunt trauma to the chest wall. On examination, there was hypotension, muffled heart sounds and increased jugular venous pressure. HR was 120 bpm, and RR was 40 cpm. A differential diagnosis of cardiac tamponade was made. Which of the following is the most likely cause of shock in this patient?

A. Impaired ventricular filling
B. Myocardial hypertrophy
C. Impaired ventricular emptying
D. Abnormal cardiac rhythm

13. Which of the following is not a cause of cardiogenic shock?

A. Abnormal cardiac rhythm
B. Decreased intravascular volume
C. Impaired ventricular filling
D. Impaired cardiac contractility

14. A 67-year-old female who presents to the ER with chest pain, diaphoresis and headaches is being managed with procainamide for supraventricular tachycardia. The attending nurse must be aware of which of the following side effects?

A. Tachycardia
B. Hypotension
C. Pruritus
D. Visual disturbances

15. Which of the following is not a clinical feature of cauda equina syndrome?

A. Saddle anesthesia
B. Urinary retention
C. Urinary incontinence
D. Brisk deep tendon reflexes

16. Which of the following is most appropriate in eliciting ankle clonus in a 35-year-old male who presents to the ER with a spinal cord injury secondary to a road traffic accident?

A. Flicking the nail on the middle finger
B. Rapid dorsiflexion and plantar flexion of the ankle joint
C. Extension of the knee when the hip is flexed
D. Stroking the sole of the foot

17. Which of the following is not a clinical feature of transection of the spinal cord at C8?

A. Flaccid paralysis
B. Horner's syndrome
C. Respiratory failure
D. Absent deep tendon reflexes

18. Which of the following is not a clinical feature of Brown-Séquard syndrome?

A. Contralateral loss of pain
B. Contralateral loss of temperature sensation
C. Ipsilateral spastic paralysis
D. Preserved proprioception

19. A 35-year-old female is being managed in the ER for Horner's syndrome due to a spinal cord injury. The lesion is most likely to be in which of the following nerve roots?

A. T1
B. C5
C. C7
D. L4

20. Which of the following differentiates neurogenic shock from spinal shock?

A. Bradycardia
B. Hypotension
C. Peripheral neuropathy
D. Autonomic neuropathy

21. Which of the following is not a clinical presentation of lesions around L1?

A. Erectile dysfunction
B. Urinary retention
C. Constipation
D. Abnormal anal wink reflex

22. Which of the following modalities is contraindicated for acute treatment in a 55-year-old male being managed for left hemispheric ischemic stroke secondary to malignant hypertension?

A. Anticoagulants
B. IV crystalloids
C. Diuretics
D. Antipyretics

23. Reduction of blood pressure is usually not a priority in the acute management of ischemic stroke. Which of the following best explains the reason?

A. It increases the risk of rebound hypertension.
B. Cerebral autoregulation is lost.
C. It increases the risk of hemorrhagic transformation.
D. Hypertension maintains cardiac output.

24. A patient with an ischemic stroke in the posterior cerebral artery is unlikely to present with which of the following symptoms?

A. Cortical blindness
B. Aphasia
C. Memory loss
D. Hemiballismus

25. A 57-year-old male presents to the ER with weaknesses of the left side of the body and an inability to form intelligible words. He is, however, able to understand words. A differential diagnosis of ischemic stroke is made. What type of speech disorder does this patient have?

A. Wernicke's aphasia
B. Motor aphasia
C. Global aphasia
D. Dysarthria

26. A 56-year-old male who is being managed in the ER for an ischemic stroke is unable to form comprehensible sentences. He is, however, not aware of this and is upset that no one understands what he is saying. What form of speech disorder is this?

A. Global aphasia
B. Dysarthria
C. Motor aphasia
D. Wernicke's aphasia

27. Which of the following best describes a patient with dysarthria?

A. Inability to use intelligible words
B. Inability to perform previously learned activities
C. Slurred speech
D. Inability to understand spoken words

28. Which of the following is not an indication of commencement of antihypertensives in a patient with ischemic stroke?

A. MAP greater than 130 mmHg
B. Acute renal failure
C. Use of tPA
D. Hyperthermia

29. Which of the following drugs is unsuitable for monotherapy in controlling blood pressure in a patient with ischemic stroke?

A. Labetalol
B. Nitroglycerin
C. Nicardipine
D. Hydralazine

30. A 66-year-old female with ischemic stroke is being managed with alteplase. Which of the following best describes the mechanism of action of this drug?

A. Plasmin activator
B. Plasminogen antagonist
C. Plasminogen activator
D. Plasmin antagonist

31. Which of the following management options is not useful in a 35-year-old male who is being managed for a TIA secondary to cocaine abuse?

A. Antipyretics
B. IV fluids
C. Enteral feeding
D. Anticoagulants

32. Which of the following is an unusual cause of stroke in a young adult?

A. Hypercoagulability
B. Hemoglobinopathy
C. Drug abuse
D. Hypertension

33. Which of the following is not a finding on brain CT suggestive of ischemic stroke?

A. Cortical hyperdensity
B. Effacement of the gyra
C. Loss of differentiation of gray-white matter
D. Effacement of the sulci

34. Which of the following treatment modalities is contraindicated in the management of a 55-year-old male with hemorrhagic stroke?

A. Dabigatran
B. IV labetalol
C. IV acetaminophen
D. IV diazepam

35. A 56-year-old male who was admitted with ST elevated myocardial infarction was discharged with oral dabigatran. Which of the following best describes the mechanism of action of this drug?

A. Inhibits platelet aggregation
B. Inhibits thrombin
C. Cleaves plasminogen
D. Inhibits vitamin K epoxide reductase

36. Which of the following IV fluids is most suitable for use in a five-year-old male admitted to the ER with severe dehydration caused by acute gastroenteritis?

A. Normal saline
B. Dextrose saline
C. Ringer's lactate
D. Dextrose water

37. Which of the following IV fluids is most suitable in resuscitating a 45-year-old male who presents with traumatic brain injury following a road traffic accident?

A. 0.9% normal saline
B. Half-strength Darrow's
C. Mannitol
D. 4.3% dextrose saline

38. Which of the following is a complication of administering hypotonic fluid?

A. Dehydration
B. Cell lysis
C. Oliguria
D. Hyperthermia

39. A 56-year-old male who presents to the ER with malignant hypertension is being managed with a hypertonic solution for cerebral edema. Which of the following is the nurse expected to monitor the patient closely for?

A. Dehydration
B. Pulmonary edema
C. Fever
D. Oliguria

40. A 67-year-old male who presents to the ER with pedal and sacral edema is being managed with a solution that can cause movement of water from the cellular to the extracellular space. What type of fluid is this?

A. Hypertonic
B. Isotonic
C. Hypotonic
D. Crystalloids

41. Which of the following cases is suitable for management with a hypotonic fluid?

A. Cerebral edema
B. Diabetic ketoacidosis
C. Severe burns
D. Hypovolemic shock

42. Which of the following is not a hypertonic fluid?

A. 5% dextrose water
B. 3% normal saline
C. 10% dextrose water
D. Full-strength Darrow's

43. You are to administer 50% dextrose through a central line in a 56-year-old female. It is important to monitor the central line to prevent which of the following?

A. Thrombosis
B. Phlebitis
C. Infiltration
D. Extravasation

44. Which of the following is not a short-term complication in a 56-year-old male receiving red blood cells for acute hemorrhagic shock?

A. Febrile nonhemolytic reaction
B. Post-transfusion purpura
C. Fluid overload
D. Reduced oxygen affinity

45. Which of the following is not a complication of massive blood transfusion?

A. Hyperthermia
B. Coagulopathy
C. Hypercalcemia
D. Hyperkalemia

46. Which of the following drugs is most suitable in managing a 56-year-old female with primary pulmonary hypertension caused by increased vascular resistance?

A. Sildenafil
B. Losartan
C. Amlodipine
D. Propranolol

47. Which of the following is a characteristic chest X-ray finding specific to pulmonary embolism?

A. Kerley B lines
B. Westermark sign
C. Pleural effusion
D. None of the above

48. Which of the following investigations is not necessary for confirming a diagnosis of pulmonary embolism?

A. V/Q scan
B. D-dimer
C. CT angiography
D. Chest X-ray

49. A 56-year-old obese female who presents to the ER with chest pain, dyspnea, cough and hemoptysis is suspected of having pulmonary fibrosis. Serum D-dimer is markedly elevated. Which of the following statements is correct?

A. Pulmonary embolism is confirmed.
B. CT angiography should be done.
C. V/Q scan is more sensitive than CT angiography.
D. Duplex ultrasonography should be done to locate emboli in the lungs.

50. A 76-year-old woman is being managed in the ER with pulmonary embolism. For the initial anticoagulation, the attending physician decides to use IV unfractionated heparin over low-molecular-weight heparin. Which of the following best explains the rest of his decision?

A. Decreased risk of bleeding
B. Short half-life
C. Improved bioavailability
D. Weight-based dosing

51. Which of the following is not a complication of pulmonary hypertension?

A. Heart failure

B. Raynaud's syndrome

C. Ortner's syndrome

D. Bartter syndrome

52. A 56-year-old female is placed on mechanical ventilation for respiratory failure secondary to acute exacerbation of COPD. Which of the following is a target used in measuring effective ventilation?

A. Respiratory rate >12 cpm

B. PaO2 >55mm Hg

C. Tidal volume of 6 mL/kg

D. PaCo2 <45 mmHg

53. Which of the following is not a pathophysiologic process involved in acute respiratory distress syndrome?

A. Pulmonary hypertension

B. Increased alveoli capillary permeability

C. Increased alveoli hydrostatic pressure

D. Airspace collapse

54. A patient presents to the ER with dyspnea, cough and anemia. On examination, the patient is pale, tachycardic and tachypneic. An emergency chest X-ray reveals diffuse alveolar infiltrates in both lungs. Which of the following investigations is required in diagnosing diffuse alveolar hemorrhage?

A. CT scan
B. Bronchoscopy
C. Spirometry
D. CT angiography

55. In which of the following conditions is the prone position for mechanical ventilation contraindicated?

A. Pulmonary embolism
B. Raised intracranial pressure
C. Aspiration pneumonitis
D. Epiglottis

56. Which of the following principles is false when liberating a patient from mechanical ventilation?

A. Daily breathing exercises should be done with a T piece.
B. The patient is capable of spontaneous ventilation when breathing deeply and slowly without a ventilator.
C. There should be a progressive withdrawal of sedatives.
D. Chest physiotherapy should be commenced.

57. Which of the following is not a cause of Eisenmenger syndrome?

A. Tetralogy of Fallot
B. Ventricular septal defect
C. Truncus arteriosus
D. Patent ductus arteriosus

58. Which of the following will not be assessed by a left heart catheterization?

A. Aortic blood pressure
B. Aortic valve function
C. Anatomy of the coronary arteries
D. Pulmonary artery pressure

59. A patient who presents to the ER with prelabor contractions is being managed with salbutamol. Which of the following best describes the function of this drug in this patient?

A. Bronchodilation
B. Tocolytic
C. Cervical dilatation
D. Anxiolytic

60. You are to discharge a patient who was admitted with acute cystitis. Which of the following measures is not useful in reducing the risk of recurrence?

A. Wiping from front to back
B. Cranberry juice
C. Avoid tampons
D. Use of antiseptic soaps

61. Nurse T is about to measure the fetal heart rate in an obstetric patient who presents with antepartum hemorrhage. Which of the following is false about the measurement of fetal heart rate?

A. The normal range is 120 to 160 bpm.
B. Fetal heart rate is mostly heard at the fundus of the uterus.
C. Continuous fetal heart rate monitoring is done via a cardiotocograph.
D. A Pinard is less sensitive than a Sonicaid.

62. A patient who is being managed in the ER with premature rupture of membranes is noted to have a fetal heart rate of 110 bpm. Which of the following interventions is most appropriate?

A. Give oral salbutamol.
B. Increase rate of IV drips
C. Encourage the patient to lie on the left side.
D. Perform pulse oximetry.

63. Which of the following patients will not benefit from Fowler's position?

A. A 56-year-old female with pulmonary edema
B. A 45-year-old male with a head injury
C. A 25-year-old male with GERD
D. A 55-year-old postop appendectomy patient

64. A patient who presents to the ER was placed in the Trendelenburg position. Which of the following describes the purpose of this position?

A. Reduces cerebral swelling
B. Relieves pulmonary congestion
C. Increases venous return
D. Reduces pedal edema

65. A 35-year-old male who had a lumbar puncture is counseled to stay in the supine position for an hour to reduce the risk of spinal headaches. Which of the following best describes the cause of spinal headaches after lumbar puncture?

A. Irritation of the nerve plexus in the spinal canal
B. A side effect of the local anesthetic
C. Redistribution of CSF
D. Bleeding into the spinal canal

66. After controlling and monitoring hemodynamic function in a patient with postpartum hemorrhage, the most appropriate stepwise action is:

A. Uterine evacuation
B. Balloon tamponade
C. B-Lynch suture
D. Hysterectomy

67. Which of the following drugs is unsuitable in inducing labor in a 35-year-old known asthmatic with preeclampsia at 36 weeks gestation?

A. Misoprostol
B. Prostaglandin
C. Mifepristone
D. Oxytocin

68. A 26-year-old gravid patient at 18 weeks gestation is being managed for hyperemesis gravidarum. She is at risk for all of the following except:

A. Wernicke encephalopathy
B. Mallory-Weiss tear
C. Liver disease
D. Gestational diabetes mellitus

69. Which of the following methods is most appropriate in stimulating a newborn with an Apgar score of six in the first minute of life?

A. Suctioning
B. Sternal rub
C. Flicking the soles of the feet
D. Depressing the nail beds

70. You are to commence chest compressions in a 34-week-old infant with an Apgar score of five in the fifth minute. Which of the following is the appropriate compression-to-ventilation ratio?

A. 1:3
B. 1:4
C. 3:1
D. 4:1

71. You are anticipating resuscitating a fetus delivered at 30 weeks gestation. Which of the following is not an expected physical feature?

A. Lanugo hair
B. Dry skin
C. Little body fat
D. Curly ears

72. Which of the following is not a risk factor for placenta previa?

A. Older maternal age
B. Prior caesarean section
C. Multiparity
D. Hypertension

73. A 25-year-old female who is being managed for antepartum hemorrhage secondary to third-degree placenta previa has the placenta located in which of the following?

A. Completely covering the internal os
B. Encroaching on the internal os
C. Asymmetrically covering the internal os
D. Encroaching on the lower uterine segment

74. Which of the following is not a usual characteristic of antepartum hemorrhage secondary to placenta previa?

A. Abdominal cramps
B. Scarlet blood
C. Normal fetal heart rate
D. Maternal tachycardia

75. A 35-year-old lactating female presented to the ER with fever, redness, induration and tenderness of her left breast. She is still in the puerperium. What is the most implicated bacteria?

A. Streptococcus
B. Staphylococcus
C. Actinobacteria
D. Corynebacteria

76. You are to discharge a lactating mother who was managed for mastitis. To reduce the risk of recurrence, you advise the mother to do which of the following?

A. Wear a tight bra
B. Apply warm compression pads on the nipples daily
C. Break suction after each feed by placing a finger between the baby's mouth and the nipple
D. Commence formula feeds

77. You are to discharge a patient who had an emergency caesarean section for prelabor rupture of membranes at 34 weeks gestation. You are to discharge her on ferrous sulfate. To increase the absorption of this drug, you should counsel this patient to take the drug with which of the following?

A. Milk
B. Orange juice
C. Warm water
D. Fatty meals

78. A patient is being managed with magnesium sulfate for severe preeclampsia. Which of the following best describes the rationale behind the use of this drug?

A. Tocolytic
B. Antihypertensive
C. Anticonvulsant
D. Anticoagulant

79. Which of the following is an early sign of magnesium sulfate toxicity in a patient being managed for severe preeclampsia?

A. Tinnitus
B. Hyporeflexia
C. Bradypnea
D. Oliguria

80. Which of the following is the most appropriate method of administering the loading dose of magnesium sulfate that comes in an ampule of 5 g/10mL?

A. Withdraw 4 ml of magnesium sulfate and dilute in 12 ml of normal saline
B. Withdraw 6 ml of magnesium sulfate and dilute in 14 ml of normal saline
C. Withdraw 10 ml of magnesium sulfate and dilute in 10 ml of normal saline
D. Withdraw 8 ml of magnesium sulfate and dilute in 12 ml of normal saline

81. Which of the following best describes the intramuscular regimen of giving a maintenance dose of magnesium sulfate in the Pritchard's regimen?

A. 10 g IM, 5 g every four hours
B. 10 g IV, 5 g every four hours
C. 10 g IM, 4 g every four hours
D. 10 mg IM, 4 g every four hours

82. In a patient being managed with IV labetalol for severe preeclampsia, which of the following statements is false?

A. 20 mg IV is given as a bolus.
B. The maximum dose in 24 hours is 350 mg.
C. The dose is increased sequentially to a maximum of 80 mg.
D. Fatigue is a side effect of its administration.

83. You are assessing clotting time in a 34-year-old female with severe preeclampsia. Her prothrombin time is prolonged. Which of the following is not the pathophysiology of her coagulopathy?

A. Hepatitis
B. Low platelets
C. Vitamin K deficiency
D. Fibrinolysis

84. A patient at 33 weeks gestation is being prepped for emergency caesarean section due to prelabor rupture of membranes and chorioamnionitis. To improve the respiratory function of the fetus, the woman is given which of the following?

A. Surfactant
B. Naltrexone
C. Magnesium sulfate
D. Dexamethasone

85. Which of the following aspects of an examination is used to differentiate threatened abortion from inevitable abortion?

A. Bimanual examination
B. Cervical motion tenderness
C. Fetal heart rate
D. Cervical os

86. A patient who presents to the ER with inevitable abortion is being managed with methotrexate. Which of the following describes the mechanism of action of this drug?

A. Cervical dilatation
B. Induction of labor
C. Contraction of the uterus
D. Cytotoxic

87. A patient who presents to the ER with inevitable abortion at 18 weeks will be managed with which of the following evacuation methods?

A. Suction curettage
B. Manual vacuum aspiration
C. Misoprostol
D. Oxytocin

88. Which of the following is not a clinical presentation of a hydatidiform mole?

A. Doughy uterus
B. Uterine bleeding
C. Severe vomiting
D. Jaundice

89. An obstetric patient who presents to the ER with vaginal bleeding has a fundal size that is smaller than the gestational age. Which of the following is not a likely cause?

A. Anemia
B. Potter's syndrome
C. Gestational diabetes
D. Young maternal age

90. Which of the following statements is false in the management of a patient in the active phase of labor?

A. Cervical dilatation is more than 4 cm.
B. Fetal heart rate should be monitored continuously with a Sonicaid.
C. Amniotomy is avoided in patients with HIV.
D. Cervical examinations are done every four hours.

91. In the management of abrasions, it is important that the wounds be prevented from drying out because dryness interferes with which of the following?

A. Clotting
B. Re-epithelization
C. Debridement
D. Asepsis

92. Which of the following is not an intervention in the management of abrasions?

A. Irrigation
B. Suturing
C. Antibiotics
D. Dressing

93. Which of the following sutures is unsuitable for the repair of the epidermis?

A. Nylon
B. Silk
C. Polyester
D. Polyglycolic acid

94. Which of the following is a disadvantage of nylon sutures?

A. Risk of infection
B. Tissue reactivity
C. High memory
D. High tensility

95. Which of the following is unlikely to slow down wound healing?

A. Hyperglycemia
B. Hypoproteinemia
C. Hypertriglyceridemia
D. Hypokalemia

96. Which of the following dressings is unsuitable for the primary dressing of a wound created by a pressure ulcer?

A. Transparent films
B. Gauze
C. Hydrocolloids
D. Foam dressings

97. Which of the following is a disadvantage of an alginate wound dressing?

A. Desiccation
B. Adhere to the wound
C. Tissue reaction
D. Requires frequent changing

98. Which of the following is a disadvantage of using a hydrocolloid dressing?

A. Desiccation
B. Adheres to the wound
C. Leaves residue on the wound bed
D. Requires frequent changing

99. Which of the following is not a function of a sitz bath in a patient who had an episiotomy?

A. Increases blood flow
B. Reduces edema
C. Cleans the perineum
D. Antiseptic properties

100. Which of the following is not a risk factor for pressure ulcers?

A. Urine incontinence
B. Immobility
C. Diabetes
D. Dementia

101. Which of the following measures is not useful in reducing the risk of pressure ulcers in a patient with cervical spine injury?

A. Two-hourly turning
B. Use of cotton sheets
C. Padding bony prominence
D. Use of petroleum jelly on friction areas

102. In the management of a patient with pressure ulcers, the wound should be cleaned with which of the following?

A. Povidone-iodine

B. Normal saline

C. Hydrogen peroxide

D. Chlorhexidine

103. Which of the following is an example of mechanical wound debridement?

A. Wet-to-dry dressings

B. Sterile scalpel

C. Hydrocolloid dressings

D. Use of sterile maggots

104. Which of the following is an example of autolytic wound debridement?

A. Transparent films

B. Sterile maggots

C. Use of collagenase

D. Wet-to-dry dressings

105. Which of the following is not a factor contributing to pressure ulcers?

A. Shearing

B. Pressure

C. Heat

D. Friction

106. Which of the following microorganisms is most implicated in erysipelas?

A. Staphylococcus aureus
B. Haemophilus influenzae
C. Streptococcus spp
D. Klebsiella pneumoniae

107. Which of the following interventions is most appropriate in the treatment of cutaneous abscesses?

A. Warm compresses
B. IV antibiotics
C. Incision and drainage
D. Topical antibiotics

108. Which of the following clinical features help differentiate cellulitis from deep vein thrombosis?

A. Peau d'orange
B. Tenderness
C. Edema
D. Ulcer

109. Which of the following groups is most at risk for scalded skin syndrome?

A. Infants
B. Elderly
C. Males
D. Females

110. Which of the following interventions is most appropriate for impetigo?

A. Wet-on-dry dressing
B. Incision and drainage
C. Warm compress
D. Topical antibiotics

111. Which of the following substances is least likely to cause physical dependence?

A. Nicotine
B. Alcohol
C. Heroine
D. Cannabis

112. A patient with symptoms of withdrawal from alcohol will be managed with which of the following?

A. Disulfiram
B. Bupropion
C. Naloxone
D. Diazepam

113. Which of the following is not a chronic complication of alcohol abuse?

A. Delirium tremens
B. Wernicke encephalopathy
C. Korsakoff psychosis
D. Enlarged parotid glands

114. A false positive result can be obtained for all of the following substances except:

A. Heroin
B. Amphetamine
C. Marijuana
D. Cocaine

115. A patient who presents to the ER with acute lead poisoning will be managed with any of these chelating agents except:

A. Succimer
B. Dimercaprol
C. BAL
D. Deferoxamine

116. A patient who presents to the ER with acute aspirin poisoning is being managed with IV sodium bicarbonate. Which of the following justifies the use of this drug?

A. Inhibits absorption of aspirin
B. Inhibits metabolism of aspirin
C. Increases excretion of aspirin
D. Stimulates enterohepatic circulation

117. A patient who presents to the ER with acute acetaminophen poisoning is being managed with Mucomyst. The emergency nurse knows that this drug is most effective if given within how many hours of acetaminophen ingestion?

A. 6
B. 8
C. 4
D. 2

118. The emergency nurse is to commence gastric lavage on a four-year-old male who presents to the ER with acute poisoning. Which of the following is the most likely complication of this procedure?

A. Prolonged vomiting
B. Abdominal distension
C. Aspiration
D. Hematemesis

119. A patient who presents to the ER with heavy metal poisoning is being managed with polyethylene glycol via an NGT. Which of the following best describes the action of this drug?

A. Saline laxative
B. Cathartic
C. Emollient
D. Osmotic laxative

120. The relatives of a patient with third-degree burns present to the ward with flowers. Which of the following responses is most appropriate?

A. Accept the flowers and place them on the patient's bedside table
B. Accept the flowers and place them at the reception
C. Inform the attending physician
D. Ask the caregivers to take the flowers away

121. A patient presents to the ER with third-degree burns. Which of the following statements is false?

A. Burns have extended into subcutaneous fat.
B. Treatment will include skin grafting.
C. Healing will start from the hair follicles.
D. Hypothermia is an immediate complication.

122. Which of the following interventions is inappropriate in a patient who presents to the ER with second-degree burns on the lower extremities?

A. IV analgesia
B. Assess airway
C. Insert a line with a size 18G cannula
D. Place the patient in a supine position

123. Which of the following best describes the use of the Parkland formula in burns management?

A. Determines total surface area with burns
B. Determines fluid management in the first 24 hours of the burn
C. Determines the degree of burns
D. Determines the amount of analgesic to be given

124. A patient with third-degree burns will be managed with which of the following fluids?

A. IV normal saline
B. IV dextrose saline
C. IV dextrose water
D. IV Ringer's lactate

125. Which of the following is not a characteristic of a first-degree burn?

A. May present as vesicles
B. Blanches easily
C. Intact pain sensation
D. Appears red

126. Which of the following animals is most implicated in the transmission of rabies in the United States?

A. Bats
B. Dogs
C. Raccoons
D. Skunks

127. Which of the following is the treatment modality in the management of rabies?

A. Sedatives
B. Rabies vaccine
C. Immunoglobulin
D. Ribavirin

128. Which of the following is not a clinical feature of heat exhaustion?

A. Dizziness
B. Nausea
C. Tachycardia
D. Delirium

129. During fluid correction in a patient with third-degree burns, the nurse must be alert to which of the following side effects?

A. Hyponatremia
B. Hypoglycemia
C. Hypokalemia
D. Hypoproteinemia

130. An emergency nurse is attending to a patient who presents to the ER with third-degree burns secondary to a fire incident. During the examination, the nurse notices that the mucous membranes of this patient are cherry red. Which of the following should the nurse suspect?

A. Inhalational injury
B. Carbon monoxide poisoning
C. Cyanosis
D. Shock

131. Which of the following interventions is suitable to be assigned to an LPN in the management of a patient with pulmonary embolism?

A. Serving the patient small, semisolid food
B. Auscultation of the lungs
C. Administering IV morphine
D. Assessing blood gases

132. You are to discharge a patient who was admitted with abdominal bloating, flatulence and dyspepsia. As you educate the patient on food choices, you encourage her to eat only little amounts of:

A. Yogurt
B. Cabbage
C. Corn
D. Radishes

133. Which of the following is not a right offered by EMTALA?

A. Right to medical screening
B. Right to resuscitation and stabilization
C. Right to transfer
D. Right to health insurance

134. Which of the following is a significant consequence of EMTALA on health-care organizations?

A. Increased working hours
B. Uncompensated care
C. Sepsis
D. Misdiagnosis

135. The privacy rule is enforced by which of the following bodies?

A. State nursing board
B. State law
C. Joint commission
D. Federal law

136. Which of the following bodies is not required to follow HIPAA regulations?

A. Health-care providers

B. Churches

C. Employers

D. Health insurance companies

137. Which of the following is not protected health information?

A. Billing address

B. Radiologic reports

C. Prescription forms

D. Educational data

138. HIPAA gives patients the right to do all of the following except:

A. Request a copy of their health records

B. Request corrections to their health records

C. Refuse treatment for their medical conditions

D. Refuse permission to use their health information

139. Which of the following is not a requirement for informed consent?

A. Competence

B. Voluntariness

C. Patient education

D. Financial ability

140. A 16-year-old married Muslim presents to the ER with acute appendicitis. For the patient to have an emergency appendectomy, informed consent must be obtained from?

A. Her father
B. Her husband
C. Her employer
D. Herself

141. You are preparing to examine a Muslim patient who presents to the ER with symptoms of acute PID. In the examining room, which of the following is most appropriate?

A. Ask the patient to remove her hijab and clothes and drape herself with a sheet.
B. Ask the patient to remove all her clothes and keep her hijab on.
C. Ask the patient to remove her hijab but keep her clothes on.
D. Expose only the parts that need to be examined.

142. Nurse P, a male CEN, is about to perform a cervical position on a married Muslim female. Nurse P is expected to first do which of the following?

A. Seek permission from the patient's husband
B. Get a chaperone
C. Get a female nurse to attend to the patient
D. Obtain consent

143. Nurse P has just withdrawn a sample from a venipuncture. To reduce the risk of needle injuries, he is expected to do which of the following?

A. Separate the needle from the syringe before discarding it
B. Cap the needle after withdrawing the sample
C. Disinfect his hands with hand sanitizer
D. Dispose of the syringe with the needle

144. Nurse M is attending to a patient from a road traffic accident. To reduce the risk of wound contamination, she is expected to do which of the following?

A. Use sterile gloves
B. Wear a drape
C. Work from uncontaminated to contaminated areas
D. Dress wounds with isopropyl alcohol

145. Nurse A has just had an accidental needle-prick injury. Which of the following should be her first action?

A. Dab the site with povidone-iodine
B. Run the affected site under tap water
C. Suck the puncture site
D. Commence HIV PEP

146. You are attending to a patient with meningococcal meningitis. Which of the following precautions should you employ?

A. Contact precautions
B. Airborne precautions
C. Droplet precautions
D. Bloodborne precautions

147. A patient who presents to the ER with a fracture of the wrist with no other injuries will be triaged as:

A. Urgent
B. Delayed
C. Expectant
D. Immediate

148. A patient who presents to the ER with Beck's triad following blunt trauma to the chest will be triaged as:

A. Delayed
B. Urgent
C. Immediate
D. Expectant

149. The emergency physician requests that the START protocol be used to attend to the mass casualty patients in the ER. Nurse P will assess patients with which of the following?

A. Chest auscultation and GCS
B. Respiration, pulse and mental status
C. GCS, respiration and blood pressure
D. Mental status, respiration and blood pressure

150. What is another name for the decontamination corridor?

A. Hot zone
B. Cold zone
C. Warm zone
D. Neutral zone

151. A 45-year-old homeless patient is being managed for Wernicke encephalopathy. This patient will need management with which of the following micronutrients?

A. Thiamine
B. Folic acid
C. Cobalamin
D. Ascorbic acid

152. Which of the following is not a clinical feature of generalized anxiety disorder?

A. Shortness of breath
B. Dizziness
C. Urinary frequency
D. Constipation

153. A patient with generalized anxiety disorder is being treated with citalopram. Which of the following describes the mechanism of action of this drug?

A. Norepinephrine reuptake inhibitor
B. Serotonin reuptake inhibitor
C. Serotonin receptor antagonist
D. Norepinephrine receptor antagonist

154. In which of the following disorders is a patient likely to have a fictitious illness for personal gain?

A. Conversion disorder
B. Munchausen's
C. Malingering
D. Hypochondriasis

155. A female patient who is being managed for schizophrenia attempts to converse with the nurse attending to her. Her speech is rambling, although fluent. Which of the following terms describes this phenomenon?

A. Glossolalia
B. Logorrhea
C. Aphasia
D. Apraxia

156. A 15-year-old female who presents to the ER with major depressive disorder is placed on an SSRI. Which of the following is the patient most at risk of developing?

A. Hallucination
B. Obesity
C. Suicidal ideation
D. Anorexia nervosa

157. Which of the following drugs is unlikely to cause neuroleptic malignant syndrome?

A. Haloperidol
B. Olanzapine
C. Droperidol
D. Citalopram

158. To reduce the risk of hypertensive crises in a patient placed on phenelzine, the patient must be counseled on the effects of taking certain foods with the drug. Which of the following foods is not implicated?

A. Cheese
B. Grapes
C. Cured meat
D. Raisins

159. Which of the following is not a feature of serotonin syndrome?

A. Hyperthermia
B. Metabolic acidosis
C. Acute kidney injury
D. Hypokalemia

160. A 27-year-old female who presents to the ER says people can hear her thoughts. Which of the following best describes this phenomenon?

A. Thought insertion
B. Delusion of persecution
C. Thought broadcasting
D. Delusion of grandeur

161. A patient who is being treated with buspirone is likely to have which of the following?

A. Schizophrenia
B. Alcohol dependence
C. Generalized anxiety disorder
D. Bipolar disorder

162. A patient who is being managed with olanzapine is likely to complain of reduced libido due to the drug's antagonistic effect on which of the following?

A. Norepinephrine
B. Dopamine
C. Serotonin
D. Acetylcholine

163. A patient who presents to the ER with agitation and psychosis is given haloperidol. Sedation is a side effect of this drug because of its action on which of the following receptors?

A. Serotonin
B. Dopamine
C. Histamine
D. Acetylcholine

164. A 54-year-old woman who presents to the ER with insomnia and anxiety says that she sees images of snakes on her bed as soon as she wakes up from sleep. What form of hallucination is this?

A. Hypnopompic
B. Hypnagogic
C. Gustatory
D. Tactile

165. A patient who presents to the ER is noticed to imitate the speech of the attending nurse. Which of the following best describes this occurrence?

A. Echopraxia
B. Apraxia
C. Echolalia
D. Aphasia

166. A client is being managed with warfarin for transient ischemic attacks. Which of the following is required to evaluate the therapeutic level of warfarin?

A. Platelet count
B. Partial thromboplastin time
C. Bleeding time
D. Prothrombin time

167. A toddler who presents to the ER has just been diagnosed with shaken child syndrome from child abuse. Which of the following signs most supports this diagnosis?

A. Fracture of the clavicle
B. Dislocation of the wrist
C. Retinal hemorrhage
D. Battle's sign

168. Which of the following is the most common cause of postpartum hemorrhage?

A. Cervical laceration
B. DIC
C. Uterine atony
D. Retained placenta

169. Which of the following is the primary cause of anemia in a patient with end-stage renal disease?

A. Increased lysis of the red blood cells
B. Erythropoietin deficiency
C. Poor iron absorption
D. Hyperplasia of the bone marrow

170. A patient who presents to the ER with angina is being managed with nitroglycerin. Which of the following best describes the mechanism of action of this drug?

A. Reduces preload
B. Reduces afterload
C. Reduces heart rate
D. Dilates the coronary arteries

171. A patient who is being managed for hyperemesis gravidarum is at risk of all these except:

A. Dehydration
B. Wernicke encephalopathy
C. Liver failure
D. HELLP

172. A patient who presents to the ER with antepartum hemorrhage at 34 weeks is being worked up for emergency CS. For prophylaxis of Rh sensitization, she is to receive RhoGAM at which of the following times?

A. Within one week of delivery
B. Within 72 hours of delivery
C. Within one month of delivery
D. Within 48 hours of delivery

173. A woman who presents to the ER with hyperemesis gravidarum at 34 weeks has just had an amniotomy for augmentation of labor. Which of the following actions must be prioritized by the nurse?

A. Assess cervical dilatation
B. Assess fetal heart rate
C. Assess maternal pulse
D. Assess contractions

174. A 67-year-old female is being managed for a fracture of the neck of the femur secondary to osteoporosis. Which of the following is the most common risk factor of osteoporosis in women?

A. Insufficient calcium intake
B. Estrogen depletion
C. Hypertension
D. Genetics

175. Which of the following is correct about the blood group AB?

A. It is a universal donor.
B. It has both A and B antibodies.
C. It has no A and B antigens.
D. It has both A and B antigens.

Test 4: Answers and Explanations

1. (B) Smoking history.
This patient most likely has Buerger's disease, a peripheral arterial disease seen in young adults. It is commonly seen in tobacco smokers, with a high prevalence in Asians and people from the Middle East. Buerger's disease is also called thromboangiitis obliterans.

2. (C) The short onset of action.
Heparin is used in acute and emergency settings because of its short onset of action compared to warfarin. The therapeutic effect of warfarin starts about five days after the commencement of therapy. The goal of treatment in this patient will include initial treatment with low molecular-weight heparin, then long-term management with warfarin and other oral anticoagulants.

3. (B) Unfolding of the aorta.
The unfolding of the aorta is not a characteristic chest X-ray finding in aortic disruption. It is seen in hypertensive heart disease. Classic findings on chest X-ray are widened mediastinum, obliterated aortic knob, tracheal or esophageal deviation, apical or pleural cap, pneumothorax, pulmonary contusion, hemothorax and depressed bronchus.

4. (A) Pericardiocentesis.
Emergency subxiphoid pericardiocentesis must be performed in patients with suspected cardiac tamponade secondary to trauma to the chest. During the procedure, the cardiac activity must be monitored with an ECG for ST elevation. Pericardiocentesis is therapeutic even when as little as 10 mL of blood is

withdrawn. Definitive treatment is thoracotomy with pericardiotomy. This is done on patients with confirmed cardiac tamponade. It must be done by trained and qualified personnel.

5. (A) Fluid input.
Pulmonary capillary wedge pressure determines the amount of fluid used in fluid management. Pulmonary capillary wedge pressure is done to assess the end-diastolic pressure in the left ventricle. The high pressure causes backflow of blood from the intravascular space into the tissue space. This causes pulmonary effusion and worsens the patient's symptoms.

6. (C) Measurement of pulmonary wedge pressure.
The Swan-Ganz catheter is also known as the pulmonary artery catheter. It is used to monitor and measure pressures in the pulmonary artery, right atrium, right ventricle and the wedge pressure of the left atrium. Unlike right cardiac catheterization, it does not diagnose occlusion of coronary arteries and valvular insufficiency.

7. (D) Expect low-grade fever one to two weeks after surgery.
This statement is false because fever is a sign of ongoing infection. The patient should be instructed to check his temperature regularly and report any temperature spikes, bleeding from the wound site, erythema or pus drainage.

8. (A) Capillary refill.
Capillary refill should be assessed on the nail beds of the toes to assess tissue perfusion of the lower limbs.

9. (B) Deflate the balloon quickly.
To prevent obstruction of blood flow to the lung, the balloon must be quickly deflated as soon as the pulmonary capillary wedge pressure is obtained.

10. (B) Liberal IV fluids.
In this patient, IV fluids must be used cautiously to avoid worsening pulmonary function. Already, there is increased hydrostatic pressure in the pulmonary bed leading to pulmonary edema and congestion. Liberal IV fluids can raise this pressure and further congest the lungs. Treatment modalities include IV vasopressors like dobutamine or dopamine, or a combination of both; balloon pumps for temporary support; and emergency angiography or coronary artery bypass grafting.

11. (B) Beta-agonist.
Dobutamine is a beta-agonist. It is a vasoconstrictor that works by stimulating the beta-agonist receptors in the heart. This stimulation increases heart rate, cardiac output and stroke volume. Dobutamine is given intravenously.

12. (A) Impaired ventricular filling.
This patient has obstructive shock caused by impaired ventricular filling. Accumulation of blood within the pericardial sac prevents expansion of the heart during diastole and sufficient ventricular filling. Treatment in this patient is the immediate removal of the accumulated blood via either a pericardiocentesis or pericardiotomy.

13. (B) Decreased intravascular volume.
This is a cause of hypovolemic shock, not cardiogenic shock. Decreased intravascular volume leads to reduced preload, diminished ventricular filling and

reduced stroke volume. Causes of decreased intravascular volume include acute blood loss from accidents; surgeries; upper or lower gastrointestinal bleeding; or other fluid losses like dehydration, severe burns, vomiting, diarrhea and others.

14. (B) Hypotension.
Procainamide is a sodium channel blocker and a class 1 antiarrhythmic drug. Particular side effects are hypotension, bradycardia and shock. High doses also cause lupus erythematosus that manifests as pleurisy, myalgia and arthralgia. These side effects are caused by the acetylation of procainamide.

15. (D) Brisk deep tendon reflexes.
The symptoms of cauda equina syndrome are a result of compression of a segment of the lumbar section of the spinal cord. Clinical features are paresis of the distal leg; saddle anesthesia (loss of sensation around the perineum); dysfunction of the bladder and bowel, which manifests as erectile dysfunction, urinary frequency and incontinence; urinary retention; and loss of anal wink reflexes and rectal tone. Deep tendon reflexes and muscle tone are decreased in the distal limbs.

16. (B) Rapid dorsiflexion and plantar flexion of the ankle joint.
Ankle clonus is elicited by rapidly plantar flexing and dorsiflexing the ankle joint. A positive reflex involves rapid and involuntary movement of the ankle. It is a sign of an upper motor neuron disease. Some causes are spinal cord injury, cerebral palsy, multiple sclerosis, epilepsy, stroke and hepatic encephalopathy. Option A describes Hoffman's reflex. Options C and D describe the Kernig sign and Babinski sign respectively.

17. (C) Respiratory failure.
Respiratory failure occurs in spinal cord transections at or above C5. This is because of loss of innervation to the muscles involved in respiration. Transections that are higher up at C3 cause dysfunction in the autonomic regulation of respiration and blood pressure. This leads to neurogenic shock.

18. (D) Preserved proprioception.
Brown-Séquard syndrome is caused by unilateral hemisection of the spinal cord. Clinical features include ipsilateral loss of proprioception and spastic paralysis below the lesion and contralateral loss of temperature and pain sensation below the lesion.

19. (A) T1.
Horner's syndrome is caused by a transverse lesion of the C8 or T1 nerve roots. Clinical features include ptosis, miosis, anhidrosis, enophthalmos and hyperemia. Transections at C5 cause respiratory failure and quadriplegia, transection at C7 causes quadriplegia and transections at L4 cause cauda equina syndrome.

20. (D) Autonomic neuropathy.
Neurogenic shock is an autonomic neuropathy caused by a disruption of the sympathetic nervous system. It is caused by lesions around the C3-C5 spinal cord. Spinal shock is a peripheral neuropathy caused by loss of response of the peripheral nerves to stimuli from the brain. It is temporal. Clinical features of neurogenic and spinal shock overlap. They are hypotension, bradycardia, flaccid paralysis and absent bulbocavernosus reflex.

21. (C) Constipation.

Constipation is not a clinical presentation of lesions around L1. Such lesions cause conus medullaris syndrome. Clinical features of this syndrome are saddle anesthesia; paresis of the distal leg; urinary retention, frequency or incontinence; hypotonic anal sphincter leading to fecal incontinence; abnormal anal wink and bulbocavernosus reflexes.

22. (A) Anticoagulants.

Anticoagulants are generally not used in the acute treatment of ischemic stroke due to the risk of hemorrhagic transformation, which can worsen the outcome of the patient. This risk is higher in patients with large infarcts.

23. (B) Cerebral autoregulation is lost.

Reduction of blood pressure is usually not a priority in the acute management of ischemic stroke because cerebral autoregulation is lost. This means that cerebral perfusion in patients with ischemic stroke is dependent on cerebral arterial pressure. Reducing the blood pressure can cause hypoperfusion and worsen the patient's outcome.

24. (B) Aphasia.

Aphasia is an inability to comprehend or use previously learned words. It is a sign of ongoing pathophysiology in the speech center of the brain, which is located in the frontal lobe of the cerebral cortex and supplied by the middle cerebral artery. The posterior central artery supplies the occipital lobe, the posterior limb of the internal capsule, the thalamus and the inferior part of the temporal lobe. An infarct in this artery causes dysfunction in vision, memory, movement and balance.

25. (B) Motor aphasia.
Also known as Broca's aphasia, motor aphasia occurs as a result of an infarct to the Broca's area in the frontal lobe of the brain. This is commonly seen in infants, involving the middle cerebral artery. In this condition, the patient is unable to form intelligible words. The person is, however, able to understand words.

26. (D) Wernicke's aphasia.
This speech disorder is caused by an infarct in the Wernicke area in the temporal lobe of the brain. Patients who have this disorder can speak but are unable to use comprehensible words. They also cannot understand others when they speak and do not seem to know that their listeners cannot comprehend their words.

27. (C) Slurred speech.
Dysarthria is also called slurred speech. It is a motor speech disorder characterized by paralysis of the muscles responsible for speech. The vocal cords can also be affected.

28. (D) Hyperthermia.
Reduction of blood pressure is usually not required in the acute management of ischemic stroke. However, some indications warrant the use of antihypertensives. Some of these are MAP that is greater than 130 mmHg, features of end-organ failure (e.g., acute renal failure, aortic dissection, pulmonary edema and hypertensive encephalopathy)and use of tPa, thrombolytics or thrombectomy.

29. (B) Nitroglycerin.
Nitroglycerin is a potent vasodilator, useful in reducing both preload and afterload in patients with high blood pressure. It is a short-acting drug and unsuitable for monotherapy due to the risk of rebound hypertension.

30. (C) Plasminogen activator.
Alteplase is thrombolytic that binds to fibrin and activates plasminogen. It cleaves plasminogen into plasmin. Plasmin is a fibrinolytic that breaks down fibrin polymers and thereby dissolves blood clots.

31. (C) Enteral feeding.
Patients with TIA have focal neurologic deficits that last less than an hour. Enteral feeding with a feeding tube is inappropriate since acute correction for hypoglycemia can be done with oral fluids. Treatment options in TIA are focused on eliminating risk factors to reduce the risk of reoccurrence.

32. (D) Hypertension.
Hypertension is an unusual cause of stroke in a young adult. Usual causes of stroke include hypercoagulability, hemoglobinopathy, drug abuse, heart disorders, vasculitis, cigarette smoking, psychosocial stress and others.

33. (A) Cortical hyperdensity.
This statement is false because cortical hypodensity is a CT finding of ischemic stroke. Other features are hypoattenuation of the deep nuclei, flattening of the sulci and gyri due to cerebral edema, loss of gray-white matter differentiation and changes in the lentiform nucleus.

34. (A) Dabigatran.
Anticoagulants are contraindicated in all cases of hemorrhagic stroke. This is due to the high-risk bleeding and worsening of the patient’s outcome. Patients with prior antiplatelet use before presentation are treated with fresh frozen plasma,

platelet, hemodialysis, vitamin K or prothrombin complex concentrate, whichever is appropriate.

35. (B) Inhibits thrombin.
Dabigatran is an anticoagulant that works by directly inhibiting the action of thrombin (Factor IIa). In the clotting cascade, thrombin cleaves fibrinogen into fibrin. These fibrin fibers are then added to the platelet plug to reinforce blood clots.

36. (C) Ringer's lactate.
Ringer's lactate or Hartman's solution is a potassium-rich isotonic fluid used for managing pediatric patients with severe dehydration caused by gastroenteritis. It is also used for managing patients with metabolic acidosis.

37. (A) 0.9% saline.
Normal saline is the fluid of choice in resuscitating a patient with traumatic brain injury. It is an isotonic fluid; therefore, most of the fluid is contained in the intravascular space. It increases blood pressure and cerebral perfusion. Although mannitol is used in treating cerebral edema, it is not used for resuscitation.

38. (B) Cell lysis.
Cellular edema and cell lysis are complications of using hypotonic fluids. Hypotonic fluids cause the movement of water from the intravascular space into the extracellular space. This is because the osmolality in the fluids is less than the osmolality in the cells. These fluids are used in patients with cellular dehydration (diabetic ketoacidosis and hyperglycemic hyperosmolar state).

39. (B) Pulmonary edema.
Hypertonic solutions have a higher osmolality than those in the cells. As a result of this differential gradient, water moves from the cell into the intravascular space. Hypertonic solutions are useful for patients with cellular edema and increased intracranial pressure. However, these patients must be monitored for fluid overload (pulmonary edema). IV diuretics like furosemide are usually used along with hypertonic fluids.

40. (A) Hypertonic.
Hypertonic solutions have a higher osmolality than those in the cells. As a result of this differential gradient, water moves from the cell into the intravascular space. Hypertonic solutions are useful for patients with cellular edema and increased intracranial pressure. Examples are 3% saline, 10% dextrose water, 5% dextrose in 0.9% saline, 5% dextrose in Ringer's lactate and 50% dextrose water.

41. (B) Diabetic ketoacidosis.
Hypotonic solutions are used to manage patients with cellular dehydration. They must be avoided in patients with cellular edema and intravascular hypovolemia.

42. (A) 5% dextrose water.
Five percent dextrose water is an isotonic solution that may be considered a hypotonic (not hypertonic) fluid. When administered, it acts as a hypotonic fluid, but after the dextrose is used up, it acts as an isotonic fluid. It is used to treat hypoglycemia and hypovolemic shock. It is also used as a maintenance fluid.

43. (D) Extravasation.
Extravasation occurs when vesicant fluids or drugs infiltrate a line and cause tissue injury. Examples of vesicant drugs and fluids are 50% dextrose water,

calcium gluconate, valium chloride, dopamine, phenytoin, promethazine, vasopressin, sodium bicarbonate, epinephrine and dobutamine. These drugs must never be given IM or SC.

44. (B) Post-transfusion purpura.
This is a long-term (not short-term) complication that arises about 4 to 14 days after transfusion of red blood cells. It causes moderate to severe thrombocytopenia. At-risk groups are multiparous women who receive red blood cells during surgery.

45. (A) Hyperthermia.
Massive blood transfusion is transfusion of blood that is more than one blood volume in 24 hours, or transfusion of more than 10 units of blood in an adult weighing 70 kg. Complications of massive transfusion are hypothermia (not hyperthermia), hyperkalemia, hypercalcemia and coagulopathy.

46. (A) Sildenafil.
Patients with familial and idiopathic pulmonary arterial hypertension are managed with drugs like oral phosphodiesterase 5 inhibitors (sildenafil), prostacyclin analogs (epoprostenol), soluble guanylate cyclase inhibitors (riociguat)and endothelin receptor antagonists (bosentan).

47. (D) None of the above.
All these signs have low specificity for pulmonary embolism. Chest x-ray is a nonspecific test for diagnosing pulmonary embolism. Tests that are used for diagnosing pulmonary embolism include D-dimer testing, V/Q scanning, CT angiography, and Duplex ultrasonography.

48. (D) Chest X-ray.
Chest X-ray findings are nonspecific for pulmonary embolism. Relevant investigations include CT angiography, D-dimer, V/Q scanning and duplex ultrasonography.

49. (B) CT angiography should be done.
CT angiography is fast, highly specific and sensitive for pulmonary embolism. It can also assess the severity of the embolism. Option A is incorrect because elevated D-dimers do not confirm the diagnosis of pulmonary embolism. Pulmonary embolism is, however, excluded if D-dimer is normal. Option C is incorrect because CT angiography is more sensitive than VQ scanning. Option D is incorrect because duplex ultrasonography is used to detect thrombi in the upper and lower limbs.

50. (B) Short half-life.
Although low-molecular-weight heparin has certain favorable characteristics (e.g., improved bioavailability, weight-based dosing, reduced risk of bleeding and thrombocytopenia, ease of administration and others), unfractionated heparin has a short half-life and is readily reversible with protamine sulfate.

51. (D) Bartter syndrome.
Bartter syndrome is a generic renal disease characterized by potassium, sodium, hydrogen ions and chloride loss via the urine, which leads to hyperaldosteronism and metabolic alkalosis. Right-sided heart failure is a common complication of chronic pulmonary hypertension. Raynaud's syndrome is a rare complication seen mostly in women. Ortner's syndrome is a rare complication characterized by hoarseness due to compression of the laryngeal nerve by an enlarged artery.

52. (C) Tidal volume of 6 mL/kg.

The target respiratory function in a person who is placed on mechanical ventilation for respiratory failure is tidal volume of 6 mL/kg of predicted weight, plateau alveolar pressures that are less than 30 cm H30 and FIO2 that is low to maintain oxygen saturation.

53. (C) Increased alveoli hydrostatic pressure.

The pathophysiologic process involved in ARDS is the onset of inflammation, which activates the release of macrophages, neutrophils and other inflammatory mediators; increased capillary permeability that leads to edema and movement of proteins and other cellular debris into the alveoli space; surfactant disruption; airspace collapse; and pulmonary hypertension.

54. (B) Bronchoscopy.

Bronchoscopy with bronchoalveolar lavage (BAL) is needed to make a diagnosis of diffuse alveolar hemorrhage.

55. (B) Raised intracranial pressure.

In mechanical ventilation, prone positioning creates better oxygenation and ensures uniform ventilation of all lung fields. However, it is contraindicated in patients with spinal injury (to avoid damage to the cervical part of the spinal cord) and in patients with raised intracranial pressure (it is important to elevate the head of the bed to about 30° to increase venous return and reduce cerebral edema).

56. (D) Chest physiotherapy should be commenced.

Chest physiotherapy is not a requirement for liberating a patient from mechanical ventilation. Indications for chest physiotherapy are orthostatic pneumonia, COPD, neuromuscular diseases affecting muscles of respiration, cystic fibrosis and bronchiectasis. Chest physiotherapy improves mobilization and clearance of secretions in the airway.

57. (A) Tetralogy of Fallot.
Eisenmenger syndrome is caused by chronic and untreated left-to-right blood shunts, as seen in cyanotic congenital heart defects. When these heart defects are not corrected, there is an increase in pulmonary resistance, which leads to right-to-left shunting of blood. Clinical features are cyanosis, finger clubbing and features of heart failure.

58. (D) Pulmonary artery pressure.
Left heart catheterization is used to assess the anatomy of the coronary arteries, systemic vascular resistance, the function of the mitral and aortic valves, aortic blood pressure and left ventricular pressure. Right heart catheterization is used to assess the pressure in the right atrium, right ventricle and pulmonary arteries.

59. (B) Tocolytic.
Salbutamol is a beta-agonist. It is also a tocolytic given to patients with prelabor contractions to stimulate relaxation of the uterine muscles.

60. (D) Use of antiseptic soaps.
This measure will increase (not reduce) the risk of urinary tract infections. This is because antiseptic soaps kill normal bacteria flora in the skin and vagina, allowing proliferation and unchecked growth of opportunistic bacteria and fungi.

61. (B) Fetal heart rate is mostly heard at the fundus of the uterus.
This statement is false. Fetal heart rate is mostly heard at the left or right of the midline of the abdomen.

62. (C) Encourage the patient to lie on the left side.
This should be the first response. Next, the rate of transfusion of the IV fluid is increased and oxygen is administered. If the fetal heart rate decreases or refuses to improve, the physician must be promptly informed.

63. (D) A 55-year-old postop appendectomy patient.
In Fowler's position, the patient's head and chest are elevated. The position can be a high Fowler's position at 45° or a low Fowler's position at about 30°. Patients with respiratory and cardiac conditions will benefit from high Fowler's position because they experience relief from long congestions. Patients with head injuries should be placed in the low Fowler's position to improve venous drainage of the brain and reduce cerebral swelling.

64. (C) Increases venous return.
In the Trendelenburg position, the patient's head is tilted down till it is lower than the lower limbs. This position is used in patients with hypovolemic shock to improve venous return to the brain and heart.

65. (C) Redistribution of CSF.
After lumbar puncture, cerebrospinal fluid gravitates from the ventricles into the spinal cord. This sudden shift of volume creates traction and causes spinal headaches.

66. (A) Uterine evacuation.
After obtaining hemostatic control with IV fluids and oxytocin, the uterus must be explored and evacuated of retained products of conception. The cervix is also examined for lacerations and prompt repair is done. If the bleeding persists, other control measures, like tamponade with the Bakri balloon, use of a B-Lynch suture, ligation of the hypogastric artery, or hysterectomy, can be done.

67. (B) Prostaglandin.
Prostaglandin is contraindicated in patients with asthma due to increased risk of bronchial construction, mucus formation and other hyperactive reactions of the airway.

68. (D) Gestational diabetes mellitus.
Hypoglycemia, not gestational diabetes mellitus, is a complication of this condition. Complications of hyperemesis gravidarum are dehydration, ketosis, hypoglycemia and electrolyte disorders. More severe complications are fatty liver disease, Wernicke encephalopathy and Mallory-Weiss tears.

69. (C) Flicking the soles of the feet.
This is the most appropriate method of stimulating a newborn with an Apgar score of six in the first minute of life. Another method is to rub the back when drying. Suctioning is not an appropriate method as it is recommended only for infants with airway obstruction. Prolonged suctioning can stimulate the vasovagal response and cause bradycardia. Sternal rubs and depressing the nail beds are unacceptable methods of stimulation.

70. (C) 3:1.

Chest compressions must be given in a ratio of three compressions to one ventilation in a minute. This means that in one minute, 120 events, that is 90 compressions and 30 ventilations, must be done. Heart rate is reassessed every one minute.

71. (B) Dry skin.

Dry, scaly skin is seen in post-term infants. Preterm infants are likely to present with shiny, pink, or translucent skin due to incomplete development of the dermis and insufficient deposition of adipose tissue. Other features of prematurity are lanugo hair, curly ears, weight less than 2500 g, underdeveloped genitals and poor cry and body tone.

72. (D) Hypertension.

Hypertension and other hypertensive diseases in pregnancy increase the risk of abruptio placentae, not placenta previa. Risk factors for placenta previa are prior caesarean section, prior induced abortion, myomectomy or fibroids, multiple gestation, older maternal age, smoking and multiparity.

73. (C) Asymmetrically covering the internal os.

In third-degree placenta previa, the placenta asymmetrically covers the internal os, such that during full dilation of the cervix, the placenta is away from the cervical os.

74. (A) Abdominal cramps.

The bleeding in the placenta previa is often painless. Blood loss is variable and bright red, unlike placenta abruption, which may present with abdominal cramps and passage of altered blood. The fetal heart rate in placenta previa is normal, but in abruptio placentae, the fetal heart rate reveals fetal distress. It is important to note that confirmation of diagnosis can be made only by a transvaginal ultrasound scan. Placenta previa must be ruled out or confirmed before a pelvic examination is done.

75. (B) Staphylococcus.
Staphylococcus species are the most implicated bacteria in mastitis. Treatment includes drugs targeted at treating Staphylococcus aureus, such as cephalosporins and macrolides.

76. (C) Break suction after each feed by placing a finger between the baby's mouth and the nipple.
This intervention will help reduce the risk of nipple soreness. Option A is incorrect because a tight bra is used to stop lactation in mothers who had stillbirths. Option B is not useful in reducing the risk of mastitis and Option D is not helpful to the infant.

77. (B) Orange juice.
Ascorbic acid increases the absorption of iron. Calcium impairs iron absorption. Therefore, foods like yogurt, cheese, broccoli, sardines, figs and canned salmon can impair iron absorption.

78. (C) Anticonvulsant.
Magnesium sulfate is used to treat seizures in preeclampsia and eclampsia. It reduces the risk of seizure by delaying calcium-dependent neurotransmission in the brain. Although magnesium sulfate is a tocolytic, it is not used for this effect in this patient because the goal of treatment is immediate delivery of the fetus.

79. (B) Hyporeflexia.
Hyporeflexia, which manifests as absent or slow patellar tendon reflex, is the first sign of magnesium sulfate toxicity. Respiratory failure occurs as magnesium sulfate accumulates in the blood. At higher doses, cardiac arrest occurs. To prevent these risks, urine output, deep tendon reflexes, respiratory rate and serum concentrations of magnesium sulfate are monitored.

80. (D) Withdraw 8 ml of magnesium sulfate and dilute in 12 ml of normal saline.
According to the Pritchard regimen, a loading dose of 4 g of magnesium sulfate is given intravenously. This means that in an ampule that comes as 5 g/10 mL of magnesium sulfate, 8 ml is withdrawn in a 20 mL syringe, then diluted with 12 mL of normal saline. This is then given slowly over ten minutes.

81. (A) 10 g IM, 5 g every four hours.
The intramuscular regimen of a maintenance dose of magnesium sulfate is the administration of a stat dose of 10 g IM, then 5 g every four hours on alternating buttocks for 24 hours after delivery of child or last seizure, whichever comes last.

82. (B) The maximum dose in 24 hours is 350 mg.
This statement is false because the maximum dose in 24 hours is 220 mg. IV labetalol is the drug of choice in managing severe hypertension in pregnant patients. It is a nonselective beta-blocker. A loading dose of 20 mg IV is given. This dose is increased sequentially to a maximum of 80 mg after assessing the blood pressure 10 minutes after administration.

83. (C) Vitamin K deficiency.
This is not a cause of coagulopathy in this patient. Patients with preeclampsia/eclampsia are at risk of developing HELLP syndrome, which is

characterized by elevated liver enzymes, hepatitis, hemolysis and thrombocytopenia. Also, in DIC there is a hypercoagulable state in the initial stage, which triggers fibrinolysis and consequent hemorrhage.

84. (D) Dexamethasone.
Dexamethasone is a corticosteroid given to hasten the maturity of the fetal lungs and reduce the risk of acute respiratory distress syndrome. It is indicated for use in the delivery of preterm babies who are less than 34 weeks. Surfactant is given to infants with ARDS, while naltrexone is given to infants with respiratory failure due to opioid intoxication from their mothers. Magnesium sulfate is given to reduce the risk of neurologic dysfunction in fetuses who are less than 32 weeks.

85. (D) Cervical os.
To differentiate between the two, the cervical os is examined with a cervical speculum. In inevitable abortion, the cervical os is opened.

86. (D) Cytotoxic.
Methotrexate is a cytotoxic used in induced abortion and gestational trophoblastic disease. It is cytotoxic that destroys the trophoblastic tissue. Methotrexate is often used with misoprostol to induce an abortion on pregnancies less than eight weeks.

87. (C) Misoprostol.
This is a prostaglandin used for medical induction. About 600 to 800 mcg stat dose of misoprostol is inserted into the vaginal fornix. Then every four hours 400 mcg is inserted. Abortion typically occurs within 48 hours. Dilatation and curettage are used for pregnancies less than 12 weeks; evacuation is used for

pregnancies that are 12 to 23 weeks and medical induction is used for pregnancies greater than 16 weeks.

88. (D) Jaundice.
This is not a clinical presentation of trophoblastic disease. Clinical features include severe vomiting, uterine bleeding with passage of grape-like vesicles and a doughy uterus that is bigger than the gestational age. In choriocarcinoma, patients may present with jaundice if the disease is advanced.

89. (C) Gestational diabetes.
Gestational diabetes is not a likely cause of a fundal size that is smaller than the gestational age. It increases the risk of fetal macrosomia and polyhydramnios. These conditions make the fundal height bigger than the gestational age.

90. (B) Fetal heart rate should be monitored continuously with a Sonicaid.
This statement is false because continuous monitoring of the fetal heart rate is done with a cardiotocograph. Intermittent fetal heart monitoring is done with a Sonicaid.

91. (B) Re-epithelization.
Abrasions are covered with commercial wound dressings to prevent the wounds from drying out. Drying interferes with the re-epithelization of the wound.

92. (B) Suturing.
Abrasions are not sutured because the wounds are scrapes that involve the epidermis. Suturing is not required because the wounds do not extend deep into the tissues. Healing occurs by primary intention.

93. (D) Polyglycolic acid.

Nonabsorbable sutures are used to repair cutaneous wounds. Because they can be removed, they reduce the risk of tissue reactivity. Polyglycolic acid is an absorbable suture and is therefore used for dermal repairs.

94. (C) High memory.

Nylon sutures have high memory (i.e., a tendency to coil back to their packaged shape). Because of this, there is a considerable risk of slippage of knots. To avoid this, the knots must be secured properly. Option A is incorrect because nylon sutures are monofilaments and therefore have a lower risk of infections. Option D is incorrect because the high tensile strength of nylon is an advantage in securing wounds.

95. (D) Hypokalemia.

Hypokalemia is unlikely to slow down wound healing. Factors that slow down wound healing are hypoproteinemia, obesity (hypertriglyceridemia), hyperglycemia, diabetes mellitus, radiation, vascular insufficiency, infections, alcohol, cigarette, vitamin C deficiency and others.

96. (B) Gauze.

Gauze dressings are dry-woven or nonwoven dressings. They are unsuitable for the primary dressing of moist wounds like pressure ulcers because they can stick to the base of the ulcer and interfere with re-epithelization.

97. (A) Desiccation.

Desiccation is a disadvantage of alginate wound dressings. This is because they contain salt that absorbs water from the wound. They also stimulate autolytic debridement. However, they can cause the wound to dry out excessively (desiccation) and interfere with re-epithelization.

98. (C) Leaves residue on the wound bed.
Hydrocolloid dressings contain methylcellulose, pectin or gelatin, which absorbs water from the wound. They are good adhesives, waterproof and encourage autolytic debridement. However, they can leave residue on the wound bed that can be mistaken for infection. Also, since they tend to spill into areas prone to friction, they can worsen existing pressure ulcers.

99. (D) Antiseptic properties.
This statement is false because a sitz bath does not have antiseptic properties. However, it is used to increase blood flow to the perineum, reduce edema, relieve pain and clean the perineum.

100. (D) Dementia.
Dementia is not a risk factor for pressure ulcers. Risk factors for pressure ulcers are age (usually, patients who are greater than 65 years have impaired capillary blood flow); decreased mobility from spinal injuries; cognitive impairment; chronic illnesses; prolonged hospital stay; urinary and fecal incontinence; impaired blood flow (vascular insufficiency); delayed wound healing (hypoproteinemia, hyperglycemia, hypertriglyceridemia, diabetes mellitus and others) and impaired skin sensation.

101. (D) Use of petroleum jelly on friction areas.
This measure will worsen the patient's outcome. Friction-prone areas must be kept dry and free from moisture and humidity. To do this, these areas are dusted with talcum powder and patted with moisture-protecting creams.

102. (B) Normal saline.
Cleaning should be done with normal saline during each dressing. Antiseptics can cause sloughing of granulation tissue and therefore delay healing. Normal saline can be applied with squeeze bottles or commercial syringes.

103. (A) Wet-to-dry dressings.
Wet-to-dry dressings are examples of mechanical wound debridement. In this method, a wet dressing is applied and removed when dry to strip off the necrotic tissue. This dressing is used for crusted and thickened wounds.

104. (A) Transparent films.
In autolytic wound debridement, hydrocolloid dressings or transparent film dressings are applied to the wounds to facilitate digestion of the wound by the body's enzymes. Option B is a form of biological debridement. Option C is a form of enzymatic debridement, and Option D is a form of mechanical debridement.

105. (C) Heat.
Heat is not a factor contributing to pressure ulcers. The factors that contribute to the formation of pressure ulcers are shearing forces, pressure, moisture and friction. All these factors cause skin dehiscence, occlusion of microvessels and maceration.

106. (C) Streptococcus spp.
Group A beta-hemolytic streptococcus is the most implicated bacteria in erysipelas. This bacteria commonly affects the leg and the face. It can also be caused by Staphylococcus aureus, Haemophilus influenzae, E. coli, Streptococcus pneumoniae, Klebsiella pneumoniae and Moraxella species.

107. (C) Incision and drainage.

All abscesses must be incised and drained of the exudative material. Warm compresses are used to make the abscess come to a point and drain. However, this intervention is not appropriate in patients who present to the ER. Oral antibiotics are given after the abscess is incised and drained. Topical antibiotics are not useful in this case.

108. (A) Peau d'orange.

Cellulitis often presents with a peau d'orange surface, while the surface of deep vein thrombosis is smooth. Also, the affected area of cellulitis is red and hot, while that of deep vein thrombosis is cool with normal skin color or cyanosis. Lymphangitis is also present in cellulitis and absent in deep vein thrombosis.

109. (A) Infants.

Scalded skin syndrome mostly affects infants. It is hardly seen in older patients. Epidemics among infants are typically seen in nurseries. The umbilical stump is the primary site of infection in the first few days of life. This syndrome is caused by group B coagulase-positive staphylococcus aureus.

110. (D) Topical antibiotics.

This intervention is the most appropriate for impetigo, a nonulcerative and superficial bacterial infection of the skin. The affected area is irrigated with water to remove the crusts, then topical mupirocin, ozenoxacin, fusidic acid, or retapamulin is applied.

111. (D) Cannabis.

Cannabis is least likely to cause physical dependence because withdrawal symptoms are not as intense as with the other listed substances. Physical dependence develops as a result of chronic use of drugs that induce tolerance.

112. (D) Diazepam.

Patients with withdrawal symptoms will be managed with benzodiazepines and thiamin. Diazepam can be given either intravenously or orally until the patient is sedated. Benzodiazepines are also given as prophylaxis for seizures. Disulfiram is used to encourage abstinence in motivated patients with alcoholism. Bupropion is used to blunt withdrawal symptoms in patients with nicotine addiction. Naloxone is used to treat opioid overdose.

113. (A) Delirium tremens.

Delirium tremens is an acute condition caused by withdrawal from alcohol. It begins about two to three days after alcohol withdrawal. Features are anxiety, insomnia with nocturnal illusions and nightmares, diaphoresis, depression and restlessness. Clinical features can progress to include disorientation, delirium and visual and auditory hallucinations.

114. (D) Cocaine.

False-positive results can be seen in drug testing. For example, poppy seeds can be taken to produce false positives for opioids. Ibuprofen can produce false positives for marijuana, while tricyclic antidepressants can produce false positives for amphetamines. However, testing for cocaine includes testing for its metabolite, benzoylecgonine. Other substances are unable to create this metabolite. Hence there is no risk for false-positive results.

115. (D) Deferoxamine.
Deferoxamine is a chelating agent used in the management of acute iron poisoning, not lead poisoning. Chelating drugs for lead poisoning include succimer, calcium disodium ethylenediaminetetraacetic acid and dimercaprol/BAL (British antilewisite).

116. (C) Increases excretion of aspirin.
Sodium bicarbonate is given to increase the urine pH and stimulate excretion of the metabolites via alkaline diuresis. Potassium is also given because hypokalemia can inhibit alkaline diuresis.

117. (B) 8.
Mucomyst (N-acetylcysteine) is used to treat acute acetaminophen poisoning. It is effective if it is given within eight hours of acetaminophen ingestion. The efficacy of the drug is uncertain after 24 hours of acetaminophen ingestion. However, it is still given.

118. (C) Aspiration.
Gastric lavage is used to empty the stomach of its contents. In this procedure, water is pushed into the stomach via an NGT, then aspirated with a syringe. This procedure is not routinely done for poisons due to the risk of aspiration. Other complications of this procedure are epistaxis and injury to the esophagus or oropharynx.

119. (D) Osmotic laxative.
Polyethylene glycol is a nonabsorbable sugar that exerts osmotic pressure in the lumen of the gut. It pulls water into the colon and stimulates peristalsis. Polyethylene glycol is also used to prepare the colon for abdominal surgeries.

120. (D) Ask the caregivers to take the flowers away.

Flowers and potted plants should not be kept beside a patient with severe burns. This is necessary to reduce the risk of infections and sepsis. Flowers and potted plants should also be kept away from patients with severe immunodeficiency.

121. (C) Healing will start from the hair follicles.

This statement is false. In third-degree burns, the injury extends from the dermis and deep into the subcutaneous fat. Healing will commence only from the periphery. In second-degree burns, healing commences from the hair follicles.

122. (D) Place the patient in a supine position.

This statement is false because burned extremities must be elevated to improve venous return and reduce edema.

123. (B) Determines fluid management in the first 24 hours of the burn.

The Parkland formula is used to determine fluid volume in the first 24 hours of the burn injury. It is calculated as (4 mL/kg) × %TBSA burned. It is used for second-degree and third-degree burns. Half of the estimated fluid is given in the first eight hours of management, while the remainder is given over 16 hours.

124. (D) IV Ringer's lactate.

Ringer's lactate is the fluid of choice in the management of burns. IV dextrose water is unsuitable because it is not an isotonic fluid. Although normal saline is isotonic, large volumes of this fluid can tip this patient into hyperchloremic acidosis.

125. (A) May present as vesicles.
First-degree burns are erythematous and very tender, and they blanch under pressure. They do not cause vesicles or bullae. Vesicle formation is a characteristic of superficial partial-thickness burns.

126. (A) Bats.
In the United States, vaccination of dogs has reduced the incidence of rabies. Rabies is typically transmitted via the bite of bats. Other implicated animals are raccoons, foxes and skunks.

127. (A) Sedatives.
Treatment of rabies is supportive with the use of sedatives, like ketamine and benzodiazepines, to control neuromuscular symptoms. Rabies vaccine and immunoglobulin are not useful once rabies has set in. Mortality rates are high and patients die 3 to 10 days after onset of symptoms.

128. (D) Delirium.
In heat exhaustion, there are no neurologic symptoms. The presence of confusion, delirium, or ataxia indicate heatstroke, a severe form of heat illness. Features of heat exhaustion include weakness, headaches, dizziness, malaise, tachycardia, hyperthermia, diaphoresis and orthostatic hypotension.

129. (C) Hypokalemia.
During the initial phase of the burn injury, the patient is likely to have hyperkalemia due to the destruction of cells. However, during fluid correction, there is a shift of potassium from the intravascular space into the intracellular space. This shift can cause hypokalemia.

130. (B) Carbon monoxide poisoning.
Oversaturation of hemoglobin in the red blood cells with carbon monoxide and dilatation of capillaries causes a cherry color of mucous membranes. This is a sign of carbon monoxide poisoning.

131. (B) Auscultation of the lungs.
This is the most appropriate intervention to be assigned, based on the scope of practice of the LPN. Option A is best suited for a nursing assistant. Options C and D are to be done by a registered nurse.

132. (B) Cabbage.
Cabbage can cause bloating and flatulence because it is a gas-releasing food. This patient should be encouraged to eat only small amounts or avoid it completely.

133. (D) Right to health insurance.
This right is not offered by EMTALA. EMTALA requires that all patients who present to the ER—regardless of race, sex, ethnicity, religion and socioeconomic status—be given medical screening, resuscitation and stabilization. It also requires that all patients who present to the ER be transferred to the appropriate level of health care after stabilization.

134. (B) Uncompensated care.
Because EMTALA demands that all patients who present to the ER be treated regardless of their health insurance, health workers and health organizations do not get compensated for the care they provide. This has led to the closure of some health organizations in America.

135. (D) Federal law.
The privacy rule is a federal law that gives patients rights over how their health information is used, stored and transferred. This rule covers all forms of health information whether oral, written or electronic.

136. (C) Employers.
Employers are examples of bodies not required to follow the privacy and security rules. Other bodies include child protective agencies, law enforcement agencies, schools, municipal offices and life insurers. Bodies that are expected to follow the regulations are health-care providers, health-care plans, health insurance companies and health-care clearinghouses.

137. (D) Educational data.
Educational data is held by noncovered entities and is therefore not protected health information. Protected health information includes all forms of health information held by the entities covered by HIPAA. Some of these covered entities are health care providers and health insurance plans. Other examples of nonprotected health information are employment records.

138. (C) Refuse treatment for their medical conditions.
HIPAA does not give patients the right to refuse treatment. HIPAA gives patients the right to decide how their health information is used, stored and transmitted.

139. (D) Financial ability.
Financial ability is not a requirement for informed consent. Before patients give informed consent, they must be competent to understand the importance of the education given and give consent. Also, patients must be properly educated to

make an informed decision. Consent must also be given voluntarily and not under duress or compulsion.

140. (D) Herself.
This patient is an emancipated minor and is therefore qualified to give informed consent. Other routes of emancipation include enlistment in the military and emancipation by a court declaration. Although she is Muslim, she is to give informed consent, not her husband.

141. (D) Expose only the parts that need to be examined.
This is the most appropriate action. In this case, the patient needs to be exposed only from the xiphisternum to the suprapubic line for an abdominal examination. To examine the cervix, the patient's abdomen is covered and she is positioned in the lithotomy position with a drape over her lower limbs. Options A, B and C are all inappropriate.

142. (D) Obtain consent.
Nurse P must first obtain informed consent from the patient (not her husband). In so doing, he gives the patient a choice to make requests, which could include asking for a female nurse. If the patient does not request one, Nurse P must provide a chaperone to witness the examination.

143. (D) Dispose of the syringe with the needle.
The syringe, with the needle, should be disposed of immediately in the biohazard box. Separating the needle, trying to manipulate the needle by bending it, or attempting to cap the needle can increase the risk of puncture injuries. Disinfecting his hands after the procedure does not reduce the risk of needle prick injuries. But it does reduce the risk of infection transmission.

144. (C) Work from uncontaminated to contaminated areas.
Option A is incorrect because the wounds are already contaminated and sterile gloves will confer no protection. Option B is incorrect because a drape does not reduce the risk of wound contamination. Option D is incorrect because the wound must be thoroughly irrigated and debrided before being dressed with antiseptics (in this case isopropyl alcohol is unsuitable).

145. (B) Run the affected site under tap water.
The first response is to run the puncture site under tap water. Thereafter, the nurse should make an incident report to appropriate management.

146. (C) Droplet precautions.
Transmission of meningococcal meningitis is via infected droplets from the nose and throat. Droplet precautions include the use of face masks, isolation and observation of cough etiquette.

147. (B) Delayed.
The five classifications of triage are:
Immediate – Color red. These patients require urgent treatment for life-threatening injuries. These patients have a good chance of survival if promptly treated.
Urgent – Color yellow. Treatment can be delayed for a short period due to no impending life-threatening risk.
Delayed – Color green. These patients do not require urgent treatment and are not at risk for mortality
Expectant – Color blue. These patients require extensive treatment that exceeds available resources or their conditions will not improve with life support.

Dead – Color black. These patients are in cardiac arrest that will not respond to resuscitation.

148. (C) Immediate.
See above question for the five classifications of triage.

149. (B) Respiration, pulse and mental status
The START protocol means simple triage and rapid treatment. It is a protocol used to rapidly assess and attend to mass casualty victims. After assessment, patients are triaged according to five colors. Assessment includes respiration, pulse rate and mental status.

150. (C) Warm zone.
The warm zone is another name for the decontamination corridor. In this zone, patients and exposed people are decontaminated. Emergency personnel must attend to exposed people with the appropriate PPE. The cold zone describes the clean zone and involves emergency rooms. The hot zone describes the primary site of exposure.

151. (A) Thiamine.
Wernicke encephalopathy is caused by thiamine deficiency. It is triggered in patients with chronic alcoholism, which impairs the absorption and storage of thiamine. Treatment includes IV or IM administration of 100 mg thiamine.

152. (D) Constipation.
Clinical features of generalized anxiety disorder are excessive anxiety and worry, difficulty in concentrating, diaphoresis, shortness of breath, palpitations,

diarrhea, nausea, vomiting, irritability, fatigue, restlessness, headaches and sleep disturbances.

153. (B) Serotonin reuptake inhibitor.
Citalopram is a selective serotonin reuptake inhibitor used in treating patients with major depression, anxiety disorders, obsessive-compulsive disorder, eating disorders and post-traumatic stress disorder. Apart from citalopram, other drugs include sertraline, escitalopram, fluoxetine, fluvoxamine and paroxetine.

154. (C) Malingering.
Patients with malingering disorder fake an illness for personal gain. This personal gain may be relief from work or monetary gain from concerned individuals or organizations. In Munchausen's, the patient fakes a disease but not for personal or economic gain. Patients with hypochondriasis believe that they have an illness even though this is not the case.

155. (B) Logorrhea.
This is a disorder of communication characterized by the use of repetitive words that are incoherent. It is often seen in psychiatric disorders and with brain injury. Aphasia is an inability to speak or use previously learned words. Apraxia is a difficulty in executing previously learned tasks.

156. (C) Suicidal ideation.
Suicidal ideation is a potential risk for teenagers commenced on antidepressants. The patients and their caregivers must be counseled on this risk. Caregivers must also be counseled to monitor their wards for signs of increased agitation and restlessness during the use of antidepressants.

157. (D) Citalopram.
Drugs implicated in neuroleptic malignant syndrome are traditional and new generation antipsychotics (e.g., haloperidol, chlorpromazine, loxapine, risperidone, olanzapine and clozapine) and antiemetics like droperidol, promethazine, metoclopramide and domperidone.

158. (B) Grapes.
The risk of hypertensive crisis increases when patients on monoamine oxidase inhibitors take foods rich in tyramine or dopamine. These foods include pickled, cured and fermented foods like yogurt, cheese, red wine, canned figs, raisins, caviar, banana peels, raisins, yeast extracts, soy sauce, sour cream and tenderized meats.

159. (D) Hypokalemia.
Hyperkalemia (not hypokalemia) is a feature of serotonin syndrome due to acute kidney injury, hyperthermia and rhabdomyolysis. Serotonin syndrome is characterized by malignant hyperthermia triggered by uncontrolled and excessive serotonergic activity of the CNS. It is caused by the intake of two serotonergic drugs either intentionally or accidentally.

160. (C) Thought broadcasting.
In thought broadcasting, patients believe that everyone can hear their thoughts. It is a positive symptom of schizophrenia. In delusions of persecution, patients believe that people are out to get them. In thought insertion, patients believe that their thoughts are not theirs but are being manipulated and controlled by someone else. In delusions of grandeur, patients elevate themselves to a higher status of importance.

161. (C) Generalized anxiety disorder.
Buspirone is a serotonin receptor agonist used in treating patients with generalized anxiety disorder. It is not used in the treatment of psychosis, alcohol withdrawal, barbiturate or benzodiazepine withdrawal.

162. (B) Dopamine.
Erectile dysfunction, reduced libido and infertility are side effects of antipsychotics because of their antagonistic effects on dopamine and consequently increased secretion of prolactin. Antagonistic effects on acetylcholine receptors cause constipation, blurred vision, dry mouth and extrapyramidal effects. Antagonistic effects on histamine cause sedation, drowsiness and dry mouth. Antiadrenergic effects cause postural hypotension. Hematologic side effects include agranulocytosis and thrombocytopenia; endocrine changes include weight gain, type 2 diabetes mellitus and metabolic syndrome. Cardiovascular changes include arrhythmia and stroke.

163. (C) Histamine.
Sedation is a side effect of most antipsychotics due to their antagonistic action on histamine. Other antagonistic effects on histamine include drowsiness and dry mouth. Antagonistic effects on acetylcholine receptors cause constipation, blurred vision, dry mouth and extrapyramidal effects. Antagonistic effects on dopamine cause reduced libido and gynecomastia. Antiadrenergic effects cause postural hypotension. Hematologic side effects include agranulocytosis and thrombocytopenia, endocrine changes include weight gain, type 2 diabetes mellitus and metabolic syndrome. Cardiovascular changes include arrhythmia and stroke.

164. (A) Hypnopompic.
Hypnopompic hallucinations are visual hallucinations that the patient sees when they wake up. Hypnagogic hallucinations are seen before the patient goes to sleep.

165. (C) Echolalia.
Echolalia is the involuntary repetition of another person's speech or vocalizations. Echopraxia is the involuntary repetition of another person's actions. Apraxia is a difficulty in performing previously learned tasks. Aphasia is an inability to use previously learned words.

166. (D) Prothrombin time.
Prothrombin time is used to assess the extrinsic and common pathway of coagulation. It is used along with the international normalized ratio and prothrombin ratio to measure clotting tendencies in conditions like warfarin therapy, liver disease and vitamin K deficiency.

167. (C) Retinal hemorrhage.
In shaken child syndrome, the child is shaken violently either to stop him or her from crying or as a threat. As the child is shaken, the head moves back and forth, creating a risk for internal head injuries and intracerebral hemorrhage. Retinal hemorrhage is the most specific sign of internal head injuries.

168. (C) Uterine atony.
The most common cause of postpartum hemorrhage is uterine atony. Risk factors for uterine atony are grand multiparity, multiple gestations, polyhydramnios, fetal macrosomia, congenital anomalies, precipitate labor, anesthesia and chorioamnionitis. Other causes of hemorrhage are uterine rupture, retained

products of conception, cervical tears, episiotomies, inversion of the uterus, bleeding disorders and coagulopathies, uterine fibroids and involution of the placenta.

169. (B) Erythropoietin deficiency.
Erythropoietin is a hormone that stimulates the production of red blood cells in the marrow. It is mainly produced in the kidneys, with small amounts from the liver. In end-stage renal disease, there is cellular death of the kidneys and fibrosis. This leads to erythropoietin deficiency.

170. (B) Reduces afterload.
Nitroglycerin is a potent vasodilator that dilates peripheral veins and arteries and consequently reduces afterload. Diuretics like furosemide, hydrochlorothiazide and spironolactone reduce afterload by reducing intravascular volume. Beta-blockers like atenolol reduce heart rate and cardiac output.

171. (D) HELLP.
A patient who is being managed for hyperemesis gravidarum is not at risk for HELLP. In hyperemesis gravidarum, there is severe vomiting that causes dehydration, electrolyte derangement, ketosis and weight loss. Patients present with features of hypovolemic shock. Complications are fatty degenerative changes in the liver, Wernicke encephalopathy and Mallory-Weiss tears.

172. (B) Within 72 hours of delivery.
To reduce maternal sensitization and production of antibodies in subsequent pregnancies, the Rh-negative mother must be given Rho(D) immune globulin within 72 hours of delivery or termination of pregnancy, at 28 weeks gestation, after an episode of vaginal bleeding and after amniocentesis.

173. (B) Assess fetal heart rate.
Fetal distress is a complication of amniotomy. Therefore, fetal heart rate is measured before and after amniotomy to assess the hemodynamic status of the fetus.

174. (B) Estrogen depletion.
Estrogen depletion is the most common cause of osteoporosis in women. Depletion of estrogen leads to increased resorption of bone and decreased bone density.

175. (D) It has both A and B antigens.
The AB blood group has both A and B antigens in the red blood cells but no A and B antibodies in the plasma. This quality makes it a universal recipient of blood. However, because of the A and B antigens in the red blood cell, it can donate blood only to recipients with the AB blood group.

Made in United States
North Haven, CT
04 January 2023